Heartburn Solved:

How to Reverse Acid Reflux and GERD Naturally

By Case Adams, Naturopath

Publishers Cataloging in Publication Data
Adams, Case
    Heartburn Solved: How to Reverse Acid Reflux and GERD Naturally
First Edition
1. Medicine. 2. Health.
Bibliography and References; Index

ISBN-13: 978-1936251353

Other Books by the author:

ARTHRITIS - THE BOTANICAL SOLUTION: Nature's Answer to Rheumatoid Arthritis, Osteoarthritis, Gout and Other Forms of Arthritis

ASTHMA SOLVED NATURALLY: The Surprising Underlying Causes and Hundreds of Natural Strategies to Beat Asthma

BREATHING TO HEAL: The Science of Healthy Respiration

ELECTROMAGNETIC HEALTH: Making Sense of the Research and Practical Solutions for Electromagnetic Fields (EMF) and Radio Frequencies (RF)

HEALTHY SUN: Healing with Sunshine and the Myths about Skin Cancer

NATURAL SLEEP SOLUTIONS FOR INSOMNIA: The Science of Sleep, Dreaming, and Nature's Sleep Remedies

NATURAL SOLUTIONS FOR FOOD ALLERGIES AND FOOD INTOLERANCES: Scientifically Proven Remedies for Food Sensitivities

ORAL PROBIOTICS: The Newest Way to Prevent Infection, Boost the Immune System and Fight Disease

PROBIOTICS - Protection Against Infection: Using Nature's Tiny Warriors To Stem Infection and Fight Disease

PURE WATER: The Science of Water, Waves, Water Pollution, Water Treatment, Water Therapy and Water Ecology

THE CONSCIOUS ANATOMY: Healing the Real You

THE LIVING CLEANSE: Detoxification and Cleansing Using Living Foods and Safe Natural Strategies

THE LIVING FOOD DIET: The Ultimate Diet for Increasing Vitality, Losing Weight and Preventing Disease

THE MIND, BRAIN AND SUBCONSCIOUS SELF: Unveiling the Ancient Secrets using Science

TOTAL HARMONIC: The Healing Power of Nature's Elements

Table of Contents

Introduction

Acid reflux, or gastroesophageal reflux disease (GERD) is plaguing more and more people in our modern world. Why is this? Is it stress? Is spicy foods? Is it overeating? Is it something else?

To say yes to any of these factors would not be completely incorrect, but it would be incorrect to narrow the condition down to these elements. If it were stress, then why doesn't everyone who experiences stress get GERD? If it were spicy foods or overeating, why doesn't everyone who eats spicy foods or overeat get GERD?

The fact of the matter is that heartburn, GERD or acid reflux—whatever we want to call it—is significantly more complex. This is not to say that we cannot easily understand the cause and solutions for the condition: They are easy to understand, but we must become aware of the real causes and solutions in order to understand them.

This book is intended to fulfill that objective: To cut through all the misnomers and misunderstandings, and clearly explain the real causes and the natural solutions of this condition.

The information presented here is based upon the combination of the most recent science on physiology and intestinal health, and the wisdom of traditional healers whose solutions have been proven successful among millions (likely billions) of people over thousands of years.

Some of the findings laid out here thus come from the latest scientific research, and some come from the cumulative clinical experiences of traditional physicians of the Americas, Europe, Middle East, Africa, Asia and the Pacific islands. Thus we draw upon tried and true practices by North American and South American Indian healers, Ayurvedic physicians, physicians of Chinese medicine, healers of Polynesian traditional medicine, Western and Eastern European healers, African healers and other successful healers from around the world.

The application of herbal therapy along with diet has a great tradition, and a successful tradition. For this simple reason, we did not see the explosion of GERD conditions that we seen in modern times. People of ancient times certainly suffered from GERD at times. But there were remedies known that resolved the condition.

And these remedies were passed down from generation to generation through a process called *mentorship*.

Furthermore, after decades of modern medicine telling us that their synthetic solutions were better, science is finally beginning to confirm the efficacy of these traditional remedies.

In this text we are bringing together these traditions with the modern physiology science and the clinical research that confirms these traditions. Here the tradition and the science are revived together, to clarify not only the cause of GERD and the physiology of GERD, but the tried and true remedies that have been used to resolve GERD. This tying together of modern science and traditional medicine gives the reader not only clarity, but confidence.

This is not to say that this text is an individual prescription. The information provided is intended to present the information as a reference to help both the health professional and the layperson better understand the condition and get to know some of the documented alternative therapies that have shown success. As for any particular situation or application, one should consult with their personal health professional before making any prescriptive changes to their diet, lifestyle or supplementation to avoid any potential complications.

The reader may notice redundancy in some of the information presented here. There are two purposes for this. While understanding the real causes for and solutions to GERD is not complex, we must still contend with decades—and even centuries—of misconstruence and misunderstanding among conventional medical circles. This requires not only reinforcement in terms of dialog and terminology, but a cross-referencing of the science and clinical application. This provides a blend of peer-review and practical application, enabling the reader ultimate control over the information.

Chapter One

What is GERD?

Tony

Tony is Italian. He's a good eater. Raised in New York, Tony is a little overweight, very active, and more than a little hot-headed. When he complains of heartburn, his friends and family immediately dismiss it by saying that it is a product of his spicy meals and hot-headedness.

Tony feels this way too. And it sure seems that the spicy meals and stress he feels at times gang up to give him heartburn.

Tony's GERD will often flare up after a particularly large meal, and will get worse as he stresses over something. And when he lays down to sleep after a big late-night meal, his heartburn will often worsen, making it hard to sleep.

In the beginning, Tony found relief by drinking a little milk. After that stopped working, Tony began taking antacids. One of those colorful and tasty chewable antacids took away the heartburn fast in the beginning. Soon he was taking two or three, then a small handful of tablets at a sitting to quell the burn. Soon he was pouring the antacids directly from the bottle into his mouth.

Tony has been to the doctor about his GERD many times. He now knows what to expect. Over the years, he's tried a number of types of acid-blocking medications, and these tended to work far better than the antacids. However, these medications also don't make him feel well in other ways. Sometimes Tony has excruciating headaches. Other times, he cannot digest his foods, resulting in alternating bouts of constipation and diarrhea.

Tony has also noticed that he is sick a lot more frequently since he's been on acid-blocking medications. He used to get a cold or flu about once a year—two at the most. Nowadays, it seems he's sick with a cold or flu almost once a month.

Tony has also tried to alter his diet over the past year or so. After the doctor advised cutting back on spicy foods and large helpings, Tony now includes "hold the spice" or "mild" with orders of his favorite foods at restaurants.

This was also helped for awhile. After a few months, Tony was having the same heartburn even with his new "mild" diet.

Tony has also tried to "mellow out" a bit. This helped in the beginning, but now he has the same level of burning abdominal pain even while staying mellow. But now, when he gets excited about something, the flare ups are excruciating.

Emily

Emily is an active thirty-something who works hard and plays hard. Stress? She doesn't believe in stress. She enjoys challenges. She likes competition. Work doesn't seem stressful to her, even though her job is quite demanding. As an editor of a national news magazine, Emily has her share of deadlines to meet.

Emily also has two children and a hard-working husband. The two of them juggle time commitments with baby-sitters, school hours and kids activities, together with working out and trying to have a social life. Her children are four and seven, both boys, and both very active.

Emily met her husband at a rock-climbing class. Emily was the teacher, and her now-husband, Rob, was a first-time climber. Needless to say, Emily has made some pretty challenging ascents   over the years.

Yet while not much seems to rile her, Emily has been increasingly plagued with acid reflux and heartburn symptoms. The symptoms seem to worsen after meals, and during more stressful periods, but neither of these predicators are consistent.

In fact, for weeks, Emily will feel fine. No heartburn, regardless of what she just ate or how much stress she is under. Then suddenly, the heartburn will flare up, and for the next week or more, it will follow practically every meal and occur during every stressful time.

Emily has seen her doctor several times about this. First the doctor asked if she had tried antacids. Not being a big believer in medications, she hadn't. So the doctor prescribed an acid suppressing medication. Emily did not fill the prescription at first. Then, during a bad flare up a few weeks later, she went ahead and filled the prescription, and took the medication for a few days.

Emily did find some relief from the acid suppressing medication. But she also felt tired and in a poor mood and nauseous after she took the drug. After several days of taking it, she had to stop. Emily just couldn't stand feeling that way. *She'd rather have the heartburn than that*, she thought.

The Canary in the Coal Mine

A healthy stomach is the key to a healthy body. A healthy stomach means we become nourished by eating good foods. A healthy stomach means our food gets prepared for maximum absorption.

Imagine only assimilating a small portion of the many healthy (and expensive) foods and supplements we buy. Sadly, this is the case for many of us.

A healthy stomach also means the freedom from heartburn and ulcers. Some reports state that almost a quarter of us will experience heartburn at some point. Nearly one in ten of us will get an ulcer. Some say these reports are conservative, as many cases go unreported. Then there is indigestion. Most of us experience this occasionally, if not daily.

GERD stands for gastroesophageal reflux disease. It is also called GER (without the word "disease") when there are symptoms but no chronic disorder. The term 'gastro' refers to the stomach and the acids produced by the stomach, while the term 'esophageal' refers to the esophagus. GERD goes under other names as well:

➤ acid reflux
➤ indigestion
➤ heartburn
➤ reflux
➤ and many others.

Conventional medicine typically characterizes GERD as the release of digestive acids from the stomach into the esophagus. This, according to the theory, burns the tissues of the esophagus. This, however, is an inadequate definition, because research has illustrated that many GERD sufferers do not have increased acidity (also called *hyperchlorhydria*).

In fact, many people who suffer from GERD actually have *hypochlorhydria*—or low acidity in their stomach and esophagus. This was illustrated in a study by researchers from (Ayazi *et al.* 2009) the Keck School of Medicine at the University of Southern California. This study tested the gastric pH of 54 healthy volunteers and 1,582 GERD patients using a pH catheter probe monitor. A total of 797 of the GERD patients—about half—had "abnormal esophageal acid exposure." And a full 176 of the GERD sufferers—11% or about one out of ten—had *low gastric acidity* (hypochlorhydria) within the esophagus.

The rest of the abnormal acidity among the patients was high—but this was only 39% of the whole group of 1,582 GERD sufferers. This means the majority of these GERD sufferers did not suffer from hyperchlorhydria (high acidity) in the esophagus. Over 60% of the 1,582 GERD sufferers had either normal or low gastric acidity in the esophagus.

The researchers concluded that: "Negative 24-h esophageal pH test results for a patient with hypochlorhydria may prompt a search for nonacid reflux as the explanation for the patient's symptoms."

Earlier research has shown that up to half of us over the age of 60 can suffer from hypochlorhydria—resulting in slower digestion and the increased risk of GERD. And the risk of GERD increases for those over the age of 60.

This differing paradigm has been neatly filed away into diagnostic attributions such as *alkaline reflux* or *alkaline reflux esophagitis*. Others have tucked the entire mystery as *mixed acid-alkaline gastroesophageal reflux*.

In addition, many GERD sufferers also suffer from ulcers and heartburn within the stomach or upper intestines that are related to hypochlorhydria and *Helicobacter pylori* infections. In fact, many clinical studies have documented heartburn complaints with stomach ulcers and hypochlorhydria together.

We'll discuss the science behind this later, but we find for some reason, that the conventional medical profession has all but ignored much of this research, primarily because it opens up GERD to quite a different mechanism than simply hyper-acidity. Whether this oversight is related to the focus upon particular medications, or whether the research simply has not been well-enough publicized is besides the point.

The compartmentalization of the GERD disorder by modern medicine has thoroughly confused its real causative issues, and its relationship with other metabolic activity within the body. Modern medicine tends to look at GERD and other disorders with a sterile view; as though its occurrence occurs outside of our lifestyles, diet and general health. This diagnostic approach—naming the disease and then following treatment guidelines approved by peers, clinics, health insurance and other authorities—has led to a limited view of GERD as a disease that can only be treated by lowering the production of acids in the stomach.

We'll talk more about this approach later, but for the purposes of communicating what GERD is, the real physiology of the disorder will take the reader significantly outside of this mainstream approach. For our purposes here, we will call the GERD mechanisms elaborated on here as the *metabolic approach* to the disorder.

This isn't to suggest that this metabolic approach to GERD is merely opinion, nor outside the scope of scientific evidence. We will be presenting significant research that illustrates this metabolic approach, and will scientifically establish the real nature of GERD and what causes it.

As this evidence becomes clear, the reader will find that GERD is more than just a problem of acid leaking into the esophagus. Rather, we'll find that GERD is a much broader ailment—one of a systemic nature.

When a disorder is characterized as *systemic*, this means the disorder has a deeper connection with the whole body and its overall metabolism. It means that there are deeper issues at play, and the condition of GERD itself is simply a outlying system: GERD is an indicator of the deeper issue: *A canary in the coal mine.*

And in case the reader isn't sure how a canary is to be applied to GERD: In the mining business, long before the use of technical environmental meters that determine the precise condition of the air within a mine shaft, miners would carry in and toss a canary deep into the mine shaft. If the canary flew out, they would know the mine was safe to enter. If it didn't, well, something was wrong with the mine.

Symptoms of GERD

Heartburn and GERD are separated simply by consistency. Heartburn that lasts more than two or three days in a row is typically classified as reflux, while GERD is characterized by consistently periodic or chronic heartburn and reflux symptoms.

Heartburn, reflux and GERD can produce numerous symptoms, making it sometimes difficult to ascertain with definity. Doctors also sometimes find it difficult to know for sure, and they often must resort to extensive testing. This is only the tip of the iceberg, however, because as we'll find in this book GERD is in many ways a deceptive and misunderstood condition.

Some of the more common symptoms include persistent belching, regurgitation, mucous build up in the mouth and throat and a sourness in the mouth.

The classic symptom most GERD sufferers describe is a burning feeling in the stomach, throat or chest. The burning can be located anywhere from the upper stomach region—just below the ribcage on the left side—all the way up to the top of the throat and even into the mouth, sinuses, lungs and mouth for more severe cases.

The sensation may not necessarily be feel like burning. Some feel pain, again anywhere from the upper abdomen all the way up to the throat, sinuses and mouth. This can be an aching pain, a throbbing pain or a sharp 'pins and needles' pain.

We will get into this in more detail later, but the varied response in terms of sensation has to do with the condition of the lining of these passageways, as well as the nature of the offending secretions that are coming into contact with these membranes. In other words, one person's GERD systems may be altogether different than another's.

It is precisely the type of burning pain described above that causes most to call GERD 'heartburn.' Because for many, the burning sensation feels like it is in the region of the heart, which is just above the stomach. For this reason, heartburn has often been confused with a heart attack.

In fact, it is not unusual for a person to end up in an emergency room fearing a heart attack, only to find the attack was a reflux attack. While it is better safe than sorry, we can know a heart attack from a numbing sensation in the left arm.

Acid reflux can also be cause regurgitation. Regurgitation means that mucus is coming up the esophagus and into the mouth or sinuses. This might produce the urge to spit or cough. Some adults will snort the mucus from the pharynx into the mouth, and then spit it out—sometimes referred to as 'horking a loogie.'

During sleep, this regurgitation can also result in drooling, as the body naturally seeks to eliminate the reflux mucus. When the pillow is left wet and stained in the morning

For infants, regurgitation will also result in drooling, whether awake or sleeping. This can also be accompanied by heartburn, so the baby may cry as it regurgitates. Infants may experience great pain during this regurgitation, which together with the acid reflux and heartburn feelings, result in what many refer to as a colic.

GERD can also cause vomiting, as the reflux mucus can trigger the vagus reflex, which stimulates the vomit response. Sometimes the vomit may only consist of a mouthful of mucus. This is sometimes described as a 'verp'.

Another set of symptoms can arise as a result of the reflux intruding onto the throat or airways. As for the throat region, the GERD sufferer may experience a sore throat, a raspy or hoarse throat or even a loss of voice or changed voice. This is because the acid reflux can damage the epithelial layers of the vocal cords and voice box.

As far as the airways, acid reflux can result in coughing, pain in the chest, and wheezing. Again, this results from the reflux mucus making its way into the lungs, and damaging our airways, and even the alveoli and other elements of our inner lungs.

The sinus cavities may also become inflamed as a result of contact with acid reflux mucus. This can result in a number of symptoms, including stuffy nose, irritated sinuses, sneezing and so on.

These are the more direct symptoms of immediate acid reflux. There are a number of symptoms that arise in chronic cases of GERD. These can include malnutrition, deficiencies in one or more nutrients, growth retardation, and even obesity. Digestive system symptoms can include stomach bleeding (seen when the stool is black), irritable bowels, symptoms of Crohn's disease, constipation, diarrhea and excessive gas.

Other symptoms of chronic GERD can include blood sugar issues, immunosuppression (weak immune system), headaches, aching muscles and joints, lethargy (tiredness) and many others.

GERD can be fairly easy to rectify in its early stages if we know the causes and solutions to the metabolic problems. But should those metabolic issues be ignored, and GERD advances, it can suffocate critical cells and tissue systems, setting off a wildfire of inflammation that can lead to cell mutation and cancer. For this reason, esophageal cancers, such as Barrett's disease and esophageal adenocarcinoma are seen in advanced GERD cases.

Diagnosing GERD

It is not surprising that GERD can be difficult to diagnose. Complicating this is the possibility that the patient may have an ulcer and/or and infection of *Helicobacter pylori*. Doctors can test regurgitation pH and esophageal pH to see if it contains strong gastric acids. The problem here as mentioned above is that reflux mucus can have a wide pH range, and not be abnormal at all.

Occasional heartburn is not typically classified as GERD. Gastroesophageal reflux disease is considered a chronic condition, and heartburn is one symptom of it. In other words, heartburn symptoms occurring daily or even weekly would likely be considered GERD, while monthly or less would likely not—unless this has occurred consistently over a year or two.

Diagnostic methods used by doctors to determine GERD include the history of the patient, a physical examination, and then tests that include nuclear medicine scintiscan, laryngoscopy, gastrointestinal studies, esophagogastroduodenoscopy with biopsy, and esophageal pH probe monitoring. These provide different approaches to sampling mucus and tissues of the esophagus, and analyzing the health and tone of the esophageal sphincters.

If the esophageal sphincters are weakened, do not close adequately, or if the lower esophageal sphincter has been purged by part of the stomach wall (hiatal hernia), acids from the stomach may be traveling up the esophagus.

When heartburn symptoms are not evident, the endoscopy can be negative. Sometimes, laryngoscopy and 24-hour dual channel intraesophageal pH-metry prove the GERD condition in these cases. Some clinicians use the effectiveness of proton pump inhibitor medications to diagnose GERD: If the medication helps, they figure it must be GERD.

The conventional pH testing system requires the physician to insert a catheter down the throat and into the esophagus to monitor the pH. This can cause pain and discomfort, and interferes with normal eating. The newest pH testing method uses a wireless 48 hour monitoring system.

Some research has shown the wireless system to be more accurate than the conventional probe (Carmona-Sánchez and Solana-Sentíes 2004).

Another test for pH is the Heidelberg gastric analysis. This utilizes an electronic capsule that is swallowed. The capsule emits radio frequencies to a receiver that registers the pH.

The Heidelberg test can be combined with a bicarbonate challenge, which can indicate the functionality of the stomach's parietal cells to produce gastric acids on demand.

Doctors will often measure the extent of the GERD as primary or secondary. Primary relates to the GERD being at least initially independent of another condition. Secondary GERD is often (correctly or incorrectly) pegged to genetic abnormalities and birth defects. There may also be an underlying nervous disorder in addition to the GERD condition.

The Modern Rise of GERD

Research indicates that GERD incidence has exploded in the industrial era. While heartburn has historically existed, its prevalence was greatest among the elite and governing classes of Europe and American societies. Historically, the traditional cultures of Asia and third world countries have had very little incidence of GERD outside of the occasional heartburn.

What are the differences in traditional societies and how do they contrast modern industrial societies with respect to their effects upon GERD? First let's look at a few of the lifestyle differences between modern and traditional cultures in general:

> ➤ traditional cultures spend more time out-of-doors
> ➤ traditional cultures are generally slower paced
> ➤ traditional cultures are generally less stressful
> ➤ traditional cultures do more manual work
> ➤ modern cultures are exposed to more environmental toxins
> ➤ modern cultures eat richer diets (more saturated fats and more sweets)
> ➤ modern cultures eat more fast foods
> ➤ modern cultures eat more fried foods (most fast foods are fried or fatty foods)
> ➤ modern cultures use more technology
> ➤ modern cultures sleep less (and have more nighttime activity)
> ➤ modern cultures do more sit-down work
> ➤ modern culture work is generally more stressful

We can see this in action as we compare two industrial countries today: China and the United States. China is rapidly rising out of a traditional society, while the U.S. has been entrenched in modern culture for many decades. Let's look at these two, and how GERD prevalence stacks up in general:

GERD Prevalence

Gastroesophageal reflux disease (GERD) affects 20-30% of the population in Western countries (Kandulski and Malfertheiner 2011).

North Americans suffer from even greater rates of GERD. University of North Carolina researchers (Shaheen and Ransohoff 2002) analyzed studies on GERD and associated diseases from 1968 through 2001. After sorting for randomized controlled clinical studies, they determined that 50% of American adults suffered from GERD symptoms on a monthly basis, and 20% of Americans suffered from GERD at least weekly.

Other studies have had similar findings. Friedman *et al.* 2008 found that about a third of the U.S. population experiences heartburn at least monthly, and about 10% experience heartburn daily.

Another study found that about 18-20% of Americans experience heartburn weekly (Locke *et al.* 1997).

In comparison, researchers from the University of Hong Kong (Wong *et al.* 2003) conducted a study of GERD among Chinese populations. In total, 2,209 adult volunteers participated in the study. The research discovered that 2.5% of the population experienced some heartburn weekly, 9% experienced heartburn monthly, and nearly 30% experienced some heartburn at least once in the past year.

In other words, Americans experience heartburn about 7.6 times more frequently than do the Chinese (18-20% versus 2.5%). That means that Americans have 760% more weekly heartburn than the Chinese. Furthermore, more Americans experience heartburn on a daily basis than Chinese experience monthly. This could be translated to Americans having over thirty times more GERD incidence. However it is calculated, Americans have dramatically more GERD than the Chinese.

Why is this? Many would quickly conclude that it must be diet, or it must be lower stress. These solutions are much too simplistic, however. This is because we know that slowing down a bit or changing the diet are not substantive fixes. They are assumptions. They are corrective measures to be sure, but they do not substantially get us to the point where we can understand the real issues at play in GERD, and what we can do to reverse the situation not only personally, but as a society.

Addressing other prevalence data, Spanish researchers (Ponce *et al.* 2010) studied 2,356 GERD patients, and found that older people were more likely to have severe GERD symptoms, and were most likely to have persistent cases despite medication treatments, which included proton pump inhibitors. They also found that women were more likely to have severe GERD than men, and overweight people were more likely to have severe GERD.

Others have found that as many as one in five adults over 65 years old suffer from GERD.

GERD often arises early in infancy, and can just as easily resolve itself within the first year or two among children. GERD will also occur in adolescents, but both incidence and severity is typically higher in adults (Sood and Rudolph 2004).

Childhood GERD is more prevalent than most of us have realized. Pediatric researchers from the Rady Children's Hospital in San Diego and the University of California San Diego (Doshi *et al.* 2012) studied 313 children between one and three years old who were checked into the emergency room with what the researchers refer to as an apparent life-threatening event (ALTE).

A diagnosis of GERD was most common diagnosis of the randomly-picked group. A total of 154 children, or 49%, were diagnosed with GERD. Within six months, 14 children (9% of the group) had another life-threatening emergency room visit for GERD, even after GERD treatment from the first ER visit.

Argentina researchers (Orsi *et al.* 2011) used 24 hr pH probe and Multichannel Intraluminal Impedance to test 243 infants and children with either digestive or lung symptoms relating to GERD. They found that more of the children under 22 months had GERD as compared with the older children.

GERD and Other Conditions

GERD has been found to occur alongside a variety of other conditions. We'll discuss the reasons for this in the next chapter, but let's first review ailments research has discovered occurs often among GERD sufferers:

One of the most common conditions with GERD is **gastritis**. In gastritis, the stomach wall is being damaged by gastric acids produced in the stomach.

GERD sufferers also often suffer from **ulcers.** Ulcers are a chronic and intensive form of gastritis, as the wall of the stomach becomes perforated, and begins to bleed.

Many GERD sufferers also suffer from **lung and congestive ailments.** In fact, many who suffer from airway conditions also have GERD without realizing it.

Many children who suffer from **airway conditions** also have GERD, and their airway conditions are often seen as a result of GERD.

Research from the Medical College of Wisconsin (Ulualp *et al.* 1999) found, in a study of 22 people, half of which had **chronic sinusitis**, that 7 of the 11 people with chronic sinusitis also had significant GERD symptoms. The researchers concluded that, "these findings suggest that pediatric GERD may contribute to the pathogenesis of chronic sinusitis in some adult patients."

Researchers from Houston's Baylor College of Medicine (Thakkar *et al.* 2010) found, in a review of studies that included 5,706 **asthma** patients, that 22% suffered from GERD symptoms, while 62.9% had abnormal esophageal pH, and 34.8% had esophagitis. The 22% of asthmatics having GERD was compared to control subjects. Only 5.4% of those without asthma had GERD.

Speaking of **esophagitis,** this condition—an inflammation of the esophagus—also frequently co-exists among GERD sufferers. It can prevail over GERD, or become entangled with the GERD prognosis.

Eosinophilic esophagitis (EOE) is increasingly common among infants, children and adults. Its symptoms, which include inflammation of the esophagus often correlate with GERD, and many patients have both conditions at the same time. However, treatments that typically help with GERD do not seem to help EoE sufferers.

This has been pegged to the fact that EOE is now seen as an allergic disorder, because the inflammation mediators found in EoE are similar to the antibody-allergen-antigen mechanisms seen amongst hay fever, food allergies and other types of allergic responses. EOE symptoms are often seasonal as well.

Research from the Children's National Medical Center in Washington, DC shows that eosinophilic esophagitis, which has gastroesophageal reflux disease-like symptoms, is linked to **allergies.**

Some clinicians have suggested that because eosinophilic esophagitis symptoms mimic GERD, EoE might be wrongly diagnosed as GERD by many doctors (Noel and Tipnis 2006).

As the GERD condition prevails, the cells that line the pharynx and larynx can also be damaged. This has been referred to as **laryngopharyngeal reflux** or LPR. LPR is often considered a part of a GERD diagnosis, because LPR rarely if ever does not eventually accompany chronic GERD.

Researchers from London's University College (Ayazi *et al.* 2012) found that many patients with GERD will suffer from **voice box changes,** resulting in changes in the voice **vocal cords,** and negatively effecting voice frequency and amplitude.

University of Texas research (Bresalier 2005) found that among Americans, **esophageal adenocarcinoma** incidence has grown faster than any other form of cancer since the 1970s.

Severe chronic **rhinosinusitis** sufferers also tend to suffer from GERD (Loehrl 2012).

Researchers from Brazil's Paulista University (Guaré *et al.* 2011) found that GERD contributes to **dental erosion**. This is assumed caused by stomach acids getting into the mouth, but this effect was found among those with weakened immunity. We'll discuss this relationship later.

Rett syndrome is a nervous system development condition that effects mainly women and young girls. Approximately 74% of those with Rett also suffer from gastroesophageal reflux or similar conditions (Lotan and Zysman 2006).

GERD has been linked with hyperacidity in **chronic renal failure** due to kidney disease (Fallone and Mayrand 2001).

Researchers from Japan's Osaka City University Graduate School of Medicine (Fujiwara *et al.* 2011) tested 2,680 patients with GERD, **functional dyspepsia,** or **irritable bowel syndrome.** They noted that these diseases often overlap with each other.

Their testing showed that 160 patients, or 6%, had more than one of these disorders.

Obesity is commonly seen with GERD (Reavis 2011). For this reason, bariatric surgery and/or gastric bypass have become increasingly more popular among GERD sufferers.

However, the mechanisms of GERD are different between obese people and thinner people. Obese people tend to be more sensitive to the contact of stomach acids against the esophageal lining. Also, **hiatal hernias** are more prevalent among obese people.

Obese people also tend to suffer from **intra-abdominal pressure,** which tends to weaken and open the lower esophageal sphincter. As we'll discuss further later, opening of this lower sphincter allows leakage of stomach acids from the stomach into the esophagus.

Interestingly, the vagus nervous system among obese people also tends to differ from lean people. Obese people tend to produce more bile and pancreatic enzymes. Increased amounts of bile and enzymes increases the level of irritation to the esophagus cells.

Gastroenterology researchers from Italy's University of Cagliari (Usai *et al.* 2008) studied the relationship between GERD and celiac disease. They found among a group of 105 celiac patients that 29 of them had the nonerosive version of GERD, also called **nonerosive reflux disease (NERD).**

Cystic fibrosis has also been linked with GERD. Researchers from Belgium's University of Leuven (Marteau *et al.* 2000) found among 41 patients with cystic fibrosis that 80% had increased levels of gastroesophageal reflux and 56% had a resulting dumping of stomach acids into the lungs.

Their study also tested 15 healthy people and 29 people with asthma and chronic cough. Using sputum drawn from everyone, they found that those with bile acid dumping in the lungs, neutrophil elastase was present in their sputum—linking stomach acids to their saliva.

They also found that 13% of the healthy group and 28% of the asthma group had bile acids in their sputum.

More recent studies (Pauwels *et al.* 2011) have also confirmed this finding.

A majority of people with **systemic sclerosis** also have GERD. Research has found that 80% of sclerosis patients have some sort of gastrointestinal issue, most of which involve or lead to GERD (Attar 2002).

Dysphagia—or difficulty swallowing—is often a consequence and symptom of GERD. This in turn has been linked to **malnutrition** among children.

GERD also dramatically increases the risk of **esophageal carcinoma** (Barak *et al.* 2002).

University of South Florida College of Medicine research (Nord 2004) categorized the conditions of **adenocarcinoma, erosive esophagitis, stricture** and **Barrett's esophagus** as complications of GERD.

Their clinical research found that symptoms of these sorts of complications often do not reflect classic GERD symptoms. They often involve the lungs, chest pain, and conditions of the ear, nose and throat.

Shaheen and Ransohoff (2002) found that reflux symptoms increased the risk of **adenocarcinoma** within the esophagus.

Barrett's esophagus often shows up in advance of a **cancerous lesion**.

This has led doctors to assume that Barrett's esophagus—a form of **throat cancer** - is caused by gastric acid exposure to the throat. And because Barrett's often forms **esophageal adenocarcinoma**—also a form of **cancer**—it has been suspected that the stomach acids are causing what is called dysplasia of the cells lining the throat, eventually leading to those cells undergoing mutation.

And because GERD and GERD medications will interfere with digestive processes and assimilation of nutrients, chronic GERD may be accompanied by **bacteria infections, diabetes, heart diseases, cystic fibrosis, immunosuppression, food allergies, malnutrition, and various intestinal disorders.**

We'll clarify these and other relationships with GERD later on.

Why do asthma sufferers often have GERD?

This is a good question. Many asthma sufferers also suffer from gastroesophageal reflux. Researchers are increasingly realizing that asthma's association with GERD is not merely a coincidence: The two disorders are somehow connected. However, the assumption that stomach acids are reaching into the lungs, is, well, a reach. Is this really why they are connected? Let's review the science on their relationship, and then we'll answer this question throughout the book:

In research from Sweden's Uppsala University (Uddenfeldt *et al.* 2010), it was found that among 8,150 people, contracting GERD more than doubled the incidence of adult onset asthma. Furthermore, obesity and GERD significantly increased the risk of asthma among the middle aged and the elderly.

University of Washington researchers (Debley *et al.* 2006) studied GERD symptoms and asthma among adolescents who had asthma. They studied 2,397 students from six Seattle middle schools. They found GERD in 19% of current asthmatic children, and only in 2.5% of the total student population. GERD symptoms were also more severe among the asthmatic children compared to non-asthmatic children with GERD. Asthmatic children required urgent medical treatment five times more than did the non-asthmatic children with GERD. Asthmatic children with GERD required more asthma medication than asthmatics without GERD. Asthmatic children with GERD also had more severe asthma episodes.

Researchers from Barcelona's Hospital de la Santa Creu i Sant Pau (Plaza *et al.* 2006) found that among 56 patients with persistent coughing, 21% had gastroesophageal reflux. More than one in five, in other words.

Researchers from Columbia University's College of Physicians and Surgeons (DiMango *et al.* 2009) studied 304 asthmatics and found that 38% also had GERD. While they found little difference in lung function and bronchial medication use, they did find that the GERD sufferers had significantly more severe asthma symptoms, had to use more oral steroids (typically reserved for severe asthma). GERD asthmatics also had poorer quality of life scores than the asthmatics without GERD.

Researchers from the Korea's Inha University College of Medicine (Kang *et al.* 2010) studied 85 young children with recurrent wheezing. They found that 48% had serious gastroesophageal reflux. They also found that 12% of the GERD patients were allergic to eggs or milk, while 20% of the non-GERD patients were allergic to eggs or milk. They concluded that while GERD were predisposed to asthma, GERD did not predict food allergies, as had been previously assumed.

Researchers from the University of Utah Health Sciences Center (Peterson *et al.* 2009) studied the relationships between exercise-induced asthma and gastroesophageal reflux. They studied 31 volunteers, 20 of which had asthma. They found that 73% of the asthmatic subjects had abnormal pH (pH levels associated with GERD) during treadmill tests. They commented that people may be misdiagnosed with asthma when they simply have respiratory symptoms related to exercise and GERD.

Spanish researchers (Tolín *et al.* 2011) used multichannel intraluminal impedance (MII) to test patients with severe asthma, coughing or chronic laryngitis. They found that of 49 total children tested, 25 children had acid reflux.

It is apparent that the asthma and GERD are related. Why are they related? We'll uncover this later.

The Quick "Fixes"

Time rules in modern life. And life has significantly speeded up. Just imagine how long it would take for a person to go into town and get some supplies at the general store one hundred years ago. It would be an all-day event that began with getting the horses ready, bridled up and saddled. The trip itself might take an hour, even if town was a few miles down the road. Once there, our shop at the store might take a few hours. By the time we got home, the sun would likely be setting.

Today, we can jump in our car and be at the store in minutes. The fast check out will speed our exit out of the store, and we can be stocking the fridge in a half hour. Then, of course, we must get some other things done. The store was simply a quick diversion.

Everything is speeded up in our lives today. Time is at a premium, and we must get what we are doing now done so we can get the next thing done.

Even our recreation is speeded up. Everything is on the clock, and we must keep pace with the rest of society to maintain our standard of living.

This also goes for our health. Our modern day mentality regarding health care typically revolves around the 'quick fix.' The quick fix might be compared to going into the bosses office and beginning to explain to her/him a problem that is slowing down productivity amongst the bosses employees, and having the boss respond with, "don't tell me why its happening, just fix it!"

In this situation, the result will often be a frenzied attempt to solve the problem without a long-term strategy of preventing the problem from recurring. This type of solution provides what we might call a "stop gap measure" to change the immediate outcome, but without a plan that will prevent the problem from returning. The problem here is that most problems, when not confronted with a good plan, will fester and get worse. Then suddenly they will reappear in a substantially more dangerous form than originally faced with.

This applies to the 'quick fixes' of conventional medicine, that reduce the symptoms temporarily, but do not fix the underlying problem. While the symptoms may be temporarily reduced, we keep

20

doing those things that are making the problem worsen. Soon, those 'quick fixes' don't reduce the symptoms, because the problem has grown.

Illustrating the danger of two of the most prominent "quick fixes" is a study from Stanford University researchers (Singh and Triadafilopoulos 1999) of 1,400 human subjects who had been taking antacids or H2-blockers for an extended period. The study found that the long-term users had more than double the rate of serious gastrointestinal complications.

Antacids

The perfect example of this is the use of antacids. The use of antacids for acid reflux has been going on for decades. This is driven, first, by the fact that antacids are generally easy to manufacture and sell. Secondly, it is driven by the fact that antacids generally do reduce the symptoms of GERD: by immediately neutralizing the acidic environment within the esophagus—temporarily.

And once the pain is relieved, the person feels generally that the problem is solved. They can now go about their day.

Not so fast. Not only do antacids not solve the problem. They create new ones. And over time, they exasperate the problem, and things get worse.

As we'll discuss in detail later, the stomach produces extremely strong acids in order to help digest our food, and help sterilize it. In fact, without the acidic nature of our stomach acids, we could be letting into our intestines so many dangerous microorganisms which will make our bodies sick. Our stomach's digestive acids create a strong barrier, because their hydrochloric acid (HCL) content will kill off numerous microorganisms.

In order to handle these acids, the lining of the healthy stomach and esophagus–the mucosal membranes—have a particular chemical make up that will protect the tissues of the stomach, the esophagus and the sphincter from the potent acids of our stomach.

So as the stomach's gastric cells produce these acids, the stomach's mucosal glands produce another substance that protects the stomach and esophagus: mucosal membranes.

The two work off of each other. The acids of the stomach generally drive mucosal gland secretions, and these alkaline mucosal secretions help support healthy acid production.

Eating antacids completely interferes with both processes. Antacids immediately neutralize our stomach acids. Yes, this does ease our discomfort. But it also prevents us from digesting our foods correctly. And it also allows microorganisms into our intestines.

When the region's pH is altered by antacids, the parietal cells will produce an increased amount of gastric acid in an attempt to reach the necessary acidity for digestion and sterilization. After counteracting antacids repeatedly, the parietal cells will become exhausted, and slow their all-important gastric secretions. This helps accomplish the goal of reducing acids for a short period, but over the long run can be dangerous to our body's future ability to digest and assimilate our foods.

In one study (Jancin 1996), out of 155 otherwise healthy people using antacids over a long period, 47% had esophageal erosion and 6% had Barrett's esophagitis.

Furthermore, antacids allow the underlying problem–weakened mucosal membranes–to get worse. They become even less useful and more weakened, because their need has been decreased by the addition of antacids into the picture.

The body does this all the time. For example, when people take steroid medications for a long period, the adrenal system will slow down its own production of corticosteroids. This is because the body contains various feedback loops that stimulate responses in the body, and measure the body's conditions. When conditions indicate that a particular secretion is not necessary, the body slows that secretion down.

Antacids can also produce a myriad of other adverse side effects, depending upon the type. Let's look at the main types:

Magnesium salts (Milk of Magnesia®, Gaviscon®, Gelucil®, Mylanta®, Maalox®, others)

These can contain either magnesium hydroxide, magnesium carbonate or magnesium trisilicate. While these can neutralize acids, they can also produce diarrhea, constipation and stomach upset. Dehydration and mineral imbalances can also result. Extended use can cause constipation or a dependency upon laxatives for bowel movements. Mylanta and Maalox combine magnesium with aluminum to lessen diarrhea. Some also have experienced allergic reactions.

Calcium salts (Titralac®, Rolaids®, Tums®, Alka-2®, others)

Most of these are calcium carbonates, which neutralize acids, but also can produce constipation and diarrhea. They can also produce hypercalcemia (too much calcium in the blood), leading to kidney failure and other problems. Vomiting, slowed reflexes, increased urination, appetite loss, muscle weakness and allergic reactions have also been seen.

Aluminum salts (Alternagel®, Amphogel®, Mylanta®, Maalox®, others)

Aluminum hydroxide has a variety of side effects in the body, including depleting calcium stores in the bones. Aluminum hydroxide can produce renal failure, and aluminum can deposit in the bones, joints and aluminum deposits have been found in the brains of dementia patients. They can also alter iron levels.

Antacids are just one example of the quick fix solution that has been applied to GERD. There are several others. Here are a few of them:

Bismuth Subsalicylate (Pepto Bismol®) and Bismuth Subcitrate (De-Nol®)

Bismuth is a slightly radioactive element that produces an alkaline state. Both the subsalicylate and subcitrate versions have been shown to help relieve some heartburn and ulcer pain, depending upon whether they are related to hyperacidity or hypoacidity.

One of the ways they seem to help is that they have been shown to inhibit the growth of *H. pylori* bacteria growth—which we will discuss later on. The subcitrate has been shown to yield the better benefit for *H. pylori* reduction (Rokkas and Sladen 1988).

Problems can arise from bismuth medications' side effects, however. They include: Moderate to severe allergic reactions—including rash, hives, itching, difficulty breathing, chest tightness, swelling of the mouth, face, lips, or tongue—fever, hearing loss, ringing in the ears, severe constipation, vomiting and nausea. It can also produce Reye's syndrome, and mask viral infections.

Besides these, bismuth can dramatically reduce our ability to digest our food, as it inhibits HCL and peptic enzyme production and activity.

Today, isolated bismuth subcitrate is typically only available through a compounding pharmacy. It is primarily sold as a combination therapy, together with two antibiotics. Let's discuss these:

Bismuth subcitrate potassium, metronidazole, and tetracycline (Pylera®)

This combination is typically applied for gastritis or ulcer associated with *H. pylori* infections. And as a combination, it has been shown to be very successful.

Besides altering our natural acids, enzymes and protective mucous membranes, the antibiotic cocktail of metronidazole and tetracycline depletes our healthy probiotic colonies. We'll discuss later see how important these are. By depleting our probiotic colonies, our bodies are opened up to a plethora of possible bacterial, fungal and viral infections, due to our lacking what is now considered about 75% of our gut's immunity. Knocking down both our acidic levels and our probiotic colonies is a recipe for disaster, as it invites infection with little protection.

These antibiotics also produce bacteria strains that become resistant. These 'super-bugs' are now threatening us with stronger and stronger versions of bacteria that we used to be able to fight off easily—such as MRSA. Treating *H. pylori* in this way also produces stronger, more resistant strains, and these medications and others will have little or no effect. Thus these antibiotics are the ultimate in 'quick fixes,' as they are more like ticking time bombs.

And besides these issues, the bismuth subcitrate/metronidazole/tetracycline combination is known to have other side effects: Watery or bloody diarrhea; seizures/convulsions, numbness; burning, pain, or tingling in the hands and/or feet; burning or irritation of the throat; chest or upper stomach; and fever, chills, and other negative consequences. Taking this if we have kidney or liver issues can cause still other problems.

Prokinetics - metoclopramide, domperidone and others.

Prokinetics' effectiveness, especially over the longer term, has been debated. Some of these—notably cisapride, have been withdrawn from the market. Those still on the market, like metoclopramide, come with serious side effects that include nervousness, anxiety, sleep disturbance, numbness and even Parkinson's disease and tardive dyskinesia (involuntary nervous movements)—the latter two which have occurred in as many as 25% of high dose patients and 5% of longer-term usage.

Histamine-2-receptor antagonists

Proton pump inhibitors (PPIs): omeprazole, lansoprazole and others. These by far are the most used medications, as they significantly retard the body's production of stomach acids.

A number of studies and large scale reviews have found that proton pump inhibitors were more effective than histamine-2 receptor antagonists for short term relief of GERD symptoms. And both were generally more successful than laparoscopic surgery outcomes.

However, new research has revealed that PPIs may not help severe reflux sufferers for long. In a study by researchers from 200 severe GERD patients, Medical University of South Carolina researchers (Clayton *et al.* 2012) found that those taking PPI medications were likely to suffer from nighttime reflux episodes than those not taking the PPI drugs. Those in the PPI group suffered from an average of 3.76 mean reflux episodes per night, while those severe GERD patients not taking PPIs had an average of 2.82 episodes per night. The researchers stated: "PPIs decrease the acidity of esophageal refluxate but do not decrease the relative frequency of reflux episodes in the recumbent position in patients with refractory GERD despite twice-a-day treatment with PPI therapy."

PPIs also come with a number of side effects, especially when taken on the long term.

Proton pump inhibitors have more recently been linked with heightened risk of bone fractures, and the possibility of hypomagnesemia—low levels of magnesium in the blood stream (Chen *et al.* 2012).

Other possible adverse side effects of PPIs include contracting infections of *Clostridium difficile* and other intestinal bacteria, including spontaneous bacterial peritonitis. Reduced nutrient absorption has also been documented, along with hypergastrinemia, a rebound form of high acid secretion. Increased risks of various cancers, including carcinoid tumors, have been noted as PPI side effects in the literature.

In addition to these, side effects such as rashes, headaches, diarrhea, constipation and nausea have been observed in between 1 and 5% of patients taking PPI medications (McCarthy 2010).

Acid-blocking medications prevent our gastric cells from producing the gastric pyloric acids that are necessary for breaking down food and preventing microorganisms from getting to the intestines. This means that we are removing from our body one of the most critical gatekeepers—one that blocks our body from a plethora of bacteria, viruses, fungi and toxins. Without the availability of these acids, our digestive tracts offer an attractive home for colonization of *E. coli,* salmonella, cholera and other dangerous bugs.

Acid-blocking medications also change our body's delicate pH balance among mucosal membranes elsewhere in the body. This leaves other epithelial tissues also open to invasion from microorganisms and toxins.

When our gastric acids are blocked, the production of mucosal membranes that line our sinus cavities, our mouth, throat and airways is also slowed. This leaves the body open to pollen allergens that penetrate these layers before they might otherwise be broken down.

Illustrating the ultimate damage gastric acid inhibitors can have, a study from Italy's University Federico II of Naples (Canani *et al.* 2006) followed children with GERD who took either H2 blockers or proton pump inhibitors for two months.

In this multicenter study, 91 children with GERD were prescribed ranitidine or omeprazole. After two months of use, the children were followed up for the next four months, and compared with 95 healthy children. The children taking the acid blockers had a significantly increased incidence of acute gastroenteritis and pneumonia during the four month follow up period. This increase was similar between the children taking H2 blockers and the PPIs.

The researchers concluded that "the use of GA inhibitors was associated with an increased risk of acute gastroenteritis and community-acquired pneumonia in GERD-affected children." They also stated that, "this points to the importance of gastric acid suppression as a major risk factor for infections."

Gastric acid inhibitors mess with the messaging and feedback systems that respond to fight-or-flight situations. They change our enzyme secretions, and they alter our adaptability to differing foods, which can open the door to intestinal permeability and food allergies.

We'll discuss the science behind these concepts shortly. For now, it is important that we realize why the 'quick fix' solution is not only not productive for permanently solving the problem: The 'quick fix' allows the problem to fester, and actually get worse.

Gastric banding: Banding has led to weight loss and in some cases a reduction of GERD symptoms among obese persons. However, many surgeries have to be reversed, and they can come with a number of unexpected side effects, including a lack of nutrient absorption. Vomiting and acid regurgitation can also result (Snow and Severson 2011).

Gastric bypass: As mentioned, sometimes vertical bandings do not work out so well. A common 'fix' among conventional doctors is to embark upon yet another surgery called gastric bypass. This is when the stomach is divided into two parts, with both parts being connected to the small intestine. This creates a smaller digestive area, increasing the feeling of fullness, and hopefully reducing the urge to overeat.

Other conventional treatments: Allergic eosinophilic esophagitis and gastroesophageal reflux will typically involve a TH2-dependent and IL-5 cytokine-mediated infiltration of eosinophils within the esophageal mucosa (Bax and Gupta 2006). As most other therapies have proven frustrating, diet modification has been the most successful form of treatment to date.

Researchers from The Netherlands' Erasmus University (Kastelein *et al.* 2011) tested whether acid suppression medications halted or even prevented dysplasia among patients with Barrett's esophagus—which often develops in advanced GERD cases. This and other research has shown that acid suppression medications—

leading to a reduction of stomach acid—will not necessarily prevent GERD from progressing to Barrett's or eosinophilic esophagitis.

Non-Acid Reflux and NERD

Remember earlier that we pointed out clinical research confirmeding that at least one out of ten GERD sufferers has low acidity rather than high acidity.

A newly-configured version of GERD has now been branded as *"non-acid reflux disease"* or NERD. This of course is similar to the *alkaline reflux,* it simply wipes away the relationship between gastric acidity (or lack thereof) within the esophagus and the symptoms of GERD.

This, together with alkaline reflux, virtually pulls the carpet out from underneath the assumption that GERD is simply a problem of too much acid production—or acid leaking from the stomach into the esophagus. Practically the same symptoms are produced between NERD and GERD patients. Why?

While there are other names given to try to connect the dots— such as **esophageal hypersensitivity, psychological comorbidity** and **esophageal motor dysfunction**—the core condition remains similar. In these conditions, GERD symptoms are experienced even when acid suppression medications are being taken and/or there is significantly less acid being produced—often close to nil—by the stomach's gastric cells.

This of course has mystified doctors, who wrongly assumed that because GERD is often evidenced by stomach acid leaking into the esophagus, that if the acid is blocked, GERD will go away.

We might compare this logic to a person seeing rain alongside wind, and assuming that the wind is causing the rain. While the wind may be implicated in the storm, just because it is seen concurrently at times doesn't mean that the wind causes the rain. Furthermore, there can be windless rain, just as there is non-acidic reflux.

This non-acid reflux disorder has been seen in increasing numbers according to many clinical researchers. Furthermore, several studies have shown that NERD patients treated with proton pump inhibitors continue to suffer the same symptoms. Physicians are still struggling to figure out how to treat such patients (Remes-Troche *et al.* 2011).

According to some research, the most common form of GERD is nonerosive reflux disease or NERD (this is not the same as saying that most GERD is NERD). NERD patients typically also do not respond to proton pump inhibitor medications. (Manabe *et al.* 2011).

Given these facts, it behooves not only any individual possible-GERD sufferer, but the medical institutions that are attempting to treat GERD, to not simply discern between GERD and NERD, but to unveil the real causes of GERD and NERD, and isolate those activities that can reverse the syndrome. While this supposition may seem overly simplistic, there is real evidence indicating that indeed both GERD and NERD is reversible.

(Please note: To avoid confusion, the science through the rest of this book will combine NERD with GERD reference, as we will show the two—and many others—are two symptoms of the same general disorder.)

This points to an assumption about GERD that has become standard amongst holistic health professionals: The notion that most cases of GERD and heartburn are not issues of there being too much acid as much as they are issues related to the stomach not producing enough acids.

As we will show in this book, both hypotheses are overly sim-plistic. Creating either 'smoking gun' of not enough acid or too much acid completely bypasses the complexity within which the body creates balance within the processes of breaking apart our foods and protecting itself from those very acids that accomplish these.

These balances, as we'll find, are as complex as they are beautiful, as they illustrate the fantastic miracle of human metabolism.

Chapter Two

The Physiology of GERD

Let's start with the basic physiology, then lay out the more complex metabolic aspects of GERD. While some of the key elements discussed in this chapter may appear redundant, we are trying to link multiple concepts together to gain a clearer picture of the disorder.

The Esophageal Sphincters

The esophagus is the staging area for our food. If we masticate our food well enough, our food will pass through the esophagus to the stomach within ten seconds.

At the top and bottom of the esophagus are two valves called the esophageal sphincters. These are basically muscular rings that open and close like tubular gateways. In a healthy system, these valves work in synchrony to coordinate the entry of food into and out of the esophagus with a minimum of leakage either from the top—where air and airway mucous can get in—or the bottom—where undigested food and gastric acids can leak up from the stomach.

When we swallow, the upper sphincter opens, allowing our (hopefully) chewed food and/or liquids into the esophagus, where it is staged for entry into the stomach.

In a healthy person, the lower sphincter (also called the cardia) will be closed until it is stimulated by swallowing. When we swallow, the lower esophageal sphincter also opens in a delayed-synchronous fashion to receive the masticated (chewed) food into the stomach.

This fact—that the lower sphincter valve stays closed except for when we swallow—prevents an outpouring of stomach acids from stomach into the esophagus.

The same principle goes for the upper esophageal sphincter. A tightly closed upper sphincter helps prevent pockets of air and airway mucous from getting into the esophagus.

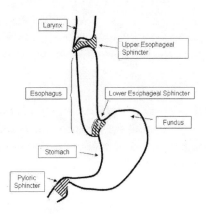

Esophageal Sphincters (with Pyloric Sphincter)

Belching or burping comes from air being trapped within the esophagus. Swallowing air is a typical cause. Trapped air can also come from the digestive process, as some foods produce gas as they are broken down. Carbonated beverages can also produce belching. Eating or drinking quickly, talking while eating and gulping fluids will also produce burps. Swallowing air during exercise, smoking or chewing gum can also produce belching.

Unhealthy sphincter valves become weakened and don't close tightly enough. A weakened upper esophageal sphincter lets more air into the esophagus. A weakened lower sphincter produces heartburn symptoms as gastric acids, undigested foods and toxins irritate the more sensitive mucous membranes of the esophagus.

And a weakened upper esophageal sphincter can allow those acids to leak up into the mouth, sinuses and airways.

Note that the lower esophageal sphincter cannot be controlled consciously except by swallowing. It is innervated by sympathetic nerves, so it is part of our autonomic system. This also means that things that affect our autonomic system—such as stress—will also affect the sphincter.

Frequently, especially as we age, the sphincter may weaken. In some cases, the top of the stomach wall may pouch through the lower esophageal sphincter. This is called a hiatal hernia. Research has suggested that up to 50% of Americans may have a hiatal hernia, although only about 5% of those with hiatal hernias suffer from GERD. This suggests two issues: First, that hiatal hernias are not always associated with GERD. And second, that stomach acids leaking into the esophagus do not necessarily produce GERD—because the hiatal hernia prevents the sphincter from closing.

Yes, many of the airway, mouth and sinus symptoms associated with GERD are the result of stomach acids leaking up. However, there are other mutual issues—related to the health of our mucosal membranes—that tend to cause multiple conditions such as GERD and asthma simultaneously.

The lower esophageal sphincter is controlled by the cricopharyngeus muscle. Just as any muscle can weaken or lose tone over time, the cricopharyngeus muscle can weaken and lose tone, causing it to not be able to tightly close the ring valve.

So what can weaken the cricopharyngeus muscle and the esophageal sphincter it supports? This will be one of the central mysteries this chapter will solve. That's because the question is not that easy to answer. There are too many confusing elements.

For example, we know that if food delivered to the sphincter comes in too fast and is not masticated enough, strain will be put on the sphincter and cricopharyngeus muscle.

While this is not necessarily the only cause for GERD, it is a fact that when this supporting muscle loses tone, the valves can weaken. But this is very simplified, as there are many reasons the muscle can lose tone.

The other mystery we will resolve in this chapter is why some GERD sufferers have high acid levels in the esophagus and some have low acid levels in the esophagus. This also goes for the stomach, as both high and low acidic levels have been found amongst GERD sufferers.

The bottom line is that GERD is not as easy as acids leaking into the esophagus.

As for acids burning the stomach, the mucosal stomach lining is specially designed to protect the wall of the stomach from acids and enzymes. The mucosal membranes that line the esophagus are also designed to protect from occasional acid leakage, and as we find from the low rates of GERD amongst hiatal hernia sufferers, acid leaking through the sphincter actually rarely produces GERD.

Still, research has validated the simplified thesis of GERD being related to a weakened lower esophageal sphincter. For example, French researchers (Zerbib *et al.* 1998) found that a relaxation of the lower esophageal sphincter was the central underlying feature of GERD among a large population of clinical patients.

So while leaking acids don't always produce GERD, a majority of GERD cases are related to a weakened sphincter. Yet not all GERD cases are related to high acid levels in the esophagus and stomach. Many are related to low acidic levels. It is quite a paradox.

But it gets more complicated than that. As the French researchers looked deeper into why this sphincter relaxed, the researchers found that cholecystokinin (also called CCK) was the key factor in this relaxation. They found out that altered levels of cholecystokinin among the muscle fibers of the sphincter altered the tone of the sphincter wall.

Cholecystokinin is stimulated by a binding with CCK-A receptors. When the CCK-A receptor is antagonized, however, the sphincter weakening is dimished.

The CCK-A receptor, however, is where things get more complicated. The CCK-A receptor is related not only to muscle tone within the sphincter valves, but also to enzyme production. This is related to the feeling of satiety (or fullness), and the release of key neurotransmitters endorphin and dopamine. So we find that the loss of muscle tone amongst the sphincters is complicated.

The Stomach Machinery

As food is dropped into the stomach, it undergoes intense churning and breakdown by the stomach's digestive juices. Special glands dispersed among the stomach cells in the stomach lining secrete a mixture of biochemicals. Mucosal cells produce an alkaline mixture, while parietal cells produce an acidic mixture.

The end result is a blend composed primarily of hydrochloric acid, sodium chloride, potassium chloride, pepsin, rennin and a special mucus—made primarily of mucopolysaccharides, glycoproteins and bicarbonate. To varying degrees, the stomach also secretes lipase, a fat-splitting enzyme, and other enzymes. The enzymes pepsin and rennin break down proteins, preparing them for intestinal assimilation. Gastric acid also facilitates the absorption of some B vitamins, calcium and iron.

Parietal cells use a network of secretion tubes called canaliculi to secrete gastric acid into the stomach. The canaliculi serves as a mixing chamber, where hydrogen and chloride ions—both secreted independently by parietal cells—come together to form the highly acidic HCl.

These parietal cells also produce significant amounts of sodium chloride (NaCl) and potassium chloride (KCl). These accelerate HCl acidity, as well as buffer and stabilize it.

This parietal process also feeds bicarbonate (CHO3) into the bloodstream. This in turn stimulates the secretion of the protective alkaline mix by the mucosal glands. This buffering formula protects the stomach wall from the harshness of the gastric acids. This feedback process allows the stomach to constantly maintain a balance of acidity and alkalinity, while generating a mucosal layer to always coat and protect the sensitive cells of the stomach wall.

The stomach has four parts, from bottom to top: the pylorus, the body; the fundus; and the cardia. The cardia lies at the top. Here lies the lower esophageal sphincter—the valve that opens and closes, allowing food from to snake in from the esophagus. As we've mentioned, should the upper sphincter not be working properly, it may regurgitate food and stomach acids back into the esophagus.

The fundus is the curvy section of the stomach and the stomach body is in the center—this section has the greatest volume. The pylorus empties churned food bolus into the top of the small intestine through the pyloric sphincter valve.

The mucosal lining of these tissue regions protect the tissues from damage due to the acidic nature of our digestive juices.

The approach that modern medicine has taken is that these digestive juices are the "bad guys." Yes, they indeed can cause tissue damage among the cells of the esophagus. And these acids do cause pain when they are in contact with these sensitive tissues.

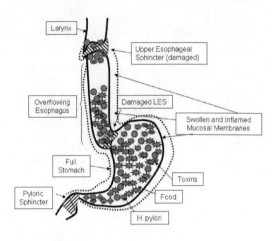

GERD and Gastritis

What conventional medicine seems to miss is the fact that these acids are necessary in order to digest our foods and prevent microorganisms from entering our intestines and our blood stream. The pH of these acids, which include hydrochloric acid, is super low—averaging a little less than 2 in a healthy body.

This low (acidic) pH will penetrate the cell membranes of most microorganisms, causing their immediate death.

This is ironic, because this is the same reason that our stomach acids will harm and damage our tissues. The low pH easily damages and penetrates the cell membranes of our own epithelial tissue cells. This damage produces inflammation, which causes the burning sensation some feel in GERD—and why its often called heartburn.

Remember, however, that many cases of GERD—more than one out of ten—are not related to high acidity. And remember the study mentioned earlier, by University of Southern California medical school researchers (Ayazi *et al.* 2009) that confirmed this. Other studies have had similar findings.

In this UC study, out of 1,582 GERD patients and 54 healthy subjects, they found the normal pH range to be 0.3 to 2.9. The average age of the GERD patients was 51 years old. Only about half (50.3%) of the patients had "abnormal esophageal acid exposure." As we mentioned earlier, a full 176 of the GERD patients, or 11%, had low gastric acidity (hypochlorhydria)—a pH over 2.9. The rest of the abnormal acidity was high—but this was only 39% of the whole group of 1,582 GERD sufferers.

This means that the majority of GERD sufferers do not suffer from hyperchlorhydria (high acidity) in the esophagus at all.

The research concluded that "the major effect of gastric pH was that the hypochlorhydric patients tended to have more reflux in the supine position than those with normal gastric pH."

Since most GERD sufferers do not have high stomach or esophageal acidity at all, we must look more deeply at the underlying conditions in GERD—as we are doing in this book. This doesn't mean we should ignore the acidity issue, however. Let's look a little more deeply first at what gastric acidity is and how it is measured.

Acids and Bases

About a third of the production of our gastric juices comes as a result of our smelling food or tasting food. This is often why the smell of food can make us hungry. The feeling of hunger comes from the production of gastric acids in the stomach.

Another two-thirds of gastric acid production is stimulated by our stomach filling up with food. The stomach is wired with nerves that sense incoming food as the sphincters open. This response also promotes an expansion of the stomach wall to accommodate food. This is called distension.

A smaller portion of acid is released through the bile duct, as churned food begins to enter the upper intestines through the pyloric sphincter. This last acidic push from the bile ducts helps clean up and boost the next phase of digestion within the intestines.

Acidity or alkalinity is measured using a logarithmic scale called pH. The term "pH" is derived from the French word *pouvoir hydrogene,* which means 'hydrogen power' or 'hydrogen potential.' pH is quantified by an inverse log base-10 scale. It measures the proton-donor potential of a solution by comparing it to a theoretical quantity of hydrogen ions (H+) or H_3O+.

The scale is pH 1 to pH 14, which converts to a range of 10^{-1} to 10^{-14} (.00000000000001) moles of hydrogen ions. This means that a pH of 14 maintains fewer hydrogen ions. pH14 is thus *less acidic* and *more alkaline* (or basic).

The pH scale has been set up based on pure water being in the middle. Using the scale, water's pH is log-7 or simply pH 7—due to water's natural mineral content. Because pure water forms the basis for so many of life's activities, and because water neutralizes and dilutes so many reactions, water was established as the standard reference point or neutral point between what is considered an acid or a base solution.

In other words, a substance having greater hydrogen ion potential (but lower pH) than water will be considered acidic, while a substance with less H+ potential (higher pH) than water is considered a base (alkaline).

Now the solution with a certain pH may not specifically maintain that many hydrogen ions. But it has the same *potential* as if it contained those hydrogen ions. That is why pH refers to hydrogen power or hydrogen potential.

As mentioned, healthy gastric juice maintains a pH between about 0.5 to 3. Hydrochloric acid (HCl) is the main component for pH control. An acidic pH is critical to sterilize our food. Without enough HCL, we run the risk of allowing unwanted bacteria into the stomach and intestines.

One of these is *Helicobacter pylori*. Recent research has connected *H. pylori* overgrowths in the stomach to a majority of ulcers and many GERD cases.

The common premise is that heartburn means too much acid in the stomach. The typical response most people have is to take antacids or another alkaline remedy (many try milk and others for example) to reduce the acid content. This may provide brief relief for those with acidic esophagus sphincter leaks. For many others, antacids don't help the pain at all. In these cases, acids aren't the problem.

In either case, antacids may make matters worse, because they drive the pH of our stomach's gastric juices too high. This shuts down the feedback loop related to submucosal gland production, effectively slowing mucosal secretion, which reduces our ability to protect the epithelial cells from contact with toxins, microorganisms, irritating foods and beverages.

The gastric acids released into the stomach environment through this parietal cell process will have a pH well below 1, but as they are buffered somewhat by the alkalinity of the mucosal secretions, the resulting pH range of a healthy stomach can get as high as 3.

This pH is sustained by a special enzyme produced by the body called ATPase. This enzyme is also called a proton pump, because it "pumps" protons ($H+$ ions) from the parietal cells in exchange for potassium ions ($K+$) produced through the production of energy: the adenosine triphosphate (ATP) cycle—which is how our cells produce energy.

This ATPase enzyme basically trades a potassium ion for a hydrogen ion, and it is these hydrogen ions that maintain the pH environment of the stomach.

The acidic pH within the stomach unfolds proteins, which exposes them to pepsin enzymes that break the aminos apart. This unfolding is also called denaturing.

Pepsin is also activated by the acids produced in the stomach. HCl is the principle acid in this process, as it converts pepsinogen to pepsin.

The quality of gastric acids within our stomach is not just acidic. It's like looking at a green forest from a distance. The closer you look, the more details you see. The stomach acids are precisely formulated with enzymes and hydrochloric acid that allows them to consume and break down foods, toxins and microorganisms.

Theses acids and enzymes that sit on top of the mucosal membranes are practically miraculous. If we were to take a drop of this mixture from the stomach and drop some of it on the floor, it would likely—depending upon the makeup of the floor—burn a hole in the floor if not leave a significant burn mark.

Eating antacids seriously compromises the strength of this important blend. When the pH of this mixture is too high, our food won't get broken down right. The enzymes will be compromised.

The stomach and the rest of the body will be left open to undigested foods, unbroken down toxins, and bacterial infection.

Acid-blocking medications such as proton-pump inhibitors (PPIs) will further exasperate this problem in many cases. While these can sometimes be helpful for temporarily easing pain or helping ulcers heal, they also can create a reduction of the very digestive juices we need to break down our foods for intestinal absorption. They also cut back HCl production, again allowing bacteria to grow among our stomach's mucosal membranes.

The *Helicobacter pylori* Connection

One of these bacteria is the *Helicobacter pylori* species. *H. pylori* infection of the stomach and upper intestines is widespread globally, but among Western countries it is linked to ulcers, GERD and gastric cancer.

This was confirmed by research from Emory University School of Medicine (Gold 2001), which found *H. pylori* overgrowths present in many patients with ulcers of the stomach and duodenal intestine, stomach cancer, intestinal tumors and GERD.

Scientists from the 2005 Canadian Helicobacter Study Group Consensus Conference (Bourke *et al.* 2005) confirmed that *Helicobacter pylori* infections are connected with gastric cancer formation. And because *H. pylori* infections also affect gastric pH, the researchers recommended that *H. pylori* testing precede the use of long-term proton pump inhibitor medications.

H. pylori infections are typically confirmed with the 13C-urea breath tests together with upper endoscopy with biopsy of the stomach to confirm the finding.

H. pylori affects stomach acid production. Researchers from Japan's Hamamatsu University School of Medicine (Furuta *et al.* 2002) studied a population of GERD sufferers who had *H. pylori* eradication (antibiotic) treatment. Elimination of *H. pylori* decreased gastric juice pH values (increasing acidity to normal levels) and increased cholesterol levels among the patients. Pancreas functions improved and protein levels were normalized after the elimination of *H. pylori*.

However, eliminating *H. pylori* wasn't necessarily the answer. After *H. pylori* was eradicated, some of the patients still suffered from or shortly developed new cases of GERD. Obese patients had the highest risk of developing GERD after *H. pylori* eradication.

The glaring issue again is the reduced mucous secretion in the stomach and esophagus. Mucous lines the cells, buffering them from the harsh stomach acids and enzymes. Typically a burning sensation in the stomach or esophagus is the result of too little mucous lining rather than too much acidity. This becomes evident in cases of ulcer, where the mucous lining is broken down, and the acids are damaging the cells of the stomach wall.

Furthermore, it is often the food itself—as it is being broken down—that actually irritates the lining of the esophagus in GERD and GERD-related disorders.

For this reason, those with GERD-related conditions often improve when they are given liquid elemental diets. Here the meal doesn't have to be staged, requiring the stomach's and intestine's enzymes and acids to break down the nutrients that nourish our bodies.

Illustrating this, researchers from the Children's Hospital of Philadelphia's Divisions of Gastroenterology and Nutrition (Markowitz *et al.* 2003) found that an elemental diet—where the patient is fed a liquid diet containing nutrients in elemental form—significantly improved symptoms of eosinophilic esophagitis.

The Mucosal Connection

Researchers from Germany's Otto-von-Guericke University (Kandulski and Malfertheiner 2011) determined that mucosal inflammation was at the root of GERD symptoms. They found that when the mucosal membranes are inflamed, characterized by IL-8 cytokines, these proinflammatory mediators infiltrate the membranes, which relaxes the lower esophageal sphincter.

In other words, advanced GERD is an inflammatory disorder caused by defective or weakened mucosal membranes.

Put simply, GERD is the result of damaged or otherwise thinned mucosal membranes that line the wall of the esophagus, the upper fundus of the stomach, and the sphincter tissues.

These walls are made up of cells called epithelial cells. Epithelial cells actually line all the passages of our body, including the mouth, nose, airways, intestines, urinary tracts, and even our skin.

Because epithelial cells throughout our body—not to mention those of our esophagus and stomach walls—come into contact with so many foreign entities, they are all lined with this special surfactant called mucosal membranes.

This surfactant contains a special ion combination, probiotic microorganisms, special phospholipids, glycoproteins, mucopolysaccharides, immune agents and other components. It is quite complex. Together, these components protect the epithelial cells from coming into contact with toxins and microorganisms from the foods we eat, the air we breathe, as well as any other foreign agents we might consume or be exposed to.

Should this mucosal membrane surfactant thin, and the cells of our epithelial tissues are exposed to these foreign agents, a cascade of events takes hold: This is called inflammation. Inflammation stimulates the production of prostaglandins, substance P and other elements that stimulate the sensation of pain.

But the pain isn't the worst problem. The pain is simply the symptom—an alarm—notifying us that our tissues are being damaged. When the cells that make up these tissues become damaged, they begin to function poorly, which endangers our ongoing health.

An example of this effect is when acids begin to harm the cells that cover the sphincter valve between the esophagus and the stomach, the sphincter valve begins to function poorly, losing its tone. It becomes weaker, and this weakness allows our stomach to regurgitate undigested foods and acids back into the esophagus.

Typically, a weakness in our mucosal membranes in one region is usually matched by weaknesses in others. For example, a weakness in the mucosal membranes of our stomach walls is also typically matched by weakened mucosal membranes among our esophagus and sphincter valve—as well as weaken mucous membranes in our airways and other epithelial areas.

This is why people who suffer from GERD also will suffer from other mucosal-related issues, such as asthma, sinusitis, allergies, ulcers, intestinal irritability and other issues. These are all metabolically related to the same issue of weakened mucosal membranes.

Conventional western medicine is not oblivious to the fact that our epithelial layers are lined with mucosal membranes. Various scientific studies have examined these membranes' chemistry and have illustrated just what they contain.

Conventional medicine is also aware of the function of the mucosal membranes—that they protect the epithelial cells and tissues from damage.

So why the disconnect? Why doesn't our doctor point out that we have defective mucosal membranes instead of giving us medication that block our body's production of important digestive acids?

There is no good answer for these questions. We might say that conventional western medicine simply has its blinders on when it comes to this issue and many others. This could be related to the short-sighted focus of modern medicine on the relief of symptoms with pharmaceutical medications.

The mucosal membranes that line our stomach and esophagus also cover just about every surface of our body that has any contact with the outside environment. Mucosal membranes line the epithelial cells of our skin, nose, throat, mouth, airways, digestive tract, urinary tract, vagina, eyes, ear canal and other surfaces are there for a reason. Some surfaces, such as the skin, have very thin mucosal membranes. Other surfaces, such as the digestive tract and airways, have thick mucosal membranes. Some surfaces are such that they are not typically referred to as mucosal, yet they are still covered with mucosal membranes.

In most parts of the body, mucous is secreted by tiny mucous glands that lie within goblet cells scattered throughout these epithelia surfaces. They are called goblets because they are shaped like little goblet glasses, except their upper surface extends through the (internal) surfaces with tiny valves.

These valves empty through gaps between the particular epithelial cells of that surface. In the intestines and airways, these epithelia are called microvilli. On skin and other surfaces, they are dermal and epidermal cells. The goblet valves between those epithelial cells that line the esophageal surface also secrete mucous membrane material into the esophagus.

The goblet cells produce mucin through a process of contraction and glycosylation within the Golgi apparatus of the cells. This glycosylation of proteins produces the glycoproteins in mucin.

43

These, together with mucopolysaccharides and lipids, provide the glueyness of mucin.

The mucosal goblet cells of the intestines, respiratory tract and many other epithelial surfaces act very similarly to those of the gastric glands of the stomach and duodenum. The central difference is that these glands produce mucous thickened to counteract the parietal cells' secretion of highly acidic gastrin. This counteractive process requires a special feedback system. This counteractivity between the goblet cells, the villi and the gastric/pyloric cells unravels the mystery surrounding the fact that many people who have GERD also suffer from disorders of other mucosal membrane regions, including asthma, ulcers, Crohn's disease, irritable bowel syndrome and others.

Let's take a moment to review the surfaces that have forms of mucosal membranes, starting from head to toe:

- Scalp
- Ears
- Eyes
- Nasal Cavity
- Sinuses
- Tongue
- Gums
- Oral cavity
- Trachea
- Esophagus
- Airways
- Alveoli
- Stomach
- Intestines
- Colon
- Rectum
- Anus
- Urethra
- Vagina
- Skin

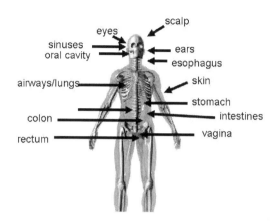

Mucosal Membrane Content

The mucosal membranes are thin layers of biochemicals produced by the body combined with probiotic bacteria. Most of our body's mucosal membranes are not the same from body region to body region either. Here is a short list of some of the ingredients in many of these regions:

- glycoproteins
- mucopolysaccharides
- enzymes (peptase, peptidase, amylase)
- probiotics
- T cells
- B cells
- macrophages
- Immunoglobulin-E antibodies
- Immunoglobulin-A antibodies
- ionic fluid, which includes ions of bicarbonate, calcium, magnesium, potassium, chloride, sodium and others

45

- many also contain antioxidant nutrients
- many contain other specialized elements specific to that particular area of the body

Each mucosal membrane provides specific tasks. However, nearly all of them will also support common tasks. Let's look at the common tasks first:

Transport

Depending upon the type of mucosal membrane, its ionic content provides a transporter medium to escort nutrients and byproducts back and forth between the epithelial cells and the surface of the mucosal membrane. These elements include oxygen, nitrogen, carbon dioxide, hydrogen carbonate and others. In the intestines and stomach, the mucosal membranes also transport nutrients such as proteins, vitamins and others across, between the epithelial microvillus cells and the mucosal membrane surface.

Some of these ions—such as the sodium, bicarbonate and chloride ions—provide the transport mechanisms into the cells and tissues of the skin surfaces. These travel through special gateways or pores among the cells. The ions attach to nutrients, oxygen and other elements—and escort them in, in other words.

This is critically important in the intestines and the stomach, where the mucosal membranes transport nutrients through the intestinal and stomach wall into the bloodstream. This is how our bodies are nourished.

But this does not mean the other membranes do not provide this service. The oral mucosal membranes also transport certain nutrients through to the bloodstream, especially under the tongue, for example. Also, the skin transports a variety of nutrients through to the epidermal layers of the skin. This goes for the other epithelial membranes as well. Each type of surface allows certain types of elements in, while blocking others.

Protection

Another most important function of the mucosal membranes is to protect the cells of the body from toxins, bacteria, fungi, viruses and any number of other elements that can harm the body. We'll focus more on the details of this function later.

Using the mucosal membranes, the body can be choosy about what kinds of elements it will allow into the epithelial cells and inner tissues. There are countless toxins, microorganisms, debris, allergens and other foreigners that the body wants kept out.

So just how does the body keep these invaders from penetrating the body's internal and external surfaces? The short answer is the mucosal membranes. This is why these membranes contain a host of immune cells. These include immunoglobulins such as IgA, B-cells, T-cells and others that are looking to trap foreigners before get any further. Once they find a foreigner, they will take it apart using a one of many immune system strategies.

Probiotic

The mucosal membranes are also mediums—also called cultures—for the survival and sustenance of many of our body's probiotic species.

The mucous membranes are thus living structures. Probiotics populate our mucosal membranes, and are an important part of the "wall" of protection provided by these membranes. These tiny protective probiotic bacteria will inhabit all healthy mucosal membranes, including the skin. Like the immune system, these bacteria are trained to protect their territory. If an invading microorganism enters the mucosal membrane, the probiotics will lead an attack on them, with the immune cells in close pursuit.

Flexibility

The mucosal membranes give the epithelial cells of the skin, scalp, oral cavity, intestines, stomach and so on their flexibility and their supple-ness. Without this, these tissues could not provide the body with the means to adjust to environmental conditions. It is critical that our skin is supple so that our internal organs and muscles can move and adjust from within.

Consider if our stomach wall was not flexible and supple. We would be restricted to eating only a small amount of food. The flexibility of the fundus allows the stomach to expand enough to hold up to four quarts of food and liquid. This is over fifty times the volume of the stomach when it is empty.

While many GERD experts will say that overeating sometimes is about the worst thing we can do, humans and most other creatures require flexible stomachs in order to handle a big meal during lean times. Being able to eat a big meal when the opportunity presents itself has been critical to the survival of most species. This is because eating is an opportunistic process. We must be flexible to the opportunity.

Of course, civilized man—especially amongst first world countries—has enough to eat, and the shelf storage to stow away what we have outside of what we can eat now. This makes it easier (and healthier) to pace ourselves as we eat, and thereby avoid overeating.

While this can reduce the stress upon our digestive tracts, our bodies were genetically designed to occasionally overeat. And most of us do—occassionally overeat now and then.

It is also critical that our digestive tract is adjustable to allow us to swallow and process our meals.

This goes for most of the other epithelial regions of the body covered with mucosal membranes. They are all, to one degree or another, flexible and supple—if in a healthy state.

We might compare this to how oil lubricates and protects an engine from overheating and dirt. The function is called viscosity. The mucosal membranes allow for viscosity, provided by the mucopolysaccharides and glycolipids. Glycolipids contain complexed fats, while mucopolysaccharides contain long chain carbohydrates that allow surfaces to glide against each other.

Epithelial Cleaning

In a well-maintained car, good motor oil will be circulated through the rods and cylinders. The oil doesn't just allow the steel parts to move with minimal friction: The motor oil also helps keep the engine clean, and prevents dirt and other contaminants from clogging up the system.

Imagine what would happen if a car were to run without oil for a few miles? The engine would surely seize up, and likely would break down completely. This may result from either a lack of lubrication, or that lack of oil allowing dirt to gunk up and jam the cylinders. While this is a crude example, there are several elements that are consistent.

This crosses over with the feature of protecting the cells as we just discussed. Killing off invaders is part of keeping the system clean. Imagine, immune cells killing off microorganisms and breaking down toxins within the mucosal membranes. What is the result? A bunch of dead bacteria parts, virus pieces, toxin portions and others floating around the region. Who wants a bunch of dead pathogen parts stuck to their skin?

Not a healthy body. This is why the mucosal membranes are fluid. Like any fluid body, mucosal membranes have motion and currents—often driven by the undulations of the epithelial cells themselves. The mucous will thus circulate through the region, dumping out the dead body parts and toxin pieces, all the while renewing the area with a clean layer of mucous.

This is what happens when we sneeze, cough, blow our nose, or even breathe or sweat. During these activities, dirty mucosal fluid is being thrown off. In the meantime, submucosal glands replenish the area with new fluid.

Quelling Reactivity

The chemistry of the mucosal membrane also buffers and calms immune response. The mucosal membrane will help transport components such as corticosteroids from the adrenals to squelch inflammatory immune responses among our epithelial tissues. In other words, a healthy mucosal membrane is calming to our digestive tract, airways, skin and other epithelial regions. And a damaged or thinned mucous membrane is a recipe for irritation of those epithelial cells, producing rashes on the skin, allergies among the sinuses, IBS among the intestines, asthma, COPD and pneumonia within the lungs, gastritis within the stomach, and of course, GERD within the esophagus.

The Stomach Lining

An adult stomach is 10 inches long, and its inside lining (fundus) will expand greatly, as we've discussed.

The mucosal membranes that make up the lining of the stomach maintain most of the benefits discussed above, along with a few others. The stomach's lining protects the stomach's epithelial cells and the parietal cells of the stomach along with the gastric pits. It keeps the stomach wall clean and healthy. It helps maintain the flexibility of the fundus and the stomach in general, allowing the stomach to stretch and shrink to the volume of the stomach's contents.

The stomach lining also houses colonies of hardy microorganisms that help protect the cells. The stomach's lining is also critical as a transport medium. The mucosal membrane lining of the stomach provides effective transport for a number of nutrients and water absorbed through the stomach's wall into the bloodstream.

The lining also helps regulate the chemistry of the stomach, which helps calm the reactivity of the stomach, allowing smooth and relaxed digestion.

Let's run through an example of how this works. When we are relaxed and hungry, our body's nervous processes stimulate the release of dopamine, serotonin, leptin and gherlin. These will stimulate the nerves along the vagus nerve pathway, which in turn switches on peristalsis and the release of gastric acid, and as we discussed, the feedback system that signals the secretion of the alkaline mucous membrane chemistry.

This balanced secretion allows us to sterilize our food and digest our meal in a healthy manner. And the mucous membrane secretions coat the cells of the stomach to prevent damage from the acids.

The most notable benefit of the stomach's gastric secretions, as we've discussed, is their acidic pH, which destroy microorganisms and in general sterilizes most of the food and liquids that get into the stomach before they get further into the body.

Consider that every bite and gulp we take will contain thousands, if not millions of microorganisms. Most food producers will pasteurize or otherwise attempt to sterilize their prepared foods and drinks; but this hardly removes all the microorganisms. There still will be hundreds of thousands of survivors, and there will also likely be addition microorganisms introduced as the package is opened and the food or drink is prepared for consumption.

The chemistry of the mucosal membrane, as we've mentioned, maintains a pH between 0.5 and 3, depending upon the health of the person. Those who take significant antacids and acid-blocking medications will likely maintain a much higher (more alkaline) pH, which could be as high as 5 or 6.

As we compare the pH to most U.S. state health departments' acceptable high pH for unpasteurized food and beverages of 4 to 5, we find that the pH of 0.5 to 3 provides significant sterilization benefits for the stomach. This means that most microorganisms—including those hundreds of thousands of microorganisms not killed by pasteurization and those billions that can be found in raw foods—will be killed off in the stomach with a healthy pH. Yet an unhealthy pH of 4-6 present in many of those who take antacids and acid-blocking medication will allow many of these microorganisms direct entry into the body.

This explains many of the side effects that have been discovered among acid-blocking medications—which we'll lay out a bit later.

Hopefully this discussion clarifies one of the more important benefits of maintaining a healthy stomach lining.

Protecting epithelial cells from gastric acids

While most of the mucosal membranes of the body will contain some acidity to repel microorganisms, the stomach and esophagus are special cases, where the pH of the entire environment is significantly lower (more acidic)—in the 0.5 to 3 pH range. The amazing thing about this is that while mucosal alkalinity balances this incredibly acidic environment, it also maintains significant barrier for the cells.

In other words, this strong acidity that sterilizes our food and beverages can also damage the gastric cells of the stomach and esophagus. That is, if the mucous membranes are damaged and the acids gain direct contact with these sensitive cells.

This is not all they are sensitive to. The epithelial cells of the stomach and esophagus are sensitive to exposure to microorganisms, allergens, toxins, free radicals, pollutants and other foreigners.

Epithelial cells have two layers of protection. In addition to the entire epithelial surface being covered by a mucopolysaccharides-glycolipid mucous membrane, each cell is covered with a phospholipid cell membrane. Should this phospholipid cell membrane come into contact with gastric acids, allergens, toxins, free radicals, microorganisms or other intruders, the bonds between the phospholipids become damaged, opening up the cytoplasm of the cell to intrusion. This is called cellular permeability, and is one of the main drivers for inflammation, and the pain symptomatic of GERD.

When these cells are part of the stomach wall, this can result in inflammatory ulcerative tissue—the beginning of an ulcer.

When they are the cells of the esophagus, the damage and inflammation produces GERD symptoms.

When this takes place among the cells making up the epithelial surface of one of the sphincters, the sphincter tissues become damaged and inflamed, weakening the ability of the sphincter to close properly. This is also called losing tone.

This inflammatory episode among the lower esophageal sphincter lies at the heart of the leakage into the esophagus, but it still is only a component. Weakened esophagus mucosal membranes are also part of the problem—and people with weakened mucosal membranes will suffer from damage to both epithelial surfaces.

Then there is inflammation caused by these mucosal-deficient epithelial surfaces being exposed to undigested food and toxins. What does undigested, radical-forming food and toxins have to do with a weakened lower esophageal sphincter and inflammation? Plenty. If we have too little acidity and enzyme power within the stomach, we are unable to properly break down and neutralize our foods. That is the purpose for these acids and enzymes: To break down and neutralize our foods into components that do not harm the body.

Should our gastric production and enzyme production be poor, the food does not move efficiently through our stomach into the intestines. This is called the *rate of emptying*, or *gastric emptying*. If our rate of emptying is too long, and we have undigested food in our stomach for an extended period, combined with a weakened sphincter valve, the undigested food, together with whatever acids and enzymes there are, will back up through the sphincter into the esophagus.

Toxins will also be found here, because a poor diet will typically contain plenty of toxins and toxic microorganisms. Healthy gastric acids will kill most of these microorganisms and will break down many toxins. But if our acids and enzyme levels are low, these will also back up in the esophagus through a weakened sphincter.

Or, if we are chronically eating too much, these undigested foods, toxins and microorganisms may simply back up before they even make it through the lower esophageal sphincter in the first place.

Heartburn Pain

GERD is symptomized, as most of us know, by pain. The pain can range from a subtle burning sensation in the abdominal area to an excruciating pain that runs all the way up the esophagus into the throat, chest and even sinuses.

Most dismiss the pain of heartburn as stomach acids, but this is not necessarily true. Many things can cause the irritation that feels like burning, including toxins, undigested foods and pathogenic microorganisms. Any of these may be irritating our epithelia, ultimately damaging them.

When epithelial cell membranes are damaged as described above, and cellular permeability is created, the immune system responds with inflammation in a desperate attempt to save the tissues. When massive inflammation erupts, pain is a byproduct. While pain doesn't feel like a byproduct of another process—because pain can be so uncomfortable—it is nonetheless. This is important to know because when we are feeling pain, pain is not the only thing going on. The body is trying to stop and heal the damage. The pain is warning us to protect the area, and begin preventative action. Pain is also nature's way of teaching us what things are good for us and what things are not so good.

While acute pain such as our hand getting burnt when we touch a hot pan is easy to respond to and prevent, chronic pain is a bit more tricky, and requires more investigative work. Still, it is chronic pain that stimulates the investigative process. It is nature's way of telling us that something is wrong. This is why pain is so important. Just imagine if we didn't feel pain. We'd probably lose a lot of appendages, and we'd be dying very quickly.

Inflammation then, inclusive of pain, is the body's way of accomplishing several objectives:

- Informing our consciousness that we need to be aware of tissue damage somewhere in our body and do something to prevent it.

- Triggering action from the immune system's warriors to fight off and hopefully remove the invading forces that are damaging the tissues.

- Repairing the damage caused by the invasion.

Before we dig deeper into the inflammatory process, let's summarize what elements (or combinations thereof) can be producing the painful inflammation of GERD:

- Epithelial exposure to gastric acids
- Epithelial exposure to digestive enzymes
- Epithelial exposure to undigested foods
- Epithelial exposure to toxins
- Epithelial exposure to microorganisms

A healthy digestive tract is designed to manage these elements. But if the system is broken, and our mucosal membranes are damaged, these will make contact with our epithelial cells, harming them and producing inflammation.

Confirming this, Gupte and Draganov (2009) found 15 different eosinophils in their biopsies of esophagus's from patients with eosinophilic esophagitis. This indicated that advanced GERD and related eosinophilic esophagitis are indeed inflammatory conditions.

Epithelial exposure is met by the immune system's launching a slew of different messengers among the damaged tissues, which include substance P and prostaglandins—which produce the sensation of pain. The epithelial damage that produces this pain is basically a wound. We might compare it to a blister on the skin. And just like a blister, if we keep rubbing against it, the wound will only get worse. With this in mind, let's look more closely at the dynamics of inflammation and wound repair:

The Process of Inflammation

Most people think of inflammation as a bad thing. Especially when they see that so many disease conditions involve inflammation. Rather, inflammation simply coordinates the various immune players into a frenzy of healing responses, along with a purge of toxins.

Our body's immune system launches inflammatory cells and factors that heal injury sites and prevent bleed-outs. This process is often stimulated by two inflammatory signalling cells called leukotrienes and prostaglandins.

This is a good thing. Imagine for a moment cutting your finger pretty badly. First you would feel pain—letting you know the body is hurt. Second, you will probably notice that the area has become swollen and red. Blood starts to clot around the area. Soon the cut stops bleeding. The blood dries and a scab forms. It remains red, maybe a little hot, and hurts for a while. After the healing proceeds, soon the cut is closed up and there is a scab left with a little redness around it. The pain soon stops. The scab falls off and the finger returns to normal—almost like new and ready for action.

Without this inflammatory process, we might not even know we cut our finger in the first place. We might keep working, only to find out that we had bled out a quart of blood on the floor. Without clotting, it would be hard to stop the bleeding. And without some continuing pain, we would be more likely to keep injuring the same spot, preventing it from healing.

Were it not for our immune system and inflammatory process slowing blood flow, clotting the blood, scabbing and cleaning up the site, our bodies would simply be full of holes and wounds. Our bodies simply could not survive injury.

Our probiotic system and immunoglobulin immune system work together to deter and kill particular invaders—hopefully before they gain access to the body's tissues. Should these defenses fail, they can stimulate the humoral immune system in a strategic attack that includes identifying antigens and recognizing their weaknesses. B-cells and probiotics coordinate through the stimulation of immunoglobulins and cytokines.

This progression also stimulates an activation of neutrophils, phagocytes, immunoglobulins, leukotrienes and prostaglandins. Should cells become infected, they will signal the immune system from paracrines located on their cell membranes. Once the intrusion and strategy is determined, B-cells will surround the pathogens while T-cells attack any infected cells. Natural killer T-cells may secrete chemicals into infected cells, initiating the death of the cell.

Leukotrienes immediately gather in the region of injury or infection, and signal to T-cells to coordinate efforts in the process of repair. Prostaglandins initiate the widening of blood vessels to bring more T-cells and other repair factors (such as plasminogen and fibrin) to the infected or injured site. Histamine opens the blood vessel walls to allow all these healing agents access to the injury site to clean it up.

Prostaglandins also stimulate substance P within the nerve cells, initiating the sensation of pain. At the same time, thromboxanes, along with fibrin, drive the process of clotting and coagulation in the blood, while constricting certain blood vessels to decrease the risk of bleeding.

Leukotrienes are molecules that identify problems and stimulate the immune system. They pinpoint and isolate areas of the body that require repair. Once they pinpoint the site of repair, one type of leukotriene will initiate inflammation, and others will assist in maintaining the process. Once the repair process proceeds to a point of maturity, another type of leukotriene will begin slowing down the process of inflammation.

This smart signalling process takes place through the biochemical bonding formations of these molecules. Leukotrienes are paracrines and autocrines. They are paracrine in that they initiate messages that travel from one cell to another. They are autocrine in that they initiate messages that encourage an automatic and immediate response—notably among T-cells, engaging them to remove bad cells. They also help transmit messages that initiate the process of repair through the clotting of blood and the patching of damaged tissues.

Leukotrienes are produced from the conversion of essential fatty acids (EFAs) by an enzyme produced by the body called arachidonate-5-lipoxygenase (sometimes called LOX). The central fatty acids of this process are arachidonic acid (AA), gamma-linolenic acid (GLA), and eicosapentaenoic acid (EPA). Lipoxygenase enzymes produce different types of leukotrienes, depending upon the initial fatty acid. The important point of this is that the leukotrienes produced by arachidonic acid stimulate inflammation, while the leukotrienes produced by EPA halt inflammation. The leukotrienes produced by GLA, on the other hand, block the conversion process of polyunsaturated fatty acids to arachidonic acid.

Prostaglandins are also produced through an enzyme conversion from fatty acids. Like leukotrienes, prostaglandins are messengers that transmit particular messages to immune cells. Their messaging is either paracrine or autocrine. Prostaglandins are critical parts of the process of injury repair. They also initiate a number of protective sequences in the body, including the transmission of pain and the clotting of blood.

Prostaglandins are produced by the oxidation of fatty acids by an enzyme produced in the body called cyclooxygenase—also called prostaglandin-endoperoxide synthase (PTGS) or COX. There are three types of COX, and each convert fatty acids to different types of prostaglandins. The central fatty acid that causes inflammation again is arachidonic acid. COX-1 converts AA to the PGE2 type of prostaglandin. COX-2, on the other hand, converts AA into the PGI2 type of prostaglandin.

The key messages that prostaglandins transmit depend upon the type of prostaglandin. Prostaglandin I2 (also PGI2) stimulates the widening of blood vessels and bronchial passages, and pain sensation within the nervous system. In other words, along with stimulating blood clotting, PGI2 signals a range of responses to assist the body's wound healing at the site of injury.

Prostaglandin E2, or PGE2, is altogether different from PGI2. PGE2 stimulates the secretion of mucus within the stomach, intestines, mouth and esophagus. It also decreases the production of gastric acid in the stomach. This combination of increasing mucus and lowering acid production keeps healthy stomach cells from being damaged by our gastric acids and the acidic content of our foods. This is one of the central reasons NSAID pharmaceuticals cause gastrointestinal problems: They interrupt the secretion of this protective mucus in the stomach.

This means that the COX-1 enzyme instigates the process of protecting the stomach, while the COX-2 enzyme instigates the process of inflammation and repair within the body. In the case of autoimmune disease, the COX-2 process often lies at the root of pain and swelling.

Cyclooxygenase also converts ALA/DHA and GLA to prostaglandins. Just as lipoxygenase converts ALA/DHA and GLA to anti-inflammation leukotrienes, the conversion of ALA/DHA and GLA by cyclooxygenase produces prostaglandins that either block the inflammatory process or reverse it.

This also means that a healthy diet with plenty of GLA and ALA/DHA fats will help buffer and balance a chronic inflammation response. ALA is found in walnuts, soybeans, flax, canola, pumpkin seeds and chia seeds. The purest form of DHA is found in certain algae, and the body produces EPA from DHA. Fish and krill also get their DHA up the food chain from algae. GLA is found in borage, primrose oil and spirulina. We'll talk more about this later.

Probiotics are often involved in the production of intermediary fatty acids used for these LOX and COX conversions, producing anti-inflammatory effects. To illustrate this, scientists from the University of Helsinki (Kekkonen *et al.* 2008) measured lipids and inflammation markers before and after giving probiotic *Lactobacillus rhamnosus* GG to 26 healthy adults. After three weeks of probiotic supplementation, the subjects had decreased levels of intermediary inflammatory fatty acids such as lysophosphatidylcholines, sphingomyelins, and several glycerophosphatidylcholines. The probiotics also reduced inflammatory markers TNF-alpha and CRP in this study.

The arachidonic acid conversion process that produces prostaglandins also produces thromboxanes. Thromboxanes stimulate platelets in the blood to aggregate. They work in concert with platelet-activating factor or PAF. Together, these biomolecules drive the process of clotting the blood and restricting blood flow. This is good during injury healing, but the inflammatory process must also be slowed down as the injury heals.

One of the elements most scientists miss in inflammation—especially among the mucosal membranes—is the role of probiotics.

Probiotics help modulate the inflammatory process. In the research from Poland's Pomeranian Academy of Medicine (Naruszewicz *et al.* 2002) mentioned earlier, scientists found that giving *Lactobacillus plantarum* 299v to 36 volunteers resulted in a 37% decrease in inflammatory F2-isoprostanes. Isoprostanes are similar to prostaglandins, formed outside of the COX process.

The probiotic and immunoglobulin immune system work together to deter and kill particular invaders—hopefully before they gain access to the body's tissues. Should these defenses fail, they can stimulate the humoral immune system in a strategic attack that includes identifying antigens and recognizing their weaknesses. B-cells and probiotics coordinate through the stimulation of immunoglobulins and clusters of differentiation (CDs).

This progression also stimulates an activation of neutrophils, phagocytes, immunoglobulins, leukotrienes and prostaglandins. Should cells become damaged and/or infected, they will signal the immune system using paracrines located on their cell membranes. Once the intrusion and strategy is determined, B-cells will surround the pathogens while T-cells attack any infected cells. Natural killer T-cells may secrete chemicals into infected cells, initiating the death of the cell.

This is often of no avail in many cases of GERD, simply because the damage caused by the stomach's acids and other toxins causes many cells to die and the tissue elements to begin to erode and die.

Depending upon the toxin or invader, the inflammation response will also accompany an H1-histamine response. Histamine is primarily produced by the mast cells, basophils and neutrophils after being stimulated by IgE antibodies. This opens blood vessels to tissues, which stimulates the processes of sneezing, watering of the eyes and coughing.

These measures, though sometimes considered irritating, are all stimulated in an effort to remove the toxin and prevent its re-entry into the body. As histamine binds with receptors, one of the resulting physiological responses is alertness (also why antihistamines cause drowsiness). These are natural responses to help the body and mind remain vigilant in order to avoid further toxin intake.

As macrophages continue the clean up, the other immune cells begin to retreat. Antioxidants like glutathione will attach to and transport the byproducts—broken down toxins and cell parts—out of the body. As this proceeds, prostaglandins, histamines and leukotrienes are signaled to reverse the inflammation and pain process.

That is, assuming that the cell and tissue damage does not continue. In most GERD cases, the thinned mucosal membranes produce chronic inflammation, or at best, periodic inflammation. This reflects itself in the form of feeling more burning sensation after or surrounding meals, during the nighttime, during stressful situations and so on. We'll get into these relationships more closely later on.

At the height of the repair process, swelling, redness and pain are at their peak. The T-cells, macrophages, neutrophils, fibrin and plasmin all work together to purge the allergen from the body and repair the damage.

One of the central features of the normalization process is the production of bradykinin. Bradykinin slows clotting and opens blood vessels, allowing the cleanup process to accelerate. A key signalling factor is the production of nitric oxide (NO). Nitric oxide slows inflammation by promoting the detachment of lymphocytes to the site of infection or toxification, and reduces tissue swelling. Nitric oxide also accelerates the clearing out of debris with its interaction with the superoxide anion. Nitric oxide was originally described as endothelium-derived relaxing factor (or EDRF)—because of its role in relaxing blood vessel walls.

The body produces more nitric oxide in the presence of good nutrition and lower stress. Probiotics also play a big role in nitric oxide production in a healthy body. Lactobacilli such as *L. plantarum* have in fact been shown to remove the harmful nitrate molecule and use it to produce nitric oxide (Bengmark *et al.* 1998). This is beneficial to not only reducing inflammation: Nitric oxide production also creates a balanced environment for increased tolerance.

Low nitric oxide levels also happen to be associated with a plethora of diseases, including diabetes, heart failure, high cholesterol, ulcerative colitis, premature aging, cancers and many others. Low or abnormal nitric oxide production is also seen among those with lifestyle habits such as smoking, overeating, and living around air pollution.

Nitric oxide was originally described by researchers as endothelium-derived relaxing factor (or EDRF)—because of its role in relaxing blood vessel walls.

The body produces more nitric oxide in the presence of good nutrition and lower stress. Probiotics also play a big role in nitric oxide production in a healthy body. Lactobacilli such as *L. plantarum* have in fact been shown to remove the harmful nitrate molecule and use it to produce nitric oxide (Bengmark *et al.* 1998). This is beneficial to not only reducing inflammation: NO production also creates a balanced environment for increased tolerance.

Low nitric oxide levels also happen to be associated with a plethora of conditions, including GERD, diabetes, heart failure, high cholesterol, ulcerative colitis, premature aging, cancers and many others. Low or abnormal NO production is also seen among lifestyle factors such as smoking, obesity, and environmental air pollution.

Esophageal Varices

Another possible contributing cause for increased inflammation among the esophagus tissues and GERD symptoms is esophageal varice. This can occur as a result of atherosclerosis—a hardening of the arteries and veins—which can produce venous thrombosis.

Should the submucosal veins beneath the esophagus mucosa become dilated with venous thrombosis, esophageal varice can occur. This is caused by a rise in portal blood pressure, which pushes pressure into other regions, including around the base of the esophagus. This dilation will often lead to an expansion of the esophagus submucosa, which in turn causes inflammation in the surrounding esophagus mucosa tissues.

In advanced cases, a variceal hemorrhage can also occur. This will damage the tissues, producing cell death and ulcerated tissue. This produces an inflammatory event as described above.

Reactive Mucosal Glands

The question we must ask now is why, if a little acid leaking into the esophagus is so bad, can so many people overeat, even regurgitate and not have GERD? Or how can some burp and even vurp (a burp combined with regurgitation) without getting heartburn? When people overeat, and food backs up into the esophagus, acid typically leaks into the esophagus. In fact, heartburn quite often appears among people who don't overeat. This indicates that the two—heartburn and acid leakage into the esophagus—are mutually exclusive in many cases. Why can some handle overeating while others can't?

This relates to the health of the esophagus mucosal membranes. A healthy esophagus will have a thick enough mucosal membrane to prevent leaking acids from burning the esophagus, because this mucosal membrane—while not as thick and alkaline as the mucosal membrane in the stomach—is typically thick enough and alkaline enough to buffer and protect the cells of the esophagus, throat and vocal cords from the effects of stomach acids, undigested foods, toxins and microorganisms.

In fact, the same issues that causes the mucosal membranes of the stomach wall and the surface of the sphincter to weaken and become damaged by gastric acids also weaken the mucosal membranes of the esophagus.

This is because the glands that secrete mucosal membranes around the body are connected by the same physiological and metabolic pathways. These are tied to our moods, stress levels, neurotransmitter and hormone levels, certain nutrients, and the relative state of homeostasis within the body.

Like most of the body's secretions, submucosal glands are stimulated by various messengers—notably hormones and neurotransmitters. While the location of the mucosal lining may differ, and those particular goblet cells may respond slightly differently, there is a common submucosal response to stress, anxiety, fear, the lack of certain nutrients, and systemic inflammation.

Among the hormones and neurotransmitters that stimulate the mucosal secretions of the esophagus lining are acetylcholine, dopamine, leptin, gherilin and serotonin. Key neurotransmitters/hormones that block or balance the process are PGE1 and PGE2, epinephrine/adrenaline and nor-epinephrine.

The pathways that stimulate these are supported by what is called the cyclooxegenase cycle—abbreviated COX. The COX enzymes stimulate certain aspects of the body's relative systems of metabolism. COX is a component of prostaglandin production. Prostaglandins drive mucosal secretions, and they are critical to inflammation. So there is a double-edged sword when it comes to COX, especially COX-1.

The COX-1 enzyme is specific to the mucosal secretions, and also connected to certain inflammatory responses. For this reason, when COX-1 is inhibited by non-steroidal anti-inflammatory drugs (NSAIDS) such as aspirin, acetaminophen and many others, there will be a side effect of gastric upset and gastric bleeding. The reason is that the NSAID blocks the COX-1 enzyme's prostaglandin pathway, which shuts down the secretion of mucous by submucosal glands.

While this shut-down takes place throughout the body, it is most symptomized in the esophagus and stomach because this is where the body's epithelial cells are most exposed to harsh stomach acids, undigested foods and toxins in the absence of a healthy mucosal membrane.

But the COX-1 inhibition will affect other mucosal membranes throughout the body as well—though the symptoms of these are typically more muted. For those who have exposure to more stomach acids in the esophagus—due to a weakened sphincter or overeating—they will experience more immediate GERD in reaction to COX inhibitors.

Other signs of weakened mucosal membranes occur among those who experience asthma, those who experience allergies and those with sinus issues. In all three cases, a weakening of the mucosal membrane secretions exposes the epithelial layers of the skin to toxins, allergens and/or other challenges, producing inflammation.

The Gut-Brain Axis

Stress does the same thing. When we are stressed, the body slows down its mucosal secretions.

For this reason, we can clarify emphatically that when the COX-1 pathway or any other part of the submucosal gland pathways are blocked or inhibited—either by stress, NSAIDs, dehydration, nutrition deficiency or any number of other possible causes as we'll describe—the esophagus becomes more exposed to whatever undigested foods, toxins, microorganisms and stomach acids build up within the esophagus.

The key pathways of acetylcholine, PGE (prostaglandin E), epinephrine/adrenaline and cyclooxegenase are also related to the nervous system and our state of mind. This is called the gut-brain-axis.

These pathways respond to different aspects of our nervous system and physiology. Hunger, stress, anger, fear, nutrient deficiency, dehydration and so many other states are discovered and communicated through the body using these messengers. Each of these states produces a particular type of nervous response and set of messenger.

The submucosal glands' production of mucous is tied to these messengers. It is this reason that when we become stressed or nervous, the submucosal glands slow down their production of mucous. This shut-down is the result of the nervous system focusing its energy into other, more urgent needs of the body such as muscle contraction, hearing, vision and so on.

Let's run through an example of how this works. When we are relaxed and hungry, our body's nervous processes stimulate the release of dopamine, serotonin, leptin and gherlin. Much of this release stimulates the vagus nerves, which in turn switch on peristalsis and the release of peptic acid and other gastric juices from the stomach's gastric glands.

This allows us to sterilize our food and digest our meal in a healthy manner, and also produce a alkaline balance of mucosal membranes among the airways and the esophagus.

Now should a healthy person be faced with a stressor—let's say we are being chased by a tiger on a African jungle tour—immediately the production of these digestive juices will be shut down. Adrenaline and supporting hormones/neurotransmitters effectively block the production of the body's mucosal membranes. This allows our body's energy to be focused upon those areas that allow us to get away from the tiger—such as our muscles, our eyes, and our brain cells.

We won't be wanting to stop and eat while when running from a tiger.

The body is not only diverting energy away from the mucosal glands of the stomach and esophagus. Most of the body's other mucosal glands are also blocked as energy is diverted. A prime example is how we typically develop dry-mouth when we are nervous about something. That nervousness is our body's stress-systems kicking into gear, blocking mucosal secretions—in this case, saliva.

Let's look at a cross section of the esophageal epithelia and mucosal secretion:

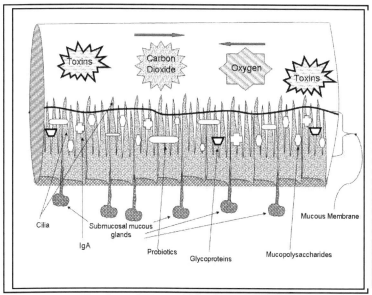

Esophageal Mucosal Membranes and Cilia

The Development of Mucosal Integrity

At birth, other than our skin—which has been covered by placenta fluid—our mucosal membranes are raw and not well developed. Gradually, as probiotics begin to colonize the sinuses, mouth, stomach and intestines—the mucosal membrane glands and their secretions begin to mature. This maturity, as we'll discuss in detail, requires good infant nutrition as well as strong probiotic populations in order to populate the mucosal membranes. As this colonization occurs, the body's epithelial cells and mucous glands provide their balance of chemistry and protective attributes.

This is the basis for the hygiene theory, a product of many studies showing that infants and children that are allowed to roam the floors, parks, soils, and those among larger families have stronger immune systems. This is because all that roaming allows our bodies to collect a variety of probiotic species, which eventually colonize and territorialize our mucosal membranes.

Then there is the transporter mechanism. The mucous membranes utilize this surfactant quality and ionic capabilities to transport nutrients among the epithelial cells, allowing them to function efficiently. It also transports toxins out of the area—assuming healthy mucosal membranes.

Should this transport mechanism not be functioning properly, the region can become laden with a thickened, toxic mucous. Instead of the mucous membranes keeping these surfaces clean, the mucous itself becomes toxic.

This thickened mucous membrane is typical in hyperreactive airway responses among COPD, asthma, and hay fever conditions. In the intestines, the condition produces irritable bowel syndrome, colitis, Crohn's and other intestinal issues. And weakened skin mucosal membranes produce eczema, dermatitis, hives and other skin irritations. And of course, in the lower esophagus and stomach, weakened mucosal membranes produce GERD and ulcers.

We have already laid out most of the significant chemical components of the mucosal membranes, specific to the esophagus and stomach. Most of these are also common amongst other mucosal membrane area, as we've discussed. Yet there are a few critical chemical elements important to the health of the esophagus and stomach mucosal membranes we should discuss further.

Water

Water is one of the most important elements to the health of the mucosal membranes. Water makes up the bulk of healthy mucous. The key physiological issue here is that the body intelligently prioritizes its water usage and availability. Here are the body's water usage priorities, beginning with the most vital:
1) Bloodstream
2) Brain
3) Lymphatic system

4) Critical organs (eyes, lungs, liver, kidneys, heart)
5) Intracellular cellular fluids (tissues)
6) Intercellular fluids (inside the cells)
7) Lacrimal systems—fluids that moisten the surface of the eyes.
8) Mucosal membranes of the airways
9) Mucosal membranes of the sinuses, throat, and mouth
10) Mucosal membranes of the esophagus
11) Mucosal membranes of the stomach
12) Mucosal membranes of the vagina and interstitial canals
13) Mucosal membranes of the skin
14) Mucosal membranes of the ears
15) Sweat glands
16) Joints
17) Ligaments and spinal disks
18) Bones

While this serves as an approximate—as few scientists have determined precisely how the body rations water—the body will make sure that the parts with the highest priority have enough water first. Those parts on the lower part of the list have the lowest priority. Thus, when the body does not get enough water, it is these parts of the body that will show symptoms of dehydration.

As we can see, the mucosal membranes are fairly low on the list of priorities.

This is why, for example, we will experience dry mouth when we are dehydrated. When we have dry mouth, the body is preserving its water content for the more critical areas of the body.

By the time we experience dry mouth, however, other parts of the body are already experiencing problems. This includes the mucosal membranes of the stomach and esophagus.

One of the central characteristics of GERD and other mucosal disorders is mucosal dehydration. When the mucosal membranes become dehydrated, the mucous is thickened and not viscous enough to provide its surfactant and transport functions. It also cannot house and feed needed probiotic populations.

Trace Elements

The mucous membrane fluids can become weakened due to a lack of trace elements—minerals, in other words.

The mucosal glands and their pores can also become blocked due to a lack of minerals—which form ions. The pores may be blocked due to an imbalance of ion chemistry in the mucosal membrane. Tests have shown that chloride ions, bicarbonate anions and other mineral-sourced elements stimulate the opening of the pores that bring liquids and nutrients into the epithelial tissues. Should the ion chemistry not allow the pores to open, the tissues will not absorb nutrients.

Having the right ion chemistry comes from our diet. Many diets are seriously lacking in trace elements and important macro minerals, such as potassium, phosphorus, magnesium and calcium and many others. Shortfalls in these can imbalance available supplies of bicarbonates, chlorides and sodium ions along with others.

Trace elements are also critical for pore opening among the various mucosal glands. Zinc, selenium and other important trace elements also work to balance the signalling process that stimulates the opening of the mucosal gland pores.

These minerals and trace elements provide crucial nutrients for all the mucosal substances around the body. Because pH is critical at each mucosal membrane site, these minerals provide the substances that control the pH.

The pH of each mucosal membrane is precisely tuned to the requirements of that region. As we've discussed, the stomach's pH ranges from 0.5 to 3, requiring significant alkalinity among the mucosal membranes of the stomach to balance these acids.

This situation is similar within the oral cavity, the esophagus, sinuses and the upper intestines, where there are strong acids and environmental toxins that must be buffered with alkalinity to prevent their damaging the epithelial cells of that region.

Alkaline Balance

On the other hand, other mucosal regions, such as the airways, the urinary tract, the colon and the skin, the risk of damage by acidity is a bit lower. This means the mucosal layer in these regions will have a pH that is not as high (alkaline) as the mucosal membranes of the stomach and esophagus or mouth have to be.

As we've mentioned, the components that provide this extra alkaline pH and buffering quality include long chain polysaccharides called mucopolysaccharides, along with delicately-balanced ionic fluids and mucin proteins.

The mucin proteins produced by the submucosal membrane glands are diluted with these ion fluids to give the mucous membrane the right balance of stickiness and fluidity. A change in this delicate balance can ruin the buffering quality of the membrane.

Exposure

Exposure to toxins, pathogenic microorganisms, cold air and any number of other triggers can result in weakened and thinned mucosal membranes among the stomach, esophagus and other mucosal regions. This depends greatly upon the condition of the body's immune system.

When the mucosal membranes are exposed to toxins, acids or other challenges in a healthy body, the production of mucous by the goblet cells is stimulated. This stimulates the quick removal of the toxin or invader, because the mucous being secreted maintains many immune cells, probiotics and other defense mechanisms that break down toxins and invaders. The excess mucous—containing the broken down parts—are swept out of the area with the movement of mucous. This might be compared to how the ocean circulates currents using the tides, the shorelines, temperatures and so on.

However, should the body be immunosuppressed or otherwise overwhelmed by the invasion of toxins or pathogens, the goblet cells will over-produce the watery elements of inflammatory mucous with too few immune cells. In other words, a unhealthy mucosal region will host toxins and unfriendly microorganisms.

This imbalance often produces an inflammatory reaction, which swamps the epithelial surfaces with immune cells and more mucous. This renders a type of war zone, leaving the region full of live and dead cell parts and toxins, and a flooding of mucous.

When these surfaces are drowning in this toxic soup of inflammatory mucous, the removal process is stifled. The lack of mucous transport, combined with the need to remove toxins, produces chronic inflammatory issues, symptomizes conditions like COPD and asthma in the lungs, and GERD and ulcers in the esophagus and stomach.

This is why medical researchers often find low acidity in some GERD cases and high acidity in other cases. The problem is not the acid—it is the inflammatory condition within the esophagus, typically created by weakened mucosal membranes.

Let's use an example. Let's say that you have a squeaky door. The hinge parts on the door are rubbing up against each other, causing the hinge to make noise. The metal is exposed to the other metal parts.

Let's say that you find a water spray bottle. You begin spraying the hinges with water. Testing the door, you find that the door does not squeak for awhile. But only for a short while.

By the time the water dries up, the door begins squeaking again, likely louder than it was squeaking before.

The problem is that the water provided little in the way of protection from the exposure between the metals that came into contact with each other.

Should you now decide to spray some silicon lubricant onto the hinges, suddenly the hinges will become quiet, and the hinge parts will easily slide against each other for months without any squeak. This is because the metal is now not exposed to the other metal parts. There is a layer of protection in between.

The mucosal membranes of our lower esophagus can either be like the water that was sprayed on the hinges or the silicone lubricant. If those mucosal membranes do not maintain a balance of ions, mucopolysaccharides, glycoproteins, probiotics and immune cells, even a little stomach acid or even some hot or acidic foods will produce a burning sensation as they get through the thin membrane and make contact with the epithelial cells of the esophagus.

But should our mucosal membranes have just the right thickness, containing all the right proportion of compounds including mucopolysaccharides, polysaccharides, probiotics, glycoproteins, bicarbonate, ions and other elements, acids leaked from the stomach, let alone undigested foods or toxins, will not have any effect upon the epithelial cells of the esophagus. Those cells will be lined with a comfy mucoid layer.

Epithelial Permeability

As we've been describing, when the mucosal membranes become defective, the epithelial cells beneath the membrane become directly exposed to numerous toxins, acids, undigested food, microorganisms and allergens. Once the epithelial layer of the esophagus is exposed to these foreigners, the foreigners will irritate and damage these epithelial cells.

As these epithelial cells are damaged by the foreigners, the cell membranes and the joints (tight junctions) between the cells become permeable. This creates a viscious cycle of chronic inflammation, because when they are permeable, foreigners can gain access to the inner tissues and the cytoplasm of the cells. And the more these cells are penetrated, the more they become inflamed. And the more they are inflamed, the more exposed they remain.

Let's look at this a bit deeper. The intercellular matrix of the esophagus epithelial layer patches together cells using a bonding system called tight junctions—also called zonula occludens. Using proteins called claudins, these tight junctions bond our esophageal cells together to create a layer of skin difficult to get through—or permeate. These junctions are aligned with proteins called zonulin, which are oriented in such a way that block the entry of the foreigners that travel through the esophagus.

These tight junctions can become damaged by repeated exposure to toxins, harsh acids and pathogens. When they are damaged, intruders are allowed access to the next layer of cells behind the epithelial cells. This is called *increased epithelial permeability* or simply *epithelial permeability.*

Epithelial permeability provokes an immediate immunity and inflammatory response. Here the tissues become inflamed and sensitive, driving the inflammation mediators including prostaglandins and cytokines, and you guessed it, pain.

Meanwhile, our cell membranes are made up of stacked phospholipids. The pores (also called ion channels) between the phospholipids that make up our cell membranes regulate what gets into the cells. These block potential intruders, keeping our cells healthy.

If the mucosal membrane becomes weakened, and epithelial permeability results, then toxins, pathogenic microorganisms, and acids from our foods and stomach acids gain access to our phospholipid cell membranes.

If these pores or the stacked phospholipid membranes become damaged, toxins and other intruders can get inside the cell. This is called *increased cellular permeability.*

Once in, these intruders will damage and even kill the cells. This provokes inflammation, which also provokes pain and the burning sensation among the esophagus in GERD.

These two issues—cellular permeability and epithelial permeability—make up the central mechanisms involved in so many conditions related to the digestive tract, the airways, the sinuses, the skin, the vagina and even many internal epithelial regions including the urinary tract and others.

As the phospholipid membranes and pores become exposed to foreigners, especially those heavy in free radicals and acidic ions, their molecular structures become altered. Depending upon the type of intruder, these will either steal electrons away from these molecules (oxidation) or will add electrons to the molecules (reduction).

The oxidation or reduction process will be accelerated in the presence of acids, because acids (H+) will easily utilize and move electrons from one molecule to another.

Regardless of whether it is an oxidation or a reduction, the reaction started by foreigners and accelerated by acids leaves the molecule's resulting state changed. This is often referred as the molecule having undergone a change in its oxidation state. Scientists will often loosely refer to this as the tissue or cells being subjected to free radical oxidation.

The instigators of this oxidation process are called reactive oxygen species, abbreviated as ROS. This is the more precise term for free radicals.

When the bonds between the molecules lining our cell membranes and those making up our intercellular are oxidized by free radicals, they become damaged. This produces inflammation and pain. And if the exposure to the offending radicals is not reversed, the damage will continue, progressing into more serious disease conditions.

Within the esophagus, this scenario progresses to conditions such as eosinophilic esophagitis and esophogeal cancer and various types of throat cancers, as we discussed in the first chapter.

This corruption of the cell membranes and intercellular matrix also results more increases in permeability—which allows more and more exposure to foreigners that present free radicals to the cells and intercellular matrix. This stirs up the immune system, which sends T-cells in to mark these cells and tissue areas as damaged. This "marking" results in a chronic inflammatory attack against those cells that have been so damaged.

This chronic inflammatory state drives the immune system to destroy and remove those cells and tissues. This allows them to be replaced by new (hopefully undamaged) ones.

This chronic inflammatory state has unfortunately been labeled by the conventional medical community as *autoimmunity*. Autoimmunity is described by conventional doctors as the body's immune system "attacking its own cells," as if the immune system has somehow gone haywire. This autoimmune thesis completely misses the actual events taking place.

While it might be true from a functional basis that the immune system is attacking its own cells, it is only because these cells have been damaged through exposure to toxins, microorganisms and/or allergens. In other words, the immune system has *not* gone haywire. It is not launching an inflammatory response against cells of the epithelial region just because it doesn't like those cells or something. The cells have been damaged, and need to be removed. The immune system is simply doing its job.

And this is where the conventional medical community gets chronic inflammation wrong. If the immune system didn't keep trying to remove these cells from the body, the damaged cells can become corrupted, resulting in genetic mutation—causing an outbreak of metastatic cancerous cells within the body.

Instead, in most cases, the immune system prevents mass metastasis by controlling the damage with inflammation. This means that trying to stop the process by introducing pain-relieving medications that also exert a toxic effect—i.e., contribute additional free radicals—is a mistake. The best approach, as we will describe in this book, is to eliminate the free radicals to the extent possible, while stimulating an increase in the immune system's repair process.

But should we allow the process to continue unabated—or simply try to slow it down by decreasing the amount of acids—the process will likely continue. This is especially if we do not curb the introduction of the offending radicals into the system.

The result of this chronic exposure to toxins, acids and so on is that the spaces in between these epithelial cells—which are supposed to protect the internal tissues and bloodstream from intruders—open up. When the gaps open up, they allow more entry of microorganisms, toxins and allergens into the body's tissues, causing the body to launch a systemic inflammatory response against these intruders, producing conditions such as allergies, allergies, asthma, infections, arthritis and others.

This permeability among the epithelial layers can occur within the linings of the mouth, the sinus cavity, the airways, the stomach, the urinary tract, the intestines and other areas. In the nasal and sinus cavity, the result is often allergies to pollens, molds and other foreigners. In the airways, the result is often COPD, asthma and other lung conditions. In the intestines, the result is often intestinal permeability, with the inflammatory condition resulting in IBS, Crohn's, polyps and other intestinal conditions.

Epithelial permability research

Does this mechanism have any scientific validation? Absolutely. Let's look at a few studies done on the topic of epithelial permeability within the esophagus, and its connection with GERD:

Researchers from Germany's Otto-von-Guericke University (Wex *et al.* 2009) studied 58 GERD patients together with 27 healthy controls. Compared with the healthy controls, the epithelial membranes of GERD patients were abnormal in that the papillae were elongated, the basal cells were swollen and inflammation and the intercellular spaces—the tight junctions—were opened— referred to as being "dilated."

Japanese researchers (Ara *et al.* 2008) found that epithelial barrier function was weakened and epithelial permeability was present among another population of GERD patients.

Researchers from Pennsylvania's Lankenau Institute for Medical Research (Mullin *et al.* 2006) found that patients with Barrett's metaplasia had increased epithelial permeability by testing with a sucrose solution and collecting urine overnight. They concluded: "Patients with Barrett's were observed to exhibit a transepithelial leak to sucrose whose mean value was threefold greater than that seen in healthy control subjects…" They also said that "Barrett's metaplasia contains dramatically more claudin-2 and claudin-3 than is found in normal esophageal mucosa, it is markedly lower in claudins 1 and 5, indicating very different tight junction barriers."

Researchers from Tulane University's School of Medicine (Tobey *et al.* 2004) used dextran to test epithelial permeability among patients with GERD. In their paper, they stated, "It has recently been established that patients with nonerosive reflux disease have on biopsy within esophageal epithelium a lesion known as dilated intercellular spaces." This is a complicated way of saying increased epithelial permeability.

The researchers then tested permeability.

In their study, they concluded: "In nonerosive acid-damaged esophageal epithelium dilated intercellular spaces develop in association with and as a marker of reduced transepithelial resistance and increased shunt permeability. This change in shunt permeability upon acid or acid-pepsin exposure is substantial, permitting dextran molecules as large as 20 kD (33 A) to diffuse across the epithelium. Also, this shunt leak enables luminal human epidermal growth factor at 6 kD to diffuse across the acid-damaged epithelium and by so doing enables it to access its receptors on epithelial basal cells."

Researchers from Japan's Hyogo College of Medicine, Nishinomiya, Japan (Chen *et al.* 2011) tested human esophageal-like squamous epithelial cell layers the laboratory. They found that treating the cell layers with taurocholic acid, glycocholic acid and deoxycholic acid resulted in increased permeability. "In conclusion, acidic bile salts disrupted the squamous epithelial barrier function partly by modulating the amounts of claudin-1 and claudin-4. These results provide new insights for understanding the role of tight junction proteins in esophagitis," the researchers stated.

Scientists from Japan's Hyogo College of Medicine (Oshima *et al.* 2011) determined that they could determine whether the tight junctions in esophageal epithelium were open (dilated and permeable) by using trans-epithelial electrical resistance (TEER) measurements.

Researchers from the University of Iowa (Squier *et al.* 2010) found that menthol together with nicotine increased esophageal permeability. This of course connects smoking with GERD.

Researchers from Japan's (Ito *et al.* 2010) Tohoku University Graduate School of Medicine found that increased permeability of the esophagus at the gastroesophageal junction could be induced using reactive nitrogen oxide species (RNOS), a type of free radical.

They also determined that free radicals can be produced with the combination of salivary nitrites and refluxed gastric acids. Salivary nitrites are formed from the consumption of foods containing nitrates. These include cured and processed meats. Some ground water sources also contain high levels of nitrates, especially near farming regions where chemical nitrogen fertilizers are used.

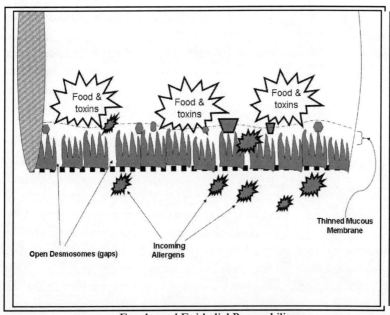

Esophageal Epithelial Permeability

Increased intestinal permeability

Another form of epithelial permeability that has been studied extensively is increased intestinal permeability (IIPS). IIPS was stumbled upon by drug researchers trying to understand drug absorption. As they tested different individuals, they found that some people will assimilate more through their intestines than others. They also found that some people also assimilate toxins more than others.

As the research progressed, it was discovered that this state of increased permeability was related to other diseased states in the body, and related to the consumption of alcohol, drugs and processed foods. Further research revealed that increased intestinal permeability was often related to other conditions involving other epithelial tissues.

French researchers (Heyman and Desjeux 2000) found that not only can intestinal permeability cause various disorders, but these conditions can also worsen intestinal permeability. The researchers found out that as undigested food antigens are transported through the intestinal wall, the immune system launches an inflammatory response.

Intact proteins and large peptides, they pointed out, stimulate inflammation among the mucosa of the intestinal wall. IFN gamma and TNF alpha are cytokines that are often part of this inflammatory response. These two—IFN gamma and TNF alpha—also so happen to increase the further opening of the tight junctions.

Researchers from Brazil's Federal Fluminense Medical School (Soares *et al.* 2004) studied the associations between IBS and food intolerance. The researchers used 43 volunteers divided into three groups: an IBS group, a dyspepsia group, and a group without gastrointestinal difficulties. All test subjects were given skin prick tests for nine food allergens. The IBS group presented the highest level of positive allergen responses. The researchers concluded that IIPS was linked to IBS.

Researchers (Forget *et al.* 1985) tested intestinal permeability using EDTA in ten normal adults, eleven healthy children, seven children with acute gastroenteritis, and eight infants with eczema. They found significantly greater intestinal permeability among those with both gastroenteritis and eczema.

This is a critical point, because both of these epithelial layers—along the intestinal wall and along the surface of the skin—are covered with mucosal membranes. This confirms that a fault in the secretion of mucous can affect different parts of the body concurrently.

This was also found by Russian researchers (Sazanova *et al.* 1992), who studied 122 children, four months old to six years old with food intolerances. Symptoms included atopic dermatitis among 52 children, and chronic diarrhea among 70 children. They found antibodies to food antigens among all the children. They also found chronic gastroduodenitis (duodenum and stomach inflammation) among every child with atopic dermatitis and among 95% of those with chronic diarrhea. They observed that lactase deficiencies and microorganism growth in the duodenum increased the levels of intestinal permeability and subsequent allergy response.

The intestinal cells are often damaged first by other toxins, resulting in an inflammatory cascade. Once the intestine's cells are damaged, macromolecules/allergens can enter the system through the damaged intestinal wall.

Thus IIPS is usually the result of two events: The first being an inflammatory process responding to an injury to the cells of the intestinal wall. These cells can be damaged by an assortment of toxins, poor dietary choices, microorganism pathogens, stress, smoking, alcohol, pharmaceuticals and toxins. Food macromolecules or allergens can also produce this damage to the cells of the intestinal walls.

Once the cells of the intestinal wall are damaged, the immune system will launch an inflammatory injury response through the T-cell system as described earlier. The T-cells will "repair" the problem by killing off these intestinal cells. This is often described as an autoimmune issue, but in reality, the T-cells are responding to real damage of toxins to these cells. They are not confusing "self" with "non-self."

While this damage and response is active, the intestinal cell wall barrier is altered. This alteration creates further increased intestinal permeability. Now large molecules (macromolecules) and/or allergens may readily enter the tissues and bloodstream, stimulating the IgE-histamine allergic immune response and/or other physiological and immune responses that produce allergies and other types of inflammation.

Again, this condition is related to the scenario of GERD because typically—but not always—when one region of mucosal membranes is not healthy, other mucosal regions will also become unhealthy. We might compare this to a rain storm that gets everything exposed wet. The submucosal glands throughout the body respond to many of the same physiological triggers because they are produced by the submucosal membranes lying beneath the epithelial layer.

This isn't to say that all mucosal membranes are exactly alike. Different submucosal glands will produce a slightly different mix, and other elements within the epithelial layers will support a different biochemical combination of elements. This in turn encourages a different mix of probiotic colonies among the different mucosal membrane regions.

Mechanical Issues and Hiatal Hernia

Hiatal hernia is often stated in the literature as a major cause for GERD, but this has not exactly proven out. As many as half of adults over 50 years old have hiatal hernia, yet only about 5% of these suffer from GERD (Murray and Pizzorno 1998). Other research (Wang *et al.* 2002) has associated hiatal hernia with GERD in older patients when looking at the inverse: Among adults over 65 years old with GERD, 65% had hiatal hernia. Similar results were found among a study of 51 GERD patients from the Lincoln County Memorial Center (Xenos 2002).

So while many people with GERD have hiatal hernia, not everyone with hiatal hernia suffers from GERD. The other statistic to ponder here is the tremendous percentage of those over 50 with hiatal hernia: *One out of two.* This quite simply means that hiatal hernia is a very common incidence as we age.

As for what causes hiatal hernia, there are numerous possibilities, mostly mechanical. These relate to pressure being put upon the stomach wall and sphincter by physical pressure—such as from obesity, wrong posture or an impact.

Some research has shown that GERD increases the likelihood of hiatal hernia. This seems to have to do with the damage to the lower sphincter by gastric acids. This was shown in a study from Canada's Queen's University (Dunne and Paterson 2000) in a study of 12 patients with hiatal hernia.

The Wang study mentioned above brings into view another element that we discussed earlier and will later—that of the relationship between GERD and obesity.

This relates to a myriad of potential relationships, but one key issue is mechanical: The pushing of fatty tissues against the lower esophageal sphincters, causing them to weaken.

This said, there is evidence—as we'll show later—that many singers, musicians and some athletes suffer from GERD simply because of the mechanical issues that relate to pressure or impact of the diaphragm against the lower esophageal sphincter. As this takes place consistently, the sphincter can weaken and lose tone, preventing it from being able to tightly close.

GERD and Airway Mucosal Conditions

The mucosal goblet cells of the respiratory tract are quite similar to the esophageal goblet cells. This similarity between the goblet cells of the two regions facilitates an understanding of the mystery of GERD-related asthma. Weakened secretions of mucosal membranes from mucosal glands can affect both regions simultaneously, because they offer more exposure to their respective epithelial layers.

In asthma, weakened mucosal membranes allow damage to the epithelial cells of the airways. Exposure to allergens, toxins, and microorganisms will penetrate the weakened mucosal membranes and damage the cells, producing epithelial permeability.

In this state, toxins, cold air and any number of other triggers can stimulate the production of thickened, inflammatory mucous. In a healthy body, this stimulates the quick removal of the toxin or invader, as the excess mucous is swept out by the cilia.

But when the epithelial cells are exposed, damaged and inflamed, the goblet cells will over-produce inflammatory mucous, which swamps the cilia along with dead cell parts and toxins. When the cilia are drowning in mucous, they cannot remove these toxins. The lack of mucous transport, combined with the need to remove toxins, is typically accompanied by the constriction of the airways stimulated by the smooth airway muscles. This restriction may protect the lungs from more toxins, but also further prevents the mucous from being cleared out. And it also restricts breathing, and produces coughing and asthma symptoms.

Restricted breathing in turn produces poorly oxygenated blood.

There are various negative consequences of having poorly oxygenated blood and/or highly acidic, carbon dioxide-rich blood. Poorly oxygenated blood can cause or contribute to brain fog, poor memory, fatigue, restlessness, nervousness, anxiety, indigestion, and cardiovascular diseases such as *cor pulmonale*, hypertension, atherosclerosis and angina. Poorly oxygenated blood can lead to low healing response, poor sleep, and increased inflammatory response—all of which can be traced back to epithelial damage to the airways caused by weakened mucosal membrane secretions.

GERD and Sore Throat

Our pharynx and larynx—like the esophagus—are lined with similar mucosal membranes that protect the cells from foreigners, including microorganisms, toxins, undigested food particles, enzymes, and allergens. This mucosal membrane is pretty resilient in a healthy body. It has elements of both the airways and the stomach, so the esophageal and throat mucosal membranes are typically pretty hardy, as they are designed to protect the epithelial layers from acidic foods and toxins as they arrive from the mouth, stomach acids as they may arise from the stomach, and toxins introduced by the air we breathe.

When the mucosal membranes in the throat and pharynx become degraded, they cannot protect our cells from these foreign particles. This exposes our epithelial area to those toxins, microorganisms and other foreigners.

As this situation progresses, and the epithelial junctions and cell membranes become more permeable, inflammation results. This produces the pain and burning sensation of heartburn.

The instigators of defective mucosal membranes in a sore throat can be many. These can include all of the elements we'll discuss in the next chapter and more. Often, it can be as simple as a pathogenic bacteria or virus that has become attached to the mucosal membranes and penetrated to the cells beneath. The body launches an immune response to rid the body of the invader, producing inflammation and the pain of the sore throat.

This process can thicken the mucosal membranes, and this thickened membrane can prevent a good clearing of the broken down invader parts. It becomes hard to clear this out, and the toxins in the membranes begin to increasingly irritate the cells—damaging them if the invasion is not stopped.

Should the throat and esophageal mucosal membranes be healthy, they will typically be able to remove the mucous and invader with little to-do. But if the mucous membranes are weak—or the invader is particularly strong—the invasion can grow quickly, producing an inflammatory response, causing the pain of a sore throat.

Often the sore throat is a sign of an oncoming cold or flu because the overloading of the virus causes the thickening of the mucosal membranes as the body works to remove the infective agent. This is a healthy response and we should not dread the sore throat. Rather, we should see it as a sign that the body's immune system is on full alert and is actively removing invaders.

In other words, the sore throat is a good sign that the immune system is doing its job.

Some bacterial invasions do not cause this sort of pain, as the bacteria have figured out how to trick the immune system in one way or another. This is why in some staph infections—especially the flesh-eating versions—will not hurt while the bacteria is eating away our tissues. The bacteria have figured out how to shut off the immune system in certain ways—allowing it to grow faster unencumbered.

Chapter Three

GERD and Probiotics

The mucosal membranes of our mouth, sinuses, throat and esophagus are all populated with probiotic bacteria in a healthy body. These serve to—along with our body's own immune cells—protect our epithelial layers from infections and toxin invasions.

Illustrating this, researchers from Italy's University of Bari (Indrio *et al.* 2011) tested 42 infants with GERD and regurgitation symptoms, together with 21 healthy control infants. They gave the infants either the probiotic *Lactobacillus reuteri* DSM 17938 (100 million CFU per day) with their formula for thirty days, or placebo.

Of the infants who completed the entire study (34) they found that those infants who consumed the probiotic had a significantly increased rate of gastric emptying. They also found that those taking the probiotic had significantly fewer regurgitations than those infants who were taking the placebo.

The mechanism is that probiotics are territorial. As such, they want to control their region. So they don't like others to intrude on their territory. This is why probiotics will colonize a particular area: because there is strength in numbers.

Here we'll discuss the various probiotics and other microorganisms that inhabit our mucosal membranes, and cover some studies that illustrate the importance of these mucosal probiotics have upon our health.

First let's review the major infections and probiotics that inhabit the mucosal membranes of our oral and nasal cavities, our intestines, airways, skin and other regions:

Probiotics and *H. pylori*

Earlier we mentioned the connection between GERD, gastritis and *H. pylori*. In both conditions, the bacteria have corrupted the ability of the mucosal membranes to provide protection to the epithelial cells from harsh stomach acids.

Repeated research has confirmed that at least 80% of all gastritis cases are associated with *Helicobacter pylori* infections.

For example, scientists from Japan's Oita University (Nguyen *et al.* 2010) studied a large population group from Vietnam. Other studies have found that *H. pylori* infections are significant in Vietnam, and this study found that 65% of the entire group were infected with *H. pylori*, and those over the age of forty were more likely to have *H. pylori*.

They also found that *all* the *H. pylori* infected people had chronic gastritis. Of these, 83% had active cases at the time of the study. The *H. pylori* infected individuals also had some form of stomach wall scarring from their gastritis.

Surprisingly, international epidemiological research has found that some other third world countries have far higher incidence of *H. pylori* infection, yet have significantly *lower* rates of gastritis among these *H. pylori*-infected populations.

Meanwhile, there is increasing evidence that *H. pylori*—like *E. coli* and *Candida albicans* microorganisms—may actually be a normal resident in a healthy intestinal tract, assuming it is properly balanced and managed by strong legions of probiotics.

In other words, a *H. pylori* infection doesn't always cause gastritis. But when *H. pylori* colonies expand, they increasingly produce gastritis as well as GERD.

The western-medicine effort to eliminate *H. pylori* isn't going too well either. As doctors and researchers have given antibiotics for *H. pylori* infections, we are finding that *H. pylori* is becoming increasingly resistant to many of the antibiotics used in prescriptive treatment.

Research from Poland's Center of Gastrology (Ziemniak 2006) investigated antibiotic use on *Helicobacter pylori* infections: 641 *H. pylori* patients were given various antibiotics typically applied to *H. pylori*. The results indicated that *H. pylori* had developed a 22% resistance to clarithromycin and 47% resistance to metronidazole. Worse, a 66% secondary resistance to clarithromycin and metronidazole was found, indicating *H. pylori*'s increasing resistance to antibiotics.

At the same time, research has indicated that probiotics have a sustained ability to control and manage *H. pylori* overgrowths. Studies have also found that probiotics have the ability to arrest ulcerative conditions together with other digestive tract epithelial conditions without side effects. Here is some of that research:

Lactobacillus brevis (CD2) or placebo was given to 22 *H. pylori*-positive GERD patients for three weeks by Italian medical researchers (Linsalata *et al.* 2004). The *L. brevis* CD2 stimulated a decrease in gastric ornithine decarboxylase activity and polyamine. The researchers concluded: "Our data support the hypothesis that *L. brevis* CD2 treatment decreases *H. pylori* colonization, thus reducing polyamine biosynthesis."

Researchers from the Academic Hospital at Vrije University in The Netherlands (Cats *et al.* 2003) gave either a placebo or *Lactobacillus casei* Shirota to 14 *H. pylori*-infected patients for three weeks. Six additional *H. pylori*-infected subjects were used as controls. The researchers determined that *L. casei* significantly inhibits *H. pylori* growth. This effect was more pronounced for *L. casei* grown in milk solution than in the DeMan-Rogosa-Sharpe medium (a probiotic broth developed by researchers in 1960).

Lactobacillus reuteri ATCC 55730 or a placebo was given to 40 *H. pylori*-infected patients for 4 weeks by researchers from Italy's Università degli Studi di Bari (Francavilla *et al.* 2008). *L. reuteri* effectively suppressed *H. pylori* infection among the patients, decreasing their gastrointestinal pain, and reducing other dyspeptic symptoms.

Mexican hospital researchers (Sahagún-Flores *et al.* 2007) gave 64 *Helicobacter pylori*-infected patients antibiotic treatment with or without *Lactobacillus casei* Shirota. *Lactobacillus casei* Shirota plus antibiotic treatment was 94% effective and antibiotic treatment alone was 76% effective.

Researchers from Switzerland's University Hospital in Lausanne (Felley *et al.* 2001) gave fifty-three patients with gastritis and *H. pylori* infections milk with *L. johnsonii* or placebo for three weeks. Those given the probiotic drink had a significant *H. pylori* density decrease, reduced inflammation and gastritis symptoms.

Scientists from the Department of Internal Medicine at the Catholic University of Rome (Canducci *et al.* 2000) tested 120 patients with gastritis and *H. pylori* infections. Sixty patients received a combination of antibiotics rabeprazole, clarithromycin and amoxicillin. The other sixty patients received the same therapy together with a freeze-dried, inactivated culture of *Lactobacillus acidophilus*. The probiotic group had an 88% eradication of *H. pylori* while the antibiotic-only group had a 72% eradication of *H. pylori*.

Scientists from the University of Chile (Gotteland *et al.* 2005) gave 182 children with *H. pylori* infections placebo, antibiotics or probiotics. *H. pylori* were completely eradicated in 12% of those who took *Saccharomyces boulardii*, and in 6.5% of those given *L. acidophilus*. The placebo group had no *H. pylori* eradication.

Researchers from Japan's Kyorin University School of Medicine (Imase *et al.* 2007) gave *Lactobacillus reuteri* strain SD2112 in tablets or a placebo to 33 *H. pylori*-infected patients. After 4 and 8 weeks, *L. reuteri* significantly decreased and suppressed *H. pylori* in the probiotic group.

In a study of 347 patients with active *H. pylori* infections and gastritis symptoms, half the group was given antibiotics and the other half was given antibiotics with yogurt (*Lactobacillus acidophilus* HY2177, *Lactobacillus casei* HY2743, *Bifidobacterium longum* HY8001, and *Streptococcus thermophilus* B-1). The yogurt plus antibiotics group had significantly more eradication of *H. pylori* bacteria, and significantly fewer side effects than the antibiotics group (Kim, *et al.* 2008).

Thirty *H. pylori*-infected patients were given either probiotics *Lactobacillus acidophilus* and *Bifidobacterium bifidum* or placebo for one and two weeks following antibiotic treatment by British researchers (Madden *et al.* 2005). Those taking the probiotics had a recovery of normal intestinal microflora, damaged during antibiotic treatment. The researchers also observed that those taking the probiotics throughout the two weeks showed more normal and stable microflora than did those groups taking the probiotics for only one out of the two weeks.

Scientists from the Department of Medicine at Lausanne, Switzerland's University Hospital (Michetti *et al.* 1999) tested 20 human adults with ulcerative *H. pylori* infection with *L. acidophilus johnsonii*. The probiotic was taken with the antibiotic omeprazole in half the group and alone (with placebo) in the other group. The patients were tested at the start, after two weeks of treatment, and four weeks after treatment. Both groups showed significantly reduced *H. pylori* levels during and just following treatment. However, the probiotic-only group tested better than the antibiotic group during the fourth week after the treatment completion.

Medical scientists from the Kaohsiung Municipal United Hospital in Taiwan (Wang *et al.* 2004) studied 59 volunteer patients infected with *H. pylori*. They were given either probiotics (*Lactobacillus* and *Bifidobacterium* strains) or placebo after meals for six weeks. After the six-week treatment period, the probiotic group "effectively suppressed *H. pylori*," according to the researchers.

In the Polish study mentioned earlier (Ziemniak 2006), 641 *H. pylori* patients were given either antibiotics alone or probiotics with antibiotics. The two antibiotic-only treatment groups had 71% and 86% eradication of *H. pylori*, while the antibiotic-probiotic treatment group had 94% eradication.

The combination of *H. pylori*, acidic foods and gastrin produced by the stomach's parietal cells have a major role in increasing the rate of inflammation among the epithelial tissues of the esophagus and stomach. However, healthy mucosal membranes that line these surfaces will contain legions of probiotics that help to create a functional barrier that prevents these from harming those epithelial cells.

Otherwise, everyone would have GERD and gastritis.

More Colonizers

Part of the barrier contributed by probiotics consists of appropriate antibiotic secretions produced by our friendly bacteria, and even some of the not-so-friendly ones who struggle to maintain their territories.

Outside of *H. pylori*, there are a number of other microorganisms that can infect the esophagus and sphincter regions. Here are some of the microorganisms that have been shown to colonize within the mucosal membranes of the esophagus, mouth, upper respiratory tract, intestines and sometimes the stomach.

While some of these may be considered pathogenic in larger colonies, they may also be part of the biotic balance that exists within the body, and are therefore necessary to maintain the protective quality of our mucosal barrier. Following is a summary of these pathogenic and sometimes symbiotic microorganisms (For references, see the author's book, *"Probiotics—Protection Against Infection"*):

Actinomyces sp.: These bacteria will live within the mouth, esophagus and the pharynx. They are tiny bacteria, and are prevalent in soils, plants, and animals. They are known to be cooperative with various other bacteria, both probiotic and pathogenic. Working in combination with Streptomyces, for example, *Actinomyces* sp. can produce antibiotics such as actinomycin.

Clostridium sp. will typically inhabit the lower intestines and colon, although they may also inhabit the esophagus, mouth and pharynx. Some of the more common species include *Clostridium difficile*, *Clostridium tetani*, and *Clostridium perfringens*. They are often implicated in various intestinal disorders.

Corynebacterium sp. are quite hardy and will inhabit the skin surfaces, the mouth, the esophagus, the nasal cavity, the pharynx, the conjunctiva of the eyes, the lower intestines and the vagina. Some species have been implicated in acne. *Corynebacterium diphtheriae* are quite common in the intestines, even to the point of being considered part of our healthy flora. When their populations become too large, however, they can cause a number of disease conditions, including diphtheria.

Escherichia coli and other Enterobacteriaceae such as *Proteus* sp. may dwell and thrive in the mouth, the esophagus, the nasal cavity, the pharynx, the eye conjunctiva, skin surfaces, the intestinal tract, the vagina and the urethra. *E. coli* are normal residents of most humans, but are still the source of disease when their populations grow. They have been known to be lethal in large populations. This illustrates the important role probiotics play in keeping populations of *E. coli* and other bacteria in control.

Enterococcus faecalis (formerly called *Streptococcus faecalis*): These mostly pathogenic bacteria are normal residents of even healthy intestines. They can also dwell within the mouth, pharynx, esophagus, urethra and vagina. They balance and strengthen our probiotics when in reasonable numbers. In larger numbers, however, they can be the cause for a number of diseases. Like other bacteria, several strains of *Enterococcus faecalis* have become antibiotic-resistant in recent years.

Haemophilus influenzae are often the cause of a number of respiratory tract infections, especially among children. They are found in the nasal cavity, the mouth, the lungs, the esophagus, the pharynx, the eye conjunctiva and the colon and lower intestines. Many strains of *Haemophilus influenzae* are now also resistant to a number of antibiotics.

Mycoplasmas: These microorganisms are known by their absence of a cell wall. They will commonly dwell in the esophagus, lower intestines, the vagina, the mouth, the pharynx, and the urethra. One of the more pathogenic species is *Mycoplasma pneumoniae*, which are known to cause a disease referred to as walking pneumonia.

Neisseria meningitides bacteria inhabit primarily the pharynx, but will also live in the esophagus, nasal cavity, the mouth and the vagina. These bacteria are the central cause for meningitis, which can be lethal. A combination of probiotics and an active immune system may readily control these bacteria, preventing serious infection while creating immunity to them.

Pseudomonas aeruginosa: These bacteria typically dwell on the skin, in the mouth, in the pharynx, in the walls of the urethra and within the colon. *P. aeruginosa* are hardy, and can live in oxygen and low-oxygen environments. Pseudomonas aeruginosa can infect wounds and enter through skin openings. They can cause lung infections, esophagus infections, urinary tract infections and kidney infections. *Pseudomonas* has also been known to cause joint infections in a condition called septic arthritis.

Spirochetes: These corkscrew-shaped bacteria of different species can live without oxygen and will embed themselves into skin, nerves, root canals, organs and various other places, including the esophagus. Spirochetes can infect the mouth, the pharynx and the lower intestines. One of the more vigorous types is the *Borrelia burgdorferi*, the bacteria implicated in lyme disease. *Treponema pallidum* is another aggressive spirochete, known for their involvement in syphilis.

Staphylococcus aureus: Most of us house these bacteria as normal residents. When controlled, they present little or no danger. They can live on skin surfaces, in the nose, in the mouth, in the vagina, in the pharynx, in the esophagus and within the intestines. They are not probiotic. However, as they compete with probiotics for territory, they will strengthen the body's probiotics, and help provide a barrier function. Many strains of *Staphylococcus aureus* are extremely pathogenic, however, especially antibiotic-resistant strains such as MRSA. Aggressive *S. aureus* can also become flesh eating, should it be allowed to grow out of control on tissue surfaces. S. aureus can be one of the most aggressive and dangerous bacteria within an immunosuppressed body with depleted probiotic colonies.

Staphylococcus epidermidis: These hardy probiotic or eubiotic organisms live on most of the body's epithelial surfaces. They thrive in the nasal cavity, in the pharynx, esophagus, on the skin, in the conjunctiva of the eyes, in the lower urethra, in the vagina and in the colon and lower intestines. In the right colony numbers, *Staphylococcus epidermidis* can aggressively protect our skin and other membranes. *Staphylococcus epidermidis* will also adapt to varying temperatures and moisture content. They will also produce unique territorial acids that provide a protective layer for our skin and membrane surfaces. This protective acidic layer repels toxins, other bacteria, fungi and viruses.

Streptococcus mitis: These bacteria live primarily within the oral cavity and the pharynx, but also can translocate to the esophagus. Streptococcus mitis are fairly normal residents of a healthy human body and help balance probiotic colonies. However, they can become pathogenic should they be allowed to outgrow our probiotic populations.

Streptococcus pyrogenes are bacteria that dwell primarily within the oral cavity, pharynx, esophagus, vagina, the conjunctiva of the eyes, and on the surface of the skin. They may also inhabit the intestines, but to a lesser degree. These bacteria are the central cause for strep throat and tonsillitis. *Streptococcus pyrogenes* can also cause pneumonia, rheumatic diseases, nephritis, and heart disease. They also stimulate inflammation, causing the swelling of tissues.

Streptococcus pneumoniae are fairly normal inhabitants of the respiratory tract and esophagus. They also can live within the mouth, the vagina, the pharynx, and the nasal cavity. *Streptococcus pneumoniae* are the central cause for most cases of pneumonia. About 50% of the human population is thought to have *S. pneumoniae* inhabitants within the upper respiratory tract. This means that for those who have not contracted pneumonia, these populations are likely under control. This is the case for numerous organisms. While we have been taught to avoid them at all costs, in reality many of us host all or many of them. In a healthy body, colonies of territorial probiotics, with the help of the immune system, keep them managed.

Streptococcus mutans thrive primarily in the oral cavity and pharynx, but can move into the esophagus. These bacteria are the central cause for plaque formation around the teeth, and the main cause for dental caries and periodontal disease. S. mutans secrete acids that break down the enamel of our teeth, which causes cavities. They also thrive off simple starches and sugars. This is the reason that refined sugars and simple carbohydrates are known to cause cavities.

Esophageal Probiotics

While the previous list contains a few microorganisms that might be considered probiotics when maintained within controlled colony sizes, these must be organized by stronger probiotics—which have been colonizing the human body for thousands of years. These organizer probiotics are needed in large enough colonies to control those numbers.

This is important, especially in the esophagus, mouth and sinuses, where those microorganisms discussed above can get out of control. Here is a summary description of some of the probiotics that are important to the health of our esophagus and upper intestines (For references, see the author's book, *"Probiotics—Protection Against Infection"*):

Streptococcus salivarius are vigorous probiotic bacteria that station themselves throughout the upper respiratory tract, but primarily inhabit the oral cavity and pharynx. *S. salivarius* are the primary and most aggressive of our oral cavity probiotic bacteria. They are extremely territorial, and produce a number of antibiotics, including salivaricin A and salivaricin B, along with a host of other antibiotic substances.

They are also permanent residents in the human body. Our resident strains are inherited from mom. Mama transfers her resident strains through a combination of birthing, breast milk and kissing; although kissing and breast milk are likely the primary means. *Streptococcus salivarius* are extremely aggressive and will be the dominant species in a healthy mouth. This means that *Streptococcus salivarius* are organizers.

To do this, they produce a number of enzymes and acids that manage the growth of other bacteria. One might conclude that

Streptococcus salivarius are one of the most important bacteria to maintaining the health of the esophagus and mouth, because they are the principal gatekeepers when it comes to preventing the entry and survival of infective microorganisms. As mentioned above, one of the mechanisms *S. Salivarius* utilize is the production of salivaricin. Salivaricin is recognized as one of the most potent group of antibiotics. While salivaricin A and salivaricin B have been isolated, it is certain that *S. salivarius* are constantly adjusting their antibiotic biochemistry to match new infective agents and their respective weaknesses.

Streptococcus thermophilus are considered subspecies of *S. salivarius*. Not surprisingly, *Streptococcus thermophilus* have been known to benefit the immune system in a number of ways. *Streptococcus thermophilus* are also commonly used in yogurt making. They are also used in cheese making, and are even sometimes found in pasteurized milk. They will colonize at higher temperatures, from 104-113 degrees F. This is significant because this bacterium readily produces lactase, which breaks down lactose. These are the only known streptococci that do this.

Like other supplemented probiotics, *S. thermophilus* are temporary microorganisms in the human body. Their colonies will typically inhabit the system for a week or two before exiting. During that time, however, they will help set up a healthy environment to support resident colony growth. Like other probiotics, *S. thermophilus* also produce a number of different antibiotic substances and acids that deter the growth of pathogenic microorganisms.

Research has determined that these S. *thermophilus* will reduce acute diarrhea (rotavirus and non-rotavirus), reduce intestinal permeability, inhibit *H. pylori*, inhibit *Clostridium difficile*, increase immune function among the elderly, restore infant microflora similar to breast-fed infants, reduce symptoms of atopic dermatitis, reduce nasal cavity infections, reduce upper respiratory tract infections from *Staphylococcus aureus, Streptococcus pneumoniae, beta-hemolytic streptococci*, and *Haemophilus influenzae*, reduce *S. mutans* in the mouth, and reduce ulcerative colitis among other things.

Lactobacillus salivarius: Lactobacilli are primarily found in the small intestines, although they will also inhabit the oral cavity, the nasal cavity, and the pharynx. Lactobacilli lower the pH of their environment by converting long-chain saccharides (complex sugars) such as lactose to lactic acid. This conversion process effectively inhibits pathogen growth and creates the appropriate acidic environment for other probiotics to colonize.

Lactobacillus salivarius are typical residents of most humans—although supplemented versions will still be transients. They are also found in the intestines of other animals. *L. salivarius* will dwell in the mouth, the nasal cavity, the pharynx, the small intestines, the colon, and the vagina. They are hardy bacteria that can live in both oxygen and oxygen-free environments. *L. salivarius* is one of the few bacteria species that can also thrive in salty environments. They can also survive many medications.

L. salivarius produce prolific amounts of lactic acid, which makes them hardy defenders of the teeth and gums. They also produce a number of antibiotics, and are speedy colonizers. Upon ingestion, they quickly combat pathogenic bacteria and defend their territory. Because of their hardiness, they will readily take out massive numbers of pathogens immediately. *L. salivarius* are also known to be able to break apart complex proteins.

Human clinical research has shown that *Lactobacillus salivarius* can inhibit *S. mutans* in the mouth, reduce dental carries, reduce gingivitis and periodontal disease, reduce risk of strep throat caused by *S. pyogenes*, reduce ulcerative colitis and IBS, inhibit *E. coli*, inhibit *Salmonella* spp., and inhibit *Candida albicans*.

Lactobacillus. reuteri is a species found residing permanently in humans. As a result, most supplemented strains attach to mucosal membranes, though temporarily, and stimulate the colony growth of resident *L. reuteri* strains. *L. reuteri* will colonize in the oral cavity, the nasal cavity, and the pharynx, stomach, duodenum and ileum regions. *L. reuteri* will also significantly modulate the immune response of the gastrointestinal mucosal membranes. This means that *L. reuteri* are effective for many of the same digestive ailments that *L. acidophilus* are used for. *L. reuteri* also have several other effects, including the restoration of our oral cavity bacteria. They also produce a significant amount of antibiotic biochemicals.

Human clinical research has shown that *L. reuteri* decrease acid reflux and GERD, as well as inhibit gingivitis, reduce pro-inflammatory cytokines, help re-establish the pH of mucosal membranes, inhibit and suppress *H. pylori,* reduce nausea, flatulence and diarrhea, reduce *Streptococcus mutans,* stimulate the immune system, reduce plaque on teeth, decrease symptoms of IBS, reduce infant colic, reduce colds and influenza, stabilize epithelial barrier function, and decrease atopic dermatitis.

Lactobacillus acidophilus primarily reside primarily in the upper intestines. But they do have a role in the esophagus and stomach, primarily in helping maintain their pH as they are temporarily colonizing. The esophagus may also host good colonies of *Lactobacillus acidophilus* in some people, and from time to time in almost every healthy person.

Lactobacillus acidophilus are by far the most familiar probiotic bacteria to most of us, and are also by far the most-studied to date. They are one of the main residents of the human gut, although supplemented strains will still be transient. They are also found in the mouth and vagina.

L. acidophilus grow best in warm (85-100 degrees F) and moist environments.

Many are facultative anaerobic, meaning they can grow in oxygen-rich or oxygen-poor environments. Probably the most important benefit of *L. acidophilus* is their ability to inhibit the growth of pathogenic microorganisms, not only in the gut, but also throughout the body. *L. acidophilus* significantly control and rid the body of *Candida albicans* overgrowth, which can invade various tissues of the body if unchecked. They also inhibit *Escherichia coli,* which can be fatal in large enough populations.

They can also inhibit the growth of *Helicobacter pylori*— implicated in ulcers; *Salmonella*—a genus of deadly infectious bacteria; and *Shigella* and *Staphylococcus*—both potentially lethal infectious bacteria. It should be noted that *L. acidophilus'* ability to block these infectious agents will depend upon the size of the pathobiotic colonization and the size of the *L. acidophilus* colonies. *L. acidophilus* produces a variety of antibiotic substances, including acidolin, acidophillin, lactobacillin, lactocidin and others.

L. acidophilus lessen pharmaceutical antibiotic side effects; aid lactose absorption; help the absorption of various nutrients; help maintain the mucosa; help balance the pH of the upper intestinal tract; create a hostile environment for invading yeasts; and inhibit urinary tract and vaginal infections.

L. acidophilus also produce several digestive enzymes, including lactase, lipase and protease. Lactase is an enzyme that breaks down lactose. Several studies have shown that milk- or lactose-intolerant people are able to handle milk once they have established colonies of *L. acidophilus*. Lypase helps break down fatty foods, and protease helps break down protein foods.

This microorganism has also been found to specifically reduce epithelial permeability, control *H. pylori*, and reduce dyspepsia in human clinical research. This means that this probiotic is critical to the health of the esophagus, stomach and small intestines.

L. acidophilus have also been found in human clinical research to lower LDL and total cholesterol, reduce stress-induced GI problems, inhibit *E. coli*, reduce infection from rotavirus, reduce necrotizing enterocolitis, inhibit and control *Clostridium* spp., inhibit *Bacteroides* spp., increase appetite, inhibit *Candida* spp. overgrowths, reduce allergic response, inhibit upper respiratory infections, inhibit tonsillitis, reduce blood pressure, and stimulate the immune system.

Lactobacillus casei are typically transient bacteria that will inhabit the esophagus, mouth, pharynx, nasal cavity and intestines. They are commonly used in a number of food applications and industrial applications. These include culturing cheese and other milk products, and fermenting green olives. *L. casei* is found naturally in raw milk and in colostrum—meaning they are typical residents of cows. *L. casei* have been reported to reduce allergy symptoms and increase immune response. This seems to be accomplished by regulating the immune system's CHS, CD8 and T-cell responsiveness. However, this immune stimulation seems to be evident primarily among immunosuppressed patients (Guerin-Danan *et al.* 1998). This of course is an indication that probiotics can somehow uniquely respond to the host's particular condition. Some strains of *L. casei* are also very aggressive, and within a mixed probiotic supplement or food, they can dominate and even remove other bacteria.

Human clinical research has shown that *L. casei* can inhibit pathogenic bacterial infections, reduce occurrence, risk and symptoms of IBS, inhibit severe systemic inflammatory response syndrome, inhibit pneumonia and other inhibit respiratory tract infections including bronchitis, inhibit *H. pylori* and ulcers, reduce allergy symptoms, support liver function, stimulate the immune system, inhibit *Clostridium difficile,* reduce asthma symptoms, reduce constipation, decrease beta-glucuronidase (associated with colon cancer), inhibit *Candida* overgrowth, decrease rotavirus infections, and decrease colds and influenza.

Lactobacillus rhamnosus was previously thought to be a subspecies of *L. casei. L. rhamnosus* is a common ingredient in many yogurts and other commercial probiotic foods. *L. rhamnosus* have also been extensively studied over the years. Much of this research has focused upon a particular strain, *L. rhamnosus* GG. *L. rhamnosus* GG have been shown in numerous studies to significantly stimulate the immune system and inhibit a variety of infections. *L. rhamnosus* will also dwell in the esophagus, mouth, pharynx and nasal cavity on a transient basis, but not for very long. This strain also has shown to have good intestinal wall adhesion properties.

Human clinical research has shown that *L. rhamnosus* can inhibit a number of pathogenic bacterial infections, reduce ear infections, reduce respiratory infections, reduce eczema, reduce colds and influenza, stimulate the immune system, increase IgA levels in the mouth and esophagus, inhibit *Pseudomonas aeruginosa* infections in respiratory tract, inhibit *Clostridium difficile,* reduce IBS symptoms, inhibit vancomycin-resistant enterococci (antibiotic-resistant), reduce the risk of colon cancer, inhibit *H. pylori,* reduce atopic dermatitis in children, reduce colic, stabilize epithelial barrier function (decrease permeability), reduce atopic eczema, reduce *Streptococcus mutans,* reduce inflammation and stimulate the immume system.

Lactobacillus rhamnosus has been part of the human diet for thousands of years, and will live in the mouth and the pharynx transiently, and the intestines on a longer-term basis. They are active in cultures of sauerkraut, gherkin and olive brines. They are used to make sourdough bread, Nigerian ogi and fufu, kocha from Ethiopia, and sour mifen noodles from China, Korean kim chi and other traditional foods. *L. plantarum* are also found in dairy and cow dung, so it is a common resident of cow intestines, which is one reason why cow dung is considered in India as being antiseptic.

L. plantarum is a hardy strain. The bacteria have been shown to survive all the way through the intestinal tract and into the feces.

Temperature for optimal growth is 86-95 degrees F. *L. plantarum* are not permanent residents, however. When supplemented, they vigorously attack pathogenic bacteria, and create an environment hospitable for incubated resident strains to expand. *L. plantarum* also produce lysine, and a number of antibiotics including lactolin.

Human clinical research has shown that *L. plantarum* can strengthen the immune system, help restore healthy liver enzymes, reduce frequency and severity of respiratory diseases, reduce epithelial permeability, inhibit various intestinal pathobiotics (such as *Clostridium difficile*), reduce Th2 (inflammatory) levels and increase Th1/Th2 ratio, reduce inflammatory responses, reduce symptoms and aid healing of multiple traumas among injured patients, reduce fungal infections, reduce IBS symptoms, reduce pancreatic sepsis (infection), reduce adhesion of vein endothelial cells by monocytes (risk of atherosclerosis), reduce risk of pneumonia, decrease flatulence

Lactobacillus bulgaricus are transients that assist *bifidobacteria* colony growth. *L. bulgaricus* stimulate the immune system and have antitumor effects. They also produce antibiotic and antiviral substances such as bulgarican and others. *L. bulgaricus* bacteria have been reported to have anti-herpes effects as well. *L. bulgaricus* require more heat to colonize than many probiotics—at 104-109 degrees F.

Human clinical research has shown that *L. bulgaricus* can reduce epithelial permeability, decrease IBS symptoms, increase immune response, inhibit viruses, and reduce *S. mutans* in the mouth.

Lactobacillus brevis are natural residents of cow intestines. They are therefore found in raw milk, colostrum, and cheese. For those who consume these frequently, *L. brevis* will temporarily inhabit the esophagus, oral cavity and pharynx. They are transient in humans, but there is also the possibility that they can reside longer-term or permanently within the human intestines.

Human clinical research has shown that *L. brevis* can reduce periodontal disease, reduce mouth ulcers and decrease *H. pylori* colonization.

Probiotics and GERD-related Conditions

There is some solid research illustrating how probiotics reduce various conditions that have been related to GERD as we've shown

97

earlier. These include asthma and other airway conditions, and various chronic digestive problems.

French researchers (Guyonnet *et al.* 2009) gave *Bifidobacterium lactis* DN-173010 with yogurt strains to 371 adults reporting digestive discomfort for 2 weeks. 82.5% of the probiotic group reported improved digestive symptoms compared to 2.9% of the control group.

Another group of French scientists (Diop *et al.* 2008) gave 64 volunteers with high levels of stress and incidental gastrointestinal symptoms either a placebo or *Lactobacillus acidophilus* Rosell-52 and *Bifidobacterium longum* for three weeks. At the end of the three weeks, the stress-related gastrointestinal symptoms of abdominal pain, nausea and vomiting decreased by 49% among the probiotic group.

Illustrating how probiotics can reduce colonization of candida fungi and other infections *remotely,* researchers from Long Island Jewish Medical Center's Division of Infectious Diseases (Hilton, *et al.* 1992) studied thirty-three patients with vulvovaginal candida infections. Infection rates decreased by a third among patients consuming an eight-ounce yogurt (orally) with *Lactobacillus acidophilus* for six months. The infection rate per person averaged 2.54 every six months in the control group versus 0.38 in the yogurt group. *Candida* spp. colonization rates were 3.23 in the control group versus only 0.84 in the yogurt group—through the six-month testing period.

Research has confirmed that probiotic bacteria inhabit the nasal cavity, the mouth and the throat. Research has also confirmed that both ingested probiotics and probiotic sprays reduce lung infections. Probiotics in the lungs does not seem so radical: Certainly not as radical as the evidence showing probiotics from the intestinal tract can somehow inhibit bacteria in the lungs and nasal cavity.

In the last chapter we showed how asthma and other lung infections are linked with GERD conditions. We attributed this primarily to the health of the mucosal membranes. Here we can add that the health of our probiotic colonies provide another link. Here is some of the clear evidence linking probiotic colonies with lung health:

Researchers from the Swiss National Accident Insurance Institute (Glück and Gebbers 2003) gave 209 human volunteers either a conventional yogurt or a combination of *Lactobacillus* GG (ATCC

53103), *Bifidobacterium* sp. B420, *Lactobacillus acidophilus* 145, and *Streptococcus thermophilus* every day for 3 weeks. Nasal microbial flora was measured at the beginning, at day 21 and at day 28 (a week after).

Significant pathogenic bacteria were found in most of the volunteers' nasal cavities at the beginning of the study. The consumption of the probiotic-enhanced milk led to a 19% reduction of pathogenic bacteria in the nasal cavity. The researchers concluded that, "The results indicate a [possible] linkage of the lymphoid tissue between the gut and the upper respiratory tract."

Scientists from Barcelona (Cobo Sanz *et al.* 2006) gave 251 children aged 3 to 12 years milk either with or without *Lactobacillus casei* for 20 weeks. The probiotic group of children experienced significantly less low respiratory tract infections, bronchitis and/or pneumonia (32% vs. 49%). The probiotic children also had a reduction in the duration of fatigue (3% vs. 13%). There was also a difference in the duration of sicknesses among the probiotic children compared to the placebo group.

French scientists (Forestier *et al.* 2008) assessed whether ventilator-associated pneumonia in intensive care units could be prevented or lessened by the use of probiotics. The 17-bed intensive care unit at the Clermont-Ferrand Teaching Hospital was used to test 208 patients with an intensive care unit stay of more than 48 hours. Patients were fed a placebo or *Lactobacillus rhamnosus* through a nasogastric feeding twice daily from their third day in the unit until discharge.

Infective *Pseudomonas aeruginosa* cultures were measured at admission, once a week, and upon discharge. Bacteriological tests of the respiratory tract also were done to determine patient infections. The study results indicated that *P. aeruginosa* respiratory colonization and/or infection was significantly reduced among the probiotic group. Ventilator-associated pneumonia by *P. aeruginosa* in the probiotic group ws reduced by more than 50% compared to the placebo group.

Researchers from the University of Arkansas' Medical School (Wheeler *et al.* 1997) studied 15 asthmatic adults in two 1-month crossover periods with placebo or yogurt containing *L. acidophilus*.

The probiotic consumption increased immune system interferon gamma and decreased eosinophilia levels.

Many other clinical research studies confirm similar findings: That the health of our lungs and the health of our esophagus are linked to the health of our probiotic populations.

So far we have presented the information and research illustrating that heartburn is not simply a problem of stomach acids leaking into the esophagus. The strength of the mucosal membranes and the makeup of our stomach acids, as well as the health of our epithelial tissues are also critical.

The research illustrates that the availability of strong colonies of probiotics among our mucosal membranes helps protect our esophagus from the damage done by acids, toxins and other foreigners.

How so? Because probiotics are living organisms that seek to protect and maintain their territories. This means that will help neutralize and balance the pH within those regions. They will produce alkaline secretions when their environment maintains too much acidity, and they will produce acidic secretions when their environment is too alkaline, or otherwise threatening.

This ability to alter their local environment is common amongst all living organisms. Our bodies are symbiotic with probiotics, as both seek to protect against invaders and other threats. Thus, our immune system works symbiotically with our probiotic colonies.

This is how organisms like *H. pylori* are controlled in the stomach. Our probiotics produce acids and antibiotic substances that control the populations of their competitors. This reduces *H. pylori* to manageable and even healthy population sizes.

This very same process is how healthy probiotic colonies keep other microorganisms—including *E. coli*, salmonella, clostridia, staph and Candida species—in check.

Should these organisms not be controlled, they can wreck havoc not only upon our intestines in the form of irritable bowel syndrome, but they can damage the epithelial integrity of our sphincters and our esophagus.

Chapter Four

GERD Precursors

So far, we've clarified the physiological basis for GERD, and we've defined the role that pathogenic and probiotic organisms play in the condition.

On a physiological basis, we've showed that GERD is a result of:

- The weakening and debilitation of our mucosal membranes;
- The absence of healthy probiotic colonies among our esophagus and digestive tract;
- The exposure of the epithelial tissues and cells of our esophagus, upper sphincter and stomach walls to acids and foreign entities;
- The opening up of the tight junctions between the cells of our epithelial tissues (increased epithelial permeability);
- The opening up of the pores within our cell membranes along the esophagus (increased cellular permeability);
- The launch of the immune system and a resulting condition of inflammation, which produces swelling and the burning pain typically described as 'heartburn.

The question now is what caused these occurences? Did they occur accidentally, or genetically? Possible, but not probable. Rather, there must be things—activities, foods or environments—that play a causative role in GERD. What are these things?

First, we should point out that it is likely that there isn't just one thing that causes all GERD conditions. Rather, there is an accumulation of research illustrating things that weaken our mucosal membranes, things that discourage healthy colonization of our probiotics, agents irritate and damage our epithelial membranes, and things that promote increased epithelial and cellular permeability.

In this chapter, we will discuss these elements, and how they produce these effects. As we consider these, however, we should note that many of us—even those without GERD—face one or more of these issues.

Instead of one particular activity or exposure, we find that GERD is typically produced by a combination of these exposures, often combined with a weakened gut immune system.

Some have termed the latter as a weak constitution. And it is often a revolving door, because a weak immune system will be caused by some of the same issues that produce GERD, and GERD is often the result of a weakened immune system. In addition, GERD inflammation can further weaken the immune system. Let's review the issues that have been shown to both weaken the immune system and produce GERD symptoms.

Toxic Chemicals

The mucosal membranes of our digestive tract and esophagus are damaged by a number of toxins, most of which are produced by the results of chemical-based manufacturing and synthetic production methods. There are several mechanisms whereby synthetic toxins damage our membranes. The most common is the oxidation of lipids, also called *lipid peroxidation.*

Many synthetic substances are toxic because they are unstable. When they come into contact with the mucosal membranes of our digestive tract, they can oxidize the phospholipids and glycolipids contained in the mucous.

And should they encounter the eipthelia of the esophagus and other parts of our digestive tract or airways, they damage our cell membranes. The cell membranes are made of stacked phospholipids.

Once oxidized, these lipids are broken down or otherwise degraded into substandard, unstable molecules. This effectively thins or damages the mucosal membranes. This damage to the mucosal membranes effectively allows these and other toxins and exposures—such as gastric acids and food acids—to penetrate the mucosal membrane barrier and irritate or damage the underlying epithelia. This then produces the symptoms of inflammation that we see around the body in the form of the mucosal conditions we discussed earlier, including GERD, asthma, COPD, eczema, allergies and so on.

Let's discuss some of the common synthetic toxins that harm practically any mucosal membrane they come into contact with.

102

Typically, the toxic exposure will need to be persistent and/or acute to have a lasting effect. In the case of an acute exposure, the immune system may repeal the damage in short order. This of course is why some short-term toxic exposures will produce gastrointestinal symptoms for a short period.

This is because our mucosal membranes are typically quite hardy. A healthy person will typically be able to resist the occasional exposure to one or a few synthetic toxins from time to time. An unhealthy person, or one with weakened probiotic colonies or otherwise suffering from immunosuppression may not be so lucky.

It is repeated toxin exposure that should concern us the most.

Clinical research by Professor John G Ionescu, Ph.D. (2009) concluded that environmental toxins are clearly associated with the development of mucosal membrane-related hypersensitivities. Dr. Ionescu's research indicated that environmental noxious agents, including many chemicals, contribute to the total immune burden, producing increased susceptibility for intolerances due to inflammation.

According to Dr. Ionescu's research, toxic inputs such as formaldehyde, smog, industrial waste, wood preservatives, microbial toxins, alcohol, pesticides, processed foods, nicotine, solvents and amalgam-heavy metals have been observed as contributing unstable radicals that damage our cells and mucosal membranes.

This is also consistent with findings of other scientists: Toxic chemicals overload the immune system and damage our mucosal membranes by contributing unstable oxidative radical species (ROS).

Some toxins are more damaging than others. Chemical toxins such as DDT, PBDEs, dioxin, formaldehyde, benzene, butane and chlorinated chemicals are all fat-soluble. Thus they can build up within the mucosal membranes and systemically ruin their structure and protective abilities.

Other compounds, such as phthalate plasticizers and parabens can also damage our membranes, but they typically do not accomplish this through lipid peroxidation. Still, they contribute free radicals that can damage our membranes and underlying epithelia.

Furthermore, as the immune system gears up to overdrive due to the overloading of multiple toxins, it becomes weaker and hypersensitive. This can cause a host of issues, including allergies, indigestion, irritable bowel syndrome and many others—all related to the weakening of the mucosal membranes.

For example, plasticizers and parabens are common amongst many of our medications, toys, foods packaged in plastic and other consumer items. Phthalates are also found in many household items. While phthalates have shorter half-lives than some toxins, they have been implicated in systemic inflammatory issues, hormone disruption, cancers and other conditions. Many cosmetics and antiperspirants contain parabens. These can thin or damage our mucosal membranes, and are thus readily absorbed into the skin where they can provoke inflammatory responses (Crinnion 2010).

These are only the tip of the toxin iceberg. Significant evidence points to the fact that our bodies are now being overloaded by synthetic toxins. For example, in conjunction with a mandate to lower toxin levels among the state's residents, in 2010 the Minnesota Department of Health compiled and released a list of the most toxic chemicals used in consumer products, building materials, pesticides, hair dyes, detergents, aerosols, cosmetics, furniture polish, herbicides, paints, cleaning solutions and many other common sources. The list also referenced research connecting the toxins to disease conditions.

The list contained 1,755 toxic chemicals.

Each of these burden the immune system. For each of these, the liver and immune system must launch a variety of macrophages, T-cells and B-cells to break them apart and escort them out of the body—if they can be escorted out. Many, especially those that are fat-soluble—will build up among our fat tissues. This means that each toxin represents an additional load the immune system must carry.

We might compare this to moving dirt. A small handful of dirt can be carried around easily, and dispersed without much effort. However, a truckload of dirt is another matter completely. What can we do with a truckload of dirt? If we dumped a truckload of dirt on our lawn, we'd have a hill of dirt that would bury the access to our front door and annihilate our lawn and/or garden.

This is a useful comparison because while our bodies can handle a small amount of toxins quite easily, modern society is increasingly dumping toxic 'dirt' into our atmosphere, water and foods, effectively inundating our bodies 'by the truckload.'

With this increased burden, our body's defenses are lowered, our mucosal membranes are weakened, and our esophagus tissues become more sensitive to irritation.

Foods that Irritate

Anyone who has suffered from GERD knows that eating certain foods will worsen the feeling of heartburn.

This is also confirmed by research. A review of research from the Mount Sinai School of Medicine (Friedman 1989) found that heartburn symptoms from gastroesophageal reflux can be reduced by eliminating fatty foods, alcohol, and chocolate from the diet. While there are many more as we'll discuss, these were the more prominent among the research through the 1980s.

In the case of fatty foods, the mechanism theorized at the time was that fatty foods slow the emptying of food from the stomach, causing food to back up. This is because fats are sometimes more difficult to break down. While this is not incorrect, this simplifies the larger mechanisms at play.

Researchers from the Chinese Academy of Medical Sciences (Chen *et al.* 2011) investigated lifestyle and diet factors among 751 cases of esophageal cancer among Chinese patients. These were compared with 2,253 randomly recruited healthy control subjects, giving them a three-to-one ratio between cancer subjects and healthy subjects.

The research found that the esophageal cancer patients were three times as likely to have suffered from GERD. They also found that the cancer patients were also more than three times more likely to prefer fried foods. The cancer patients were also more than three times more likely to have an irregular diet—verses a consistent diet—than the healthy subjects. The cancer group was 40% less likely to eat fresh vegetables daily than the healthy group. They concluded that eating fresh vegetables daily was a "protective factor."

Researchers from India's Seth G S Medical College (Bhatia *et al.* 2011), in conjunction with The Indian Society of Gastroenterology, conducted a study of 3,224 people from twelve medical centers across India. Of the total group, 245 of the people suffered from

105

GERD, with either heartburn and/or regurgitation symptoms at least once a week.

In this study, the strongest determinant of GERD was eating more fried foods and meats. Drinking carbonated beverages, black tea and coffee were also associated with GERD symptoms. The meat association was made clearer because the Indian population maintains a significant populations of vegetarians. The eating of meat could be more easily isolated among the population.

Other clinical studies have found that EOE is often mitigated to some degree by dietary change, particularly away from fried foods. (Abonia and Rothenberg 2012).

Researchers from New Jersey's Montclair State University (Navarro *et al.* 2011) utilized a large population-based study conducted in Connecticut, New Jersey, and Washington states to determine the risk factors of esophageal and gastric cancers. They determined that there were six "patterns" among those with these mucosal membrane-related cancers:

- They were more likely to eat fatty and fried foods.
- They were more likely to eat more meat, especially meat with higher nitrite levels.
- They were less likely to eat fruits and vegetables.
- They tended to be heavier—discovered through BMI levels
- They tended to have GERD
- They were more likely to smoke
- They were more likely to drink alcohol.

Thus we find clearly that the scientific evidence indicates that a variety of foods, which include fatty foods and some of the others on the list, readily form oxidative radicals. These free radicals oxidize lipids, forming harmful oxidized lipids. This process breaks down the complex lipid structures within our mucosal membranes, thinning these important protective barriers as we've discussed.

The lipids within the foods also become oxidized. These can invoke direct damage upon the epithelial cells of the esophagus, sphincter and stomach wall—especially as the mucosal membranes are weakened—as well as produce low-density lipoproteins within the intestines. As these are absorbed into the bloodstream, they damage the blood vessel walls—causing atherosclerosis, heart disease and numerous other inflammatory diseases.

Because of this resulting inflammatory nature, the foods and beverages that worsen heartburn, not surprisingly, are some of the same ones that increase asthma incidence. This of course irreparably connects asthma and GERD. These foods also happen to increase systemic inflammation around the body, again because they contribute free radicals and other toxins, stimulating inflammation.

These include foods or beverages that are:

- high in refined sugars
- highly processed (fiber removed)
- high in refined salt
- high in saturated fats
- fried
- 'fast foods'
- burnt or overcooked (including char-broiling)
- containing certain preservatives and chemical additives
- chocolate candy
- contain refined peppermint or menthol (Studies from the State University of New York, have found that eating processed foods containing peppermint tend to reduce the esophageal sphincter's holding power.)

These types of foods and beverages serve to irritate the epithelial tissues of the esophagus, spincter and stomach wall because they produce free radicals that readily deplete and weaken mucous membranes and then damage the tight junction proteins that protect the epithelial tissues, along with the membranes that protect the cells. We described these earlier as increased epithelial permeability and increased cellular permeability.

This once again is because they either directly contribute free radicals that break down the mucosal membranes and damage epithelial cells and tissues, or cause oxidation reactions that produce these free radicals.

Outside of oxidation, multiple studies have confirmed that certain types of fatty meals increase the likelihood of GERD because they slow the stomach's emptying process. When we eat repeated meals without allowing the stomach to empty—especially if we eat until we are full—there is a stronger likelihood that our esophageal sphincter valves will weaken under pressure, and our stomach acids begin to leak into the esophagus.

How we Eat

This leads directly to how we eat. Most of us wolf down our meals as if they were going to be stolen from us if we don't eat it now. Even if we don't wolf the meal down, many of us half-chew a mouthful of food and hen wash it down with a drink.

Many animals wolf food down because they have more powerful digestive enzymes. For humans, our grinding teeth allow us to fully masticate our food—and rightfully so. And because glands in our mouth secrete enzymes such as amylase that help break our foods down, a significant part of digestion for humans takes place in the mouth.

While it might be the case for some—especially in third world countries—most of us living in first and second world countries (where most of the GERD sufferers are) have little fear that our food will be stolen from us before we can eat it and swallow it. Therefore, we have time to properly masticate and begin the digestive process within the mouth.

Consistent wolfing or washing our food down puts pressure on our esophageal sphincters, on a simple mechanical basis.

We might compare this with driving through a gate. If we want to drive through a parking garage gate, typically we have to stop the car and wait for the gate to open. When open, we drive through it.

Consider what would happen if we didn't stop the car, but instead just ran into the garage gate as the gate was opening. Likely, the car would hit the gate and damage the gate as well as the car.

But take the same gate, and run five cars into it at once—or even a semi-truck—and that gate would be flattened. The weight of the impact from multiple cars or the big truck simply overwhelms the gate.

The same thing happens to our esophageal sphincters valve, which must stage food into the stomach while minimizing acid leakage back out. These valves, quite simply, can become overwhelmed when a person consistently overloads the esophagus with undigested food.

Over time, particularly when mucous membranes are weakened and the valves are not properly insulated, the overload of foods can weaken the sphincter valves—softening them. This is called a loss of tone. In other words, the amount of food and consistent ingestion both burden the esophageal sphincters.

Illustrating this, researchers from the Ohio State University College of Medicine (Jadcherla *et al.* 2011) studied gastroesophageal reflux among infants. They studied the relationship between quantity, duration and flow rates when the infants were fed. In other words, a mother can feed her infant quickly or slowly, and for short or long durations.

The researchers studied 35 infants with GERD symptoms. They used pH-impedance to determine the acidic symptoms in response to feeding. They found that longer feeding times and slower flow rates decreased GERD symptoms among the infants.

'Slow Food' anyone?

In other words, wolfing down our foods promotes heartburn symptoms and GERD. This is because chewing speeds up the food being able to empty the stomach and thus enter the stomach, due to the food being chewed into a slurry.

Chewing is also critical to our neutralizing some of the free radicals present in even the healthiest foods.

When we chew, our salivary glands produce amylase and other enzymes that serve to break apart the bonds of our foods. As they do this, they and the probiotics present in our mouth also attach unmatched ("free") electrons or protons to neutralize them.

This chewed up mix of enzymes and neutralized food particles produces a mash that is called a *bolus*. The bolus mash will allow further enzymes and probiotics to penetrate the nutrients of the foods, and continue separating them. This prepares them to become assimilated.

This breakdown process occurs within the stomach and intestines. The enzymatic neutralization process also creates what are called chelates. Chelates are nutrients attached with ions that buffer and escort their transition through the pores of the digestive tract and into the bloodstream.

These chelated nutrients, by being attached with ions, also become more alkaline in substance. This helps prevent them from infusing their free radicals directly onto the mucosal membranes and the epithelial layers beneath.

This doesn't necessarily mean that we can eat the foods mentioned earlier and simply because we chew them longer, escape their free radical-damaging effects. But chewing longer will certainly reduce their free radical effects. This is simply because some of those free radicals will no longer be free radicals. They will be neutralized.

The big takeaway is that should we eat healthy foods and take our time chewing them, we will be removing a significant burden from our esophagus, sphincters and stomach walls—reducing our risk of GERD and GERD symptoms.

Obesity

Obesity is, of course, related to not only how we eat, but how much we eat. This also typically relates to how fast we eat, since there are only so many minutes in a day, and overeaters are typically putting more calories into their bodies faster than normal eaters.

We have shown some of the science associating GERD with obesity earlier. The fact is, GERD has increased almost parallel with obesity rates, especially within the United States.

Confirming these studies, researchers from Syracuse's Upstate Medical University (Hajar *et al.* 2012) analyzed 122 human clinical studies that measured BMI, pH and GERD incidence.

They found that reflux episodes increased as BMI increased. The result was similar when analyzing recumbent incidence (GERD symptoms when sleeping or laying down). The researchers concluded: "Obesity not only increases the likelihood of reflux events, as shown in previous studies, but also makes it more likely that symptoms reported during MII-pH studies are actually due to MII detected reflux." [MII detected reflux refers to reflux that is confirmed by impedance monitoring of esophageal pH levels.]

Alcohol

Drinking alcohol—especially excessively—is a big risk factor for GERD. Why is this? Alcohol has several negative effects upon the health of our digestive tract. For one, alcohol damages the mucosal membranes of our esophagus, sphincter and stomach wall via direct contact. Once assimilated, alcohol also disrupts our submucosal secretions, as it interferes with the cyclooxygenase process—one reason people often feel less pain when they drink.

In a study from Italy's National Cancer Research Institute (Conio *et al.* 2002), 149 Barrett's esophagus and 143 patients with esophagitis were studies. Both are significantly associated with GERD as we've discussed. And alcohol consumption was significantly associated with esophagitis and to a lesser degree, Barrett's esophagus.

Alcohol (basically, ethanol) also produces dehydration amongst the cells and tissue systems, because it generates destructive reactive oxygen species (ROS)—again, free radicals. These ROS in alcohol break down water molecules in their attempts to become stable, which essentially removes water from the cells and tissues. This drying or dehydration effect of alcohol can be seen visually when using a strong alcohol such as distilled or rubbing alcohol externally. By applying the alcohol, we can see that it dries extremely quickly, effectively removing moisture and water content.

Alcohol is toxic to the body in general. The reactive oxygen species generated by alcohol damage liver cells and reduce glutathione levels. This means the liver will produce less enzymes and filter the blood poorly. This leaves the body in a state of increased toxicity. Over time this can produce severe liver disease, which can result in death.

These alcohol-produced reactive oxygen species also damage mucous membranes, epithelial cells and their intercellular bonds on contact. Just as alcohol is drying externally, it is drying internally—robbing the fluidity of our mucosal membranes. This makes alcohol highly destructive to the linings covering the esophagus wall and esophageal sphincters.

Often people consider that because wines and other spirits are made from natural ingredients, they must be healthy. For example, resveratrol from wine is touted as being healthy. Resveratrol, however, comes from the grapes themselves and is most available in the seeds and grape skins. Resveratrol also comes from red berries and is most available from the Japanese knotweed herb. While red wine certainly will also contain resveratrol, a person would need to drink a hundred bottles of wine to consume a therapeutic amount of resveratrol. And the alcohol content of the wine will do more damage than even a therapeutic amount of resveratrol can reverse.

As for those reputed to have been drinking a glass or two of wine every day while remaining seemingly healthy, yes, the liver can certainly manage a minimal amount of alcohol every day, and a little wine will not necessarily cause GERD. This doesn't mean that the alcohol is healthy for the liver or the mucosal membranes of the esophagus. And research has confirmed that even a moderate amount of wine can damage the liver.

In addition, there have been a few studies that have indicated the possibility that a drink or two of wine every day may increase longevity. This type of epidemiological research, however, is highly questionable, notably because those who have a glass or two of wine everyday may also well be doing something else—such as so-cializing while drinking or otherwise reducing stress levels—which would also account for their longevity. Other studies have shown that socializing and reducing stress levels extend life in themselves.

On the other hand, research showing that the liver is damaged by alcohol consumption, and alcohol is linked to GERD is irrefuta-ble.

Research has also confirmed that alcohol (ethanol) also damages our probiotic colonies (see the author's book, *Probiotics-Protection Against Infection*).

Other Beverage Issues

As mentioned earlier, early research found that GERD was as-sociated with carbonated soft drinks. This was confirmed by a re-view by researchers from the Yale University School of Medicine and Cancer Center (Mayne *et al.* 2006).

However, in more recent studies, this conclusion may be less clear. After a review of the research, scientists from Italy's Univer-sity of Naples (Cuomo *et al.* 2009) found the direct evidence of carbonated beverages affecting GERD to be contradictory. They did establish, however that the consumption of over 300 ml of car-bonated beverages per day was associated with "gastric mechanical distress."

In a review of the research one year later by Southern Arizona Veterans' Administration researchers (Johnson *et al.* 2010), the evidence revealed that, "carbonated beverage consumption results in a very short decline in intra-esophageal pH. In addition, carbonated beverages may lead to a transient reduction in lower esophageal sphincter basal pressure."

However, they also added that: "There is no evidence that carbonated beverages directly cause esophageal damage."

The research may be mixing drink types a bit. Sugary carbonated sodas are a completely different animal altogether than carbonated spring waters and even those mostly-European spring waters that are naturally carbonated. This type of carbonation was the subject of some of the research, while sugary sodas and even sugarless sodas have been the subject of others. In other words, the studies that tested carbonated spring waters would not produce the same results as those testing sugary sodas.

Why? Because refined sugars produce an abundance of free radicals.

Sugary sodas have been linked with heart disease and diabetes (Lustig 2012). More recent research by Harvard Medical School professor Dr. Lewis Cantley has determined that refined sugar stimulates the growth of cancer cells, producing metastatic tumors (Anastasiou *et al.* 2011).

Glucose appears to be harmful agent from both refined sugar and high-fructose corn syrup within these sodas. Because refined sugars increase glucose intolerance, and produce glycated byproducts that cause damage to arteries, it is the refined glucose contributors that provide the GERD risk from carbonated beverages. Carbonation in itself—especially spring water forms—has not proven to cause or worsen GERD.

We should also note that that refined sugars in sodas and other foods directly feed pathogenic bacteria. As pathogenic bacteria like *H. pylori* are fed more glucose, their colonies grow stronger. As they grow stronger, they increasingly damage our mucosal membranes.

The GERD Lifestyle

As we indicated in the first chapter with the epidemiological evidence and confirmed by clinical studies—GERD is significantly related to our lifestyle. This is due to what is termed by scientists as the brain-gut axis. Certain lifestyle choices stimulate this brain-gut axis in ways that reduce our body's production of healthy mucosal membranes, as well as many of the enzymes our body needs to break down and neutralize our foods. These include:

➢ Stress

➢ Anxiety

➢ Anger

➢ Lack of sunshine

As for anger and stress, when our body is stressed, our body switches to fight-or-flight metabolic mechanisms that divert our nervous energy from the processes of the sub-mucosal glands and gastric glands—to those facilities that provide for physical protection. These include pupil focus, muscle productivity, dilation of the airways and other physiological facilities that allow us to escape threats and deal with physically stressful situations.

The trick here is that the body typically responds the same regardless of whether the perceived threat is physical or mental. Decades of research shows that a threat to our position or job will invoke a similar physiological response as will being chased by a rabbid dog.

This is why a person who is nervous or anxious will also often experience a dry mouth and an upset stomach. The anxiety stimulates physiology that diverts our nervous energy away from our mucosal secretions.

While occasional stress is not a cause for great concern, it is chronic stress that is at issue. Daily stress episodes lock our physiology into a repetitive cycle of rebounding anxiety with relief. This pumps our system and pressurizes our epithelial layers with thinned mucous membranes through a good part of our day.

Worse is eating during those stressed periods, which is what many stressed people will do. We will often have a stressful meeting over lunch for example. Or we will have a stressful conversation over dinner. These reduce our mucosal secretions at the very moment we need them the most.

Eating while stressed will put those toxins and free radicals within our foods—as well as our gastric acids—in more direct contact with our epithelial surfaces. And since we produce more gastric acids when we eat, we are more prone to GERD symptoms when we are eating during stress.

Eating while stressed also increases the likelihood that we will not sufficiently chew our foods. And because we produce fewer enzymes when stressed, the rate of stomach emptying will slow down—backing food and acids into our esophagus.

GERD and the Sun

Dr. Dio Lewis, a well-known and successful Nineteenth century country doctor, was also a leading sunlight expert. He documented treating GERD, neuralia, lung infections and other diseases by exposing his patients to daily sunlight. He documented his research in his book entitled *Weak Lungs and How to Make Them Strong* (1863).

Research published in the *American Journal of Surgery* (Wei *et al.* 1984) found that vitamin D supplementation was required for 23% of patients that needed pharyngolaryngoesophagectomy and pharyngogastric anastomosis—surgeries resulting from chronic GERD.

A lack of sunshine (without supplementation) robs the body of vitamin D a key hormone-nutrient used throughout the body and nervous system.

GERD in Singers, Musicians and Athletes

A number of studies have found that professional singers suffer from GERD at greater levels than the rest of the population.

In a study by researchers from the Catholic University of Medicine and Surgery (Cannizzaro *et al.* 2007), 351 professional opera singers were compared to 578 similar subjects who were not singers. The study found that the singers had a 60% higher rate of heartburn, and 81% increased incidence of regurgitation, and higher levels of coughs and hoarse voice.

The jury seems to still be out on why this takes place. Some researchers in the above study, for example, stated that: "Future studies will be needed to clarify whether gastroesophageal reflux in professional opera choristers is stress-induced and therefore may be considered as a work-related disease."

In other words, the issue could be either stress or due to excessive pressure being put on the diaphragm while singing. This latter effect appears more probable, since many other professionals also suffer from stress, and have significantly less GERD.

This probability was confirmed by a study three years after this singing study by researchers from the same medical school (Cammarota *et al.* 2010). The research followed 1083 musicians, including 414 wind instrument players. The study found that wind instrument players—which also extensively utilize their diaphragms—had significantly more heartburn than their peers who played professional instruments other than the wind instruments.

Other research has since confirmed these same conclusions among musicians, along with, surprisingly, many athletes, especially among endurance athletes.

A study from Northwestern University's School of Medicine (Pandolfino *et al.* 2004) revealed a similar relationship as with the musicians. The researchers tested 20 people, 10 of whom had GERD. They found that exercise produced a 300% increase in stomach acid exposure in the esophagus among both groups. This, they said, was reason for GERD sufferers to be aware of the "anatomical integrity" of the sphincters as they go about their exercises and lifestyles.

The diaphragm is one of the body's strongest muscles. It lies between the abdominal cavity and the chest cavity. It contracts and its downward pressure draws air into the lungs. Supporting muscles include the pectoralis muscles, the serratus muscles, the scalenes, the levatores, and the sternocleidomastoid muscles. The prolonged exertion of these muscles is critical to a good singing voice and a sustained note on a wind instrument.

As the diaphragm contracts it moves downward, causing an increase in the rib cage volume. This lowers the atmospheric pressure in the lungs, and creates a vacuum or negative pressure within the lungs and draws in the air.

During an extended song or solo, the diaphragm of a professional singer will be engaged severely. This will put pressure on the fundus, which in turn puts the lower esophageal sphincter under pressure.

Budapest medical researchers underscored this mechanism, as they stated, "In addition to lower esophageal sphincter (LES) relaxations and decreased LES tone, increased intra-abdominal pressure can also play role in the pathogenesis of gastroesophageal re-flux disease." (Pregun *et al.* 2009).

Stress

We discussed stress in general above, but let's dig into the mechanisms a little more, because stress is one of the more critical causative elements for GERD. This of course relates directly to the epidemiological research we laid out in the first chapter that illustrated that more industrialized countries—those with more stressful lifestyles—have the most GERD cases with the most GERD frequency.

Numerous clinical studies have also linked GERD to stress. Stress increases epithelial permeability, leading to inflammation and damage to the epithelial cells (Bhatia and Tandon 2005).

As we discussed, reducing stress is critical to the health of our digestive tract. This is because of a system in the body called the "brain-gut axis." The critical mechanism uses the parasympathetic and sympathetic nerve pathways to connect moods and emotions with the production of gastric acids, digestive enzymes and mucosal membranes.

This is compounded by the fact that our nervous system governs what is called *peristalsis*—the rhythmic motions of the stomach and digestive tract that help move our food along.

When we are under stress, the body switches into emergency mode. The adrenal glands begin to produce stress hormones along with neurotransmitters that are also produced by other glands. These work together to stop most of the secretions around the body, which include the secretion of enzymes and the mucosal membranes. This is because the body is prioritizing its metabolism, and digestion is at the bottom of the list when our body's survival is at risk.

In other words, when we are feeling stressed, even if the stress offers no threat to our physical well being, the body will still respond as if its survival is threatened. The processes that relate to muscle response and sense response—such as those needed if we had to run away from a tiger while being able to look back as we are running—will take priority. The parts of our physiology that relate to protecting our epithelial cells and sphincters will meanwhile be put on hold.

This 'smart' system is of course based on our evolutionary history, as being stressed typically meant that we were under some threat of survival from some physical source. In modern societies, most of this stress response comes from mental and social stressors—which can still risk our ability to make money and thus affect our body's ability to survive.

Sleep

Several studies have connected GERD to a lack of sleep. This is because the body is stressed by a lack of sleep, and needs sleep to refresh itself.

For example, researchers from the University of Hong Kong's medical school (Zhang *et al.* 2012) studied 2,291 middle-aged adults for five years. They found that those with persistent non-restorative sleep—not enough sleep to be rested and alert throughout the day—also had twice the incidence of GERD.

As documented with more detail in the author's book, *Natural Sleep,* studies show that sleep is rejuvenating to our cells, our digestive tracts, our immune systems and our mucosal membranes. When we sleep, the immune system goes into overdrive and clears out many of the toxins that have burdened our metabolism throughout the day. This clearing effect also allows our esophagus to clear out toxins and replenish the mucosal membranes that line the epithelial region. It also allows our stomach to fully empty and refresh its mucosal lining. This is critical for ongoing protection of these cells as we've been discussing.

In addition, sleep allows our body's immune system to fix or get rid of cells that are not functioning well and toss out many of the invaders. This leaves our digestive tract stronger and able to face another day of having foods and acids slammed down it.

We'll talk about a few strategies to reduce stress and increase sleep later.

Heavy Metals

Heavy metals are metal elements that exist naturally in trace quantities within our soils, waters and foods. However, extraordinarily consolidated quantities of heavy metals such as cadmium, lead and mercury are produced by our industrial complex in the manufacturing of various consumer and commercial goods.

We can cite many studies that have associated heavy metal exposure to immunosuppression and inflammation. We simply do not have the room to do so here.

For example, in multicenter research from the Department of Medicine from the Lavoro Medical Center in Bari, Italy (Soleo *et al.* 2002), researchers studied the effects of low levels of inorganic mercury exposure on 117 workers. They compared these with 172 general population subjects. They found no difference in the white blood cell count between the two groups. However, the worker group exposed to mercury had increased levels of CD4+ and CD8+ cytokines, and CD4+ levels were particularly high. These levels indicated a state of systemic inflammation among the exposed workers. In addition, significantly lower levels of interleukin (IL-8) occurred among the exposed workers—indicating immunosuppression.

This and other research has concluded that even low levels of environmental exposure to mercury and other heavy metals (beyond the trace levels normally found in nature) suppresses the immune system and stimulates mucosal membrane defects.

Cadmium is another common heavy metal bombarding us. Among consumer products, cadmium is used in a wide range of metal coatings, batteries and colorings. Most cigarettes also contain cadmium.

A whole book can be written on the effects of heavy metal toxicity. Suffice to say that heavy metals can severely reduce the strength of our mucosal membranes and the epithelia of our esophagus.

Water Pollutants

Our industrial society has been dumping synthetic chemistry into our waters for many decades. These are responsible for what is called bioaccumulation. This means that because nature's organisms rely upon water all the way up the food chain, microorganisms, insects, fish, birds, animals and humans are now accumulating stores of these toxic chemicals, and passing them up the food chain.

Because most of these chemicals are fat-soluble, they will build up within the fat cells and other molecular lipids within these organisms.

Most of these chemicals either create free radicals as they are processed in the body or they produce free radicals among the other molecules or nutrients within the body. These effectively irritate and damage our mucosal membranes and the underlying esophageal epithelial tissues. They can also directly damage and weaken our sphincter valves, compounding the issue with stomach acid leakage.

Water contamination comes from manufacturing, household wastewater, air pollution, ship and boat waste, run-off from farms and run-of from street gutters and roadways. All of these to one degree or another end up in our drinking water supplies.

While municipalities have extensive chlorination systems in place to clear microbiological content, removal systems for chemical pollutants are still in various stages of development. For some pollutants, there is no filtration. As a result, our drinking water supplies have numerous contaminants.

Even some of the cleaning agents used in some municipal water supplies are toxic. This includes trichloroethylene. Trichloroethylene is a chlorinated hydrocarbon used to separate oil from water. The solvent was popularized in the dry cleaning business, and is a common cleansing agent in many local water municipalities.

Pharmaceutical medicines in our water supplies make for a perfect example. In 2007, researchers from Finland's Abo Akademi University (Vieno et al.) released a study showing that pharmaceutical beta-blockers, antiepileptic drugs, lipid regulators, antiinflammatory drugs and fluoroquinolone drugs were all found in river waters. The concentrations of these were well above drinking water limits.

The researchers also found that water treatment only eliminated an average of 13% of the concentration of these pharmaceuticals. This means that 87% of these pharmaceutical medicines remained in the drinking water, ready to dose each and every person drinking that water with prescription medication.

Other pollutants commonly found in our drinking water supplies include PCBs, and other biphenol compounds, dioxin, chlorine metabolites, pesticides, herbicides, petroleum byproducts, nitrates, and many others.

Agricultural runoff is a huge source of drinking water contamination. In addition, nitrogen-rich fertilizers choke rivers and oceans with extra nitrogen, causing abnormal blooms of algae. These massive algal blooms cut off oxygen supplies and lead to the die-offs of many species of marine life. *Dead zones* have been reportedly growing in many of the world's waterways. The cause is the massive use of nitrogen-based synthetic fertilizers.

The use of pesticides on agricultural land, playgrounds, parks, home lawns, and gardens throughout the United States is staggering, and it is growing. In 1964, approximately 233 million pounds of pesticides were applied in the U.S. By 1982, this amount tripled to 612 million pounds. In 1999, the U.S. Environmental Protection Agency reported that some five *billion* pounds of these chemicals were applied per year throughout America's crops, forests, parks, and lawns.

One of the more increasingly popular pesticides is imidacloprid, a neonicotinoid. Introduced by Bayer in 1994, imidacloprid is used against aphids and similar insects on over 140 different crops. Touted as a chemical with a fairly short half-life of thirty days in water and twenty-seven days in anaerobic soil, imidacloprid's half-life is about 997 days in aerobic soil. While it has a lower immediate toxicity compared with hazards like DDT, imidacloprid's use is now widespread. It is rated by the EPA and WHO as "*moderately toxic*" in small doses. Larger doses can disrupt liver and thyroid function. While this pesticide does well at killing off increasingly resistant pests, it has also been shown to decimate bee populations.

Cleaning agents are used with or rinsed by water. They will thus immediately enter our greywater systems. According to the U.S. Poison Control Centers, about ten percent of all toxin exposure is caused by cleaning products, with almost two-thirds involving children under six years old. While we might be shocked to find a child toying with a bottle of drain cleaner containing sulfuric acid, hydrochloric acid and lye, we do not think twice about feeding this same product into our waterways. We wear gloves to protect our skin from the harmful affects of ammonia and bleach while we do our cleaning but assume they disappear once poured down the sink.

An example of this is 1,4-dioxane, a common ingredient in many shampoos and other cleaning products. The California EPA documented that 1,4-dioxane is a carcinogen that can also damage kidneys, nerves and lungs. It biodegrades very slowly and is becoming a threat to drinking water supplies. This is but one of many.

In a 2002 U.S. Geological Survey report on stream water contaminants, 69% of stream samples revealed non-biodegradable detergents, and 66% of the samples contained disinfectant chemicals. Phosphates—central ingredients in many commercial laundry soaps—have been banned for dumping in over eleven states in the U.S. because of their dangerous effects upon the environment. Yet many people still use these soaps without any consideration of their effects upon our waters.

Biphenyls are considered *xenoestrogens,* or endocrine system disruptors. Long-term effects as their residues build up in the tissues of aquatic species, and bio-accumulate up the ladder to our cells, organs and tissue systems. Research has found that biphenyls have produced sexual re-orientation of fish in some water supplies.

These combined factors are increasingly problematic to a human population seeking to sustain life on the planet. Research by Slovenian researchers Tatjana Tisler and Jana Zagorc-Koncan (2003) has shown that we are drastically underestimating the effects of toxic industrial waste. Our typical method for toxicity research has been to study each individual chemical and its possible toxicity.

What we are missing with this type of research is the combined effects of the thousands of chemicals we are putting into our waters. As these chemicals mix, they create a toxic soup of new chemical combinations. Some of these are combinations are exponentially more toxic than the individual chemicals.

We'll discuss water consumption and filtration later.

Microorganisms

We have discussed this element with respect to GERD at length. Let's review it quickly here.

Pathogenic bacteria infections of *Helicobacter pylori, Clostridium* spp. and *E. coli* are known to exert damage to the mucosal membranes of our esophagus, stomach, intestines and colon. They are thus implicated in ulcers and GERD, along with many other intestinal disorders. These are only a few of the many that can infect our tissues and directly or indirectly contribute to GERD.

Destructive microorganisms can colonize the mucosal membranes. As they do this, they produce a flurry of acids and antibiotic chemical secretions set up territory within our bodies. Depending upon the species, they can be very aggressive. Their acids can break down and weaken our mucosal membranes, and they can penetrate the epithelial layers to damage our tight junctions to directly irritate our cells within the mouth, throat, esphagus, and stomach. We have talked about some of these earlier.

Bacteria can come from rotting food, plants, people and pets. Dander also can carry these creatures. Viruses can lodge within our mucosal membranes initially, eventually infecting our cells as they penetrate.

Viruses can damage DNA within the cells, and reproduce through the body via DNA mutations.

Microorganisms can grow on anything wet—especially mold. Almost any type of sitting water or dampness will grow mold, especially those in dark areas (as many fungi abhor sunlight).

Research has confirmed that infective microorganisms from viruses, bacteria and fungi can stimulate serious mucosal membrane defects.

Today we are dealing with a multitude of infections from all of these types of microorganisms. Growing infectious diseases from this list include lyme disease (*Borrelia burgdorferi*), pneumonia, staphylococcus, streptococcus, salmonella, *E. coli*, cholera, listeria, salmonella, shigella, dengue fever, yellow fever, tuberculosis, cryptosporidiosis, hepatitis, rabies and others. Many of these microorganisms are growing despite our antibiotic and antiviral medications. Some are growing because of unsafe sex, unclean water or changes in land use. Many are growing because of new opportunities arising from our destruction of nature. Many are becoming resistant to our antibiotics. These are often referred to as *superbugs.*

One of the more dangerous of these superbugs is methicillin-resistant *Staphylococcus aureus* (MRSA). MRSA rates are on the rise, and nearly every hospital—the crown jewels of our antimicrobial kingdom—is infected with MRSA. In a 2007 survey of 1200 U.S. hospitals, 46 of every 1,000 hospital inpatients are colonized or infected with MRSA, with 75% of those being infected.

Among the general population, the incidence of MRSA has skyrocketed from 24 cases per 100,000 people in 2000 to 164 cases per 100,000 people in 2005 (Hota *et al.* 2007). This means that MRSA is infecting nearly seven times the number of people it did in 2000.

Multiple pathogenic microorganisms can grow and prosper within the mouth, teeth and gums, later migrating to our esophagus. These include *Streptococcus mutans, Streptococcus pyogenes, Porphyromonas gingivalis, Tannerella forsynthensis* and *Prevotella.* Additional microbes can grow within root canals. Root canals provide protected spaces for bacterial growth. Bacteria infecting root canals can include a variety of steptococci, staphylococci, and even dangerous spirochetes such as *Borrelia burgdorferi* among many others. Just about any bacteria that can infect the body internally can hibernate inside root canals.

As these microbial populations grow, they not only can infect teeth and gums with gingivitis: They can also infect the tissues of our sinuses, throat and esophagus.

Lipopolysaccharides are common bacteria endotoxins. Lipopolysaccharides make up the cell membranes of gram negative bacteria, and they make up a significant part of their waste stream. Lipopolysaccharides also have shown in research to produce inflammation and damage our mucosal membranes.

Viral Infections

Viruses that infect the lower respiratory tract or digestive tract can produce significant inflammatory conditions. These include pneumonia, viral dysentery, influenza and so many others. They can also indirectly produce heartburn as they weaken the mucosal membranes.

An example of a serious viral infection is the respiratory syncytial virus (RSV). RSV is fairly common among premature children. As a result, doctors often give premature children anti-viral medications during infancy to help prevent an RSV infection. RSV has specifically been shown to cause wheezing in children, and as we showed earlier, wheezing is directly related to GERD, especially among children.

The human rhinovirus (HRV), which will cause the common cold in most people, can also infect the lower respiratory airways. Indeed, the association between HRV during infancy and a weakened immune system later in life is stronger with HRV than with other viruses (Jackson and Lemanske 2010).

This study confirms what other studies have indicated: An early serious viral lung infection seriously penetrates and weakens our mucosal membranes. This opens our esophagus epithelial layers to further damage.

Yeast, Molds and other Fungi

Yeast and mold are members of the fungi family. Mold spores reproduce and float through both the outdoor and indoor air. Once they land, they can begin multiplying into larger cultures. While there are several species of mold, almost all require moisture to grow and populate. A concentration of spores riding the indoor air currents can cause various sensitivities, allergies, and sickness (Sahakian *et al.* 2008).

Mold spores also produce a number of substances called mycotoxins, which can create health concerns if inhaled. Homeowners and renters should be aware of this, and make sure the houses they live in have no water entry into the basement. Moist appliances like air conditioners, bathtubs, bathroom carpets, and air ducts can also grow mold.

For these reasons, we might want to frequently check the various corners and dark places in our houses and workplaces for moisture, because the fungal populations growing on these surfaces will only get bigger with time—disbursing toxins into the air as they grow. Once found, the area should be dried, the mold or bacteria should be cleaned up. (Water with a few drops of rubbing alcohol, vinegar or chlorine will kill most mold or bacteria).

If a mold growth is over several feet, a mold specialist may need to be called in to eliminate the mold.

This was confirmed by researchers from the National University of Singapore (Tham *et al.* 2007), who found that home dampness and indoor mold is linked to an increase in asthma and allergy symptoms among children. They studied 4,759 children from 120 daycare centers. After eliminating other possible effects, home humidity was significantly associated with increased rates of allergic rhinoconjunctivitis.

As discussed earlier, these issues have also been related to GERD.

Overgrowths of yeasts like *Candida albicans* can also contribute to or overload our mucosal membranes and immune system. While Candida is a typical resident of the our body, when it is unchecked by our immune and probiotic system it can grow to incredible colony sizes. Like most other organisms, it is typically not the Candida organism that overloads the immune system: it is the endotoxins that these microscopic living beings produce.

Candida albicans can grow conjunctively with *Staphylococcus aureus*, resulting in the accelerated growth of both microorganisms. This can result in a tremendous burden for the mucosal membranes among the digestive tract.

Refluxive Pharmaceuticals

A number of pharmaceuticals can weaken the mucosal membranes and expose the epithelial layers of our esophagus, sphincter and stomach wall to stomach acids, acidic foods and toxins. This, as we've discussed, invokes the inflammatory responses that result in pain and inflammation within esophagus.

Typically, those pharmaceuticals that list a side effect of gastrointestinal bleeding or other gastrointestinal difficulties will be harmful to our digestive epithelia and mucosal membranes. This is because many pharmaceuticals, by shutting down part of the inflammatory response by inhibiting the enzyme process called cyclooxygenase (COX), also interrupt mucosal membrane secretion. Let's discuss the mechanics of this a bit more as we pinpoint some of the medications that have these effects:

NSAID COX Inhibitors

As mentioned, NSAIDs provide pain relief and reduced inflammation by interrupting the enzyme cyclooxygenase. Cyclooxygenase or COX oxidizes certain fatty acids to initiate a chain reaction that produces prostaglandins and thromboxane. These are key components involved in the process of healing wound sites and removing pathogens. The COX-1 process also stimulates the secretion of the mucins around the body that make up the bulk of our mucosal membranes. This only makes sense, because our mucosal membranes also protect healing epithelia.

The three main COX enzymes are COX-1, COX-2 and COX-3. Most NSAIDs will inhibit the activity of both COX-1 and COX-2. The problem with inhibiting the COX-1 enzyme is that this blocks the metabolic process that produces protective secretions among the mucosal membranes of our esophagus, stomach and duodenum. Without this protective lining, our stomach can be damaged by our food and the gastric acids our stomach cells produce. This blocking of our protective mucus is what causes the ulcer and GI pain characteristic of NSAID use.

When these secretions are halted, various conditions begin to pop up, including heartburn, ulcers, gastric bleeding, intestinal irritation and others. This is the reason there are so many different COX-inhibiting drugs: They each cause a number of sometimes lethal side effects, and the pharmaceutical industry keeps creating new ones in an attempt to solve the COX problem.

Let's review some of these:

Acetylsalicylic acid or aspirin (Aspirin, Ecotrin®, many others; over the counter) is a synthetic molecule designed to mimic the effects of willow bark and meadowsweet herb. For thousands of years, herbalists and ancient healers used both willow bark and meadowsweet for the relief of pain. In 1828, salicin was isolated from the bark of the willow tree by Joseph Buchner. Two years later, salicin was isolated from the flower of the meadowsweet plant by Johann Pagenstecher. In 1838, a method of isolating salicylic acid from willow extract was discovered by the Italian Raffaele Piria. Meanwhile, German chemist Karl Jacob Lowig isolated the same salicylic acid from meadowsweet extract. In 1874, salicylic acid began to be produced for commercial use.

Twenty-three years later, in 1897, Charles Garhardt, a chemist at the Friedrich Bayer & Company, synthesized a similar derivative by adding an acetyl group (OCOOH), to produce the more stable acetylsalicylic acid. The Bayer company proceeded to call it *aspirin* and began large-scale production shortly thereafter.

Aspirin's mechanism of action in the body continued to be mysterious, however. Finally, in 1971, Sir John Vane determined that aspirin's active constituent, acetylsalicylic acid, inhibited prostaglandin synthetase (later identified as cyclooxygenase and abbreviated as COX) causing its anti-inflammatory and anti-thrombosis effects. Sir John Vane received the Nobel Prize for Medicine in 1982 for this hypothesis.

Like willow and meadowsweet, aspirin has an immediate effect of reducing pain. Aspirin binds to cylooxygenase-2 within the cells. This allows it to block the pain and inflammatory process. Cylooxygenase-2 produces prostaglandins that in turn send messages to the brain that a particular part of the body is injured. When cylooxygenase-2 is blocked, the process of converting arachidonic acid to prostaglandins is halted.

Cylooxygenase-2 also stimulates the production of thromboxanes. These stimulate the process of blood clotting within the platelets—called platelet aggregation. This is again part of the healing process, because if a blood vessel were to be pierced, our blood would leak out, causing immediate death unless the vessel was sealed somehow. In other words, thromboxanes are needed for clotting, preventing our bodies from bleeding to death when injured.

This also produces the side effect that aspirin is known for—thinning the blood. Because many heart attacks, strokes and other cardiovascular problems are caused by blood clots, low-dose aspirin is used to keep the blood thinner than normal. This also creates another problem, however: This tendency to bleed slows down wound healing. And because it takes increasing amounts of aspirin to provide the same pain relief when used continuously, this adverse effect can become more dangerous.

Aspirin is also notorious for damaging the linings of the stomach and esophagus, and causing a variety of digestive issues, including acid reflux, ulcers, nausea and gastritis.

Aspirin has also been known to cause liver toxicity, Reye's syndrome (especially in children), and tinnitus—ringing of the ears. Aspirin's blood-thinning effects can create internal bleeding from a variety of injuries—reducing the body's ability to repair damage. The dangerous part of this is that the person may be bleeding internally without knowing it.

Acetaminophen or paracetamol: (many brands; over the counter) Acetaminophen, on the other hand, can in some ways be more dangerous than aspirin. A number of studies have confirmed that acetaminophen causes acute liver damage and kidney failure. Some research has indicated that more than a third of Americans take acetaminophen at least once per month.

The ubiquitous advertising by the many drug manufacturers that include acetaminophen as an active ingredient have removed much if not all consumer concern for the dangers of acetaminophen. Instead of seeing it as a potentially harmful drug, consumers have grown accustomed to acetaminophen on the bathroom shelf, ready to take at the first sign of a headache or body ache.

Current theory holds that acetaminophen works by blocking the oxidized COX enzyme, thereby blocking prostaglandin production but not thromboxane synthesis. Apparently, for this reason, acetaminophen does not produce the same level of blood thinning. Some believe the COX-3 enzyme is also blocked, but COX-3 is not connected to inflammation, so this theory is disputed.

In addition to acetaminophen, there are several other ingredients in many of the popular NSAID brands. These can include chlorpheniramine, dextromethophan, diphenhydramine, guaifenesin, pamabrom, pseudoephedrine and doxylamine. These provide antihistamine (blocking histamine production), anticholinergic (blocking the neurotransmitter acetylcholine), decongestant and diuretic properties.

One of the basic problems with acetaminophen is that it will cause acute liver failure. In a 2009 study done at the University of Maryland's School of Medicine (Mindikoglu *et al.* 2009), 661 acute

129

liver failure patients that were forced to undergo a liver transplant to survive were analyzed. The study concluded that 40% of all the liver failures were as a result of acetaminophen use. As for the other larger drug categories, 8% of the liver failures resulted from antituberculosis drugs, 7% from antiepileptic drugs, and 6% from antibiotics. In comparison with the other drugs, the acetaminophen-caused liver failure patients also required more dialysis.

Acetaminophen can also cause stomach bleeding and gastric upset. A recent study (Beasley *et al.* 2008) has also showed acetaminophen can increase asthma, eczema and conjunctivitis in young children.

Ibuprofen: (prescription and over the counter) is a fast-acting drug that provides anti-inflammatory effects and pain relief for a few hours. Brand names Advil®, Nuprin® and Motrin® use ibuprofen as the central active agent. Ibuprofen is an NSAID that inhibits both COX-1 and COX-2. This has the combined effect of reducing inflammation, reducing fever associated with inflammation, and relaxing tense muscles. Because the inflammatory process is inhibited by the blocking of the COX-2 conversion process, there is a reduction of pain associated with the inflammation. But this also is accompanied by the slowing of mucosal gland secretions.

Because ibuprofen blocks critical COX-1 enzymes, it will rob the digestive tract of healthy mucosal linings. As a result, problems associated with constant ibuprofen use include GI bleeding, ulcers, acid reflux and indigestion. These can in turn cause nausea, vomiting, diarrhea and ulcers in the esophagus—leading to cancer as we've discussed.

Side effects from ibuprofen also include a thinning of the blood, which increases the risk of bleeding. Liver enzymes are often significantly raised during ibuprofen use. This indicates possible liver damage over time. Other side effects have included dizziness, headaches, high blood pressure and loss of sexual potency. Other side effects that have been seen include heart problems, kidney damage, and lung damage. Some heart attacks have occurred with higher dosages. Ibuprofen also sometimes causes photosensitivity.

Naproxen and naproxen sodium: (OTC and prescription) These are also anti-inflammatory, pain-relieving agents. Naproxen is the active constituent in Anaprox®, Midol Extended Relief® and others. The U.S. is one of the few countries in the world that allows the sale of naproxen over the counter. Canada and Australia are one of the few others that do.

Not surprisingly, naproxen has many of the same side effects that other NSAIDs have. It has a history of causing heartburn, GI bleeding, ulcers, and complete perforations of the stomach. Naproxen has also caused circulation problems, breathing problems, liver damage, problems with blood clotting and others. Naproxen has also been implicated in heart attacks and strokes.

In addition, a 2006 study (ADAPT) of 2528 human subjects showed that naproxen has a significant risk of cardiovascular-related deaths, heart attacks and strokes. Out of 713 patients on naproxen, 8.25% suffered a heart attack, a stroke, or heart failure, while only 5.68% of the placebo group suffered any of these events.

Meloxicam: (Mobic®; prescription only) This is a COX inhibitor, but this drug requires less dosing per day because it takes longer for the body to break down. This, however, is also a possible cause for concern, as it may further burden the liver and/or kidneys.

Nevertheless, as with other COX-1 and COX-2 inhibitors, meloxicam can produce heartburn, gastrointestinal bleeding, ulcers, perforation and other intestinal difficulties. Headaches and tinnitus have also been reported.

Etodolac: (Lodine®; prescription only) This is another COX enzyme conversion inhibitor, with medium dosing required. The research has shown that etodolac can cause headaches, nausea, diarrhea, constipation, dizziness, drowsiness, kidney impairment, rashes, constipation, abdominal pain and ringing in the ears. Like the other COX inhibitors, etodolac has also been implicated in GERD, GI bleeding and ulcer issues. Anyone with a history of heart disease or asthma is warned against the product by the manufacturer.

Nabumetone: (Relafen®; prescription only) is another NSAID prescribed to relieve pain. Like the other COX inhibitors, nabumentone can produce GERD, GI bleeding, ulcers and other intestinal issues. Studies have also shown that nabumentone also can also produce nausea, liver toxicity, dizziness, abdominal pain, and the inability for the blood to clot effectively.

Research has shown that etodolac can also produce headaches, nausea, diarrhea, constipation, dizziness, drowsiness, kidney impairment, rashes, constipation, abdominal pain, lightheadedness, and ringing in the ears. Anyone with a history of heart disease or asthma is warned against the product by the manufacturer.

Sulindac: (Clinoril®; prescription only) Another nonspecific COX inhibitor. Not surprisingly, it also is associated with acid reflux, GI bleeding and ulcerous effects in the stomach, esophagus and small intestines. Also, rashes, kidney impairment, lightheadedness, ringing in the ears, weakness, internal bleeding, liver toxicity and an exacerbating of asthma and hives have been reported.

Choline magnesium salicylate: (Trilasate®; prescription only) is a salicylate, like aspirin. It thus acts the same, by blocking COX enzyme conversion. However, the risk of Reye's syndrome, compared to aspirin, is apparently slightly reduced with this drug.

Still, gastrointestinal bleeding, acid reflux and ulcers in the stomach and small intestines are side effects of all isolated salicylates. Liver toxicity, internal bleeding, and tinnitus have also been seen among users of this form of salicylate.

Ketoprofen: (prescription only, Orudis®, Oruvail®) is another NSAID that blocks the COX enzyme conversion process. This reduces pain and inflammation in the short-term, but like many of the other NSAIDs in that it can produce acid reflux, GI bleeding, intestinal cramping, ulcerations, nausea, vomiting, and diarrhea.

In addition, there are a number of other side effects with ketoprofen. These include headaches, fainting, persistent sore throats, stiff necks, rashes, itching, yellowing eyes and dark urine—indicating liver issues.

Diclofenac; (Cataflam®, Voltaren®, Arthrotec®; prescription only) **oxaprozin;** (Daypro®) **diflusinal;** (Dolobid®) **piroxicam;** (Feldene®) and **indomethicin** (Indocin®) are all COX inhibitor NSAIDs. Thus, they all block the inflammatory cascade that helps the body protect and heal itself and the production of mucosal membrane lining of the stomach and other mucosal surfaces.

Thus they all can produce gastrointestinal problems including GERD. They can all produce ulcers because they block the body's secretion of protective mucosal lining in the esophagus, stomach and intestines. They also can produce cardiovascular problems as well as potentially-dangerous bleeding issues, and to varying degrees, headaches and nausea.

Prednisone and methylprednisone: (Deltasone®, Orasone®, Prednicen-M®, Liquid Pred®, Medrol®, Depo-Medrol®; prescription only) Prednisone and methylprednisone mimic the actions of cortisol produced by the adrenal gland, and their main mechanism is to slow inflammation and suppress the immune system. Because steroids act like hormones, these drugs significantly alter mucosal gland secretions. They also affect moods and stress levels. Other side effects include headaches and gastrointestinal issues, including ulcers and bleeding.

Prednisolone: (Pediapred®, Prednisolone®, Liquid Medrol®; prescription only) The effects of prednisolone are practically identical to prednisone, because prednisone is converted to prednisolone in the liver. Thus prednisolone also significantly alters moods. This may begin with mild frustration or annoyance over trivial things. With consistent use, this can also turn into rage, depression, mania, personality change and psychotic behavior. This of course significantly affects the integrity of our sub-mucosal gland secretions. Other side effects include ulcers and other gastrointestinal issues, which can increase the risk of GERD.

In addition to these, many other pharmaceuticals will interfere with the body's production of mucosal membranes, increasing the risk of GERD, asthma, allergies and other mucosal membrane-related conditions. Here are a couple of the many studies illustrating this:

Researchers from Britain's Imperial College (Shaheen *et al.* 2008) studied the association between acetaminophen use and asthma incidence among 1,028 asthmatics and healthy matched controls. They found that the weekly use of acetaminophen was significantly related to a diagnosis of asthma. The researchers concluded that: *"These data add to the increasing and consistent epidemiological evidence implicating frequent paracetamol [acetaminophen] use in asthma in diverse populations."*

Researchers from Norway's Oslo University Hospital (Bakkeheim *et al.* 2011) studied 1,016 mothers and their children from birth until six months old, and then followed up with the children at 10 years old. They found that acetaminophen use by the mother during the first trimester significantly increased incidence of allergic rhinitis at age ten. Furthermore, girls given acetaminophen had more than double the asthma incidence at age ten.

And practically any and every synthetic pharmaceutical can add to our body's total toxin burden. This is because the body must eventually break down any synthetic chemical in order to purge it from the body. The isolated or active chemical within the pharmaceutical may have its biological effect upon the body, but it must be broken down at some point. The body rarely if ever utilizes these chemicals as nutrients, in other words. They are foreigners to the body. Thus, enzymes such as glutathione must break down these chemical molecules into forms that can be excreted in urine, sweat, exhalation or stool.

This breakdown and disposal process requires work by the body's detoxification systems. This means that they further burden or stress a system that must remove many other toxins within the body, including other environmental toxins, microorganisms and their endotoxins, inflammatory mediators, broken-down cells and other toxins the body must get rid of. In other words, pharmaceuticals can contribute to, and even become another straw that breaks the camel's back.

While these pharmaceuticals may be of concern specifically, we should look at any pharmaceutical as having the potential to increase the body's total toxic burden and damage mucosal membrane integrity leading to GERD.

Chemical Food Additives

This is a large topic, because many processed foods are full of artificial additives. These include hundreds of artificial food colors, preservatives, stabilizers, flavorings and a variety of food processing aids. A number of these additives have been found to produce sensitivities in some people, indicating they are absorbed into the body and/or have an effect upon the mucosal membranes.

A number of artificial sweeteners should be considered toxic. One is aspertame. Aspartame is a chemical combination of the amino acids phenylalanine and aspartic acid, bonded by methyl ester—a wood alcohol. Once inside the body, the wood alcohol and formaldehyde are released.

Another artificial sweetener is sucralose. This is sweet yet not readily absorbed according to manufacturers. Yet studies have found that 11-27% is absorbed, and 20-30% of that absorbed quantity can be metabolized by the body. This requires the liver and kidneys to break it down and excrete it.

While this is a huge topic, other questionable artificial sweeteners shown to break down into spurious byproducts include saccharin, acesulfame potassium and cyclamates. Stevia, mannitol and xylitol are plant-derived sweeteners that are considered by most to be relatively safe and non-toxic.

Air Pollutants

How do air pollutants effect the health of our esophagus and thus help produce GERD? When we breathe air into our lungs, that air must pass through the mouth or sinuses, the pharynx, the throat, and then to the airways. Each of these chambers maintain mucous membranes, and mucous membranes circulate through these chambers and the esophagus.

It is like asking why spilling fuel into a river will affect a nearby lake. The same waters that are flowing through the river will also flow down to a neighboring lake. When this happens, the fuel will be in the lake as well as the river.

Heartburn and other gastrointestinal symptoms are prevalent side effects among many who live in highly polluted environments. During heightened smog days, for example, many immunosuppressed people will succumb to illness. Among the illnesses will typically be increased lung infections, increased heart conditions and increased gastrointestinal symptoms—including heartburn.

Let's discuss some of the key pollution types:

Carbon Monoxide

Carbon monoxide is a substantial indoor air toxin. Carbon monoxide is released by burning gas, kerosene, or wood. It can thus arise from the use of wood stoves, fireplaces, gas stoves, generators, automobiles, kitchen stoves, and furnaces. Low concentrations of carbon monoxide in the indoor environment might cause fatigue and even chest pain and sometimes GERD symptoms.

Higher concentrations may result in headaches, confusion, dizziness, nausea, vision impairment and fever. This is due to carboxyhemoglobin formation in the bloodstream, which takes place when carbon monoxide attaches to hemoglobin instead of oxygen. This will in effect starve the body of oxygen, and higher concentrations can easily lead to death.

Acceptable carbon monoxide levels in households are about .5 to 5 parts per million. Levels near a gas stove might be 5 to 15 ppm. An improperly vented or leaking stove might cause 30 ppm or more near the stove, which becomes hazardous. The U.S. National Ambient Air Quality Standard for maximum carbon monoxide levels outside is 35 ppm for one hour and 9 ppm for eight hours. Standards for indoor carbon monoxide have not been determined.

Making sure that every appliance is vented properly is task number one in avoiding carbon monoxide poisoning. The appliance should also be checked for leaks, and those leaks should be sealed prior to use. Central heating systems should be inspected for leaks as well. Idling the car in the garage is a no-no. Open fireplaces should be avoided indoors, and wood stove doors should be kept closed. We shouldn't solely rely upon the draft up the fireplace chimney for the escape of carbon monoxide.

Nitrogen oxide

Nitrogen oxide is a gas byproduct of most engines and practically any gas-run appliance. Gas stoves, water heaters, wood stoves, gas heaters and cars are probably the biggest emitters in the home. Homes without these appliances will have very low levels of NO_2 compared to outside. Homes with these appliances may have double the levels. Nitrogen oxide can be a significant toxin if significant levels are taken in.

Researchers from Birmingham Heartlands Hospital (Tunnicliffe *et al.* 1994) tested one hour exposure to nitrogen dioxide on ten mild asthmatics with dust mite sensitivities. Forced expiratory volume (FEV1) levels were tested with non-NO_2 air, air with 100 parts per billion of NO_2, and air containing 400 ppb of nitrogen dioxide. FEV1 levels were 27% lower between the non-NO_2 air and the 400 ppb of NO_2 air. The average FEV1 among the asthmatics was nearly three times lower in the 400 ppb NO_2 air than in the clear air. The 100 ppb NO_2 air content did not seem to make a significant difference in FEV1, however. This gives us a yardstick for determining unhealthy NO_2 levels.

Cooking and Heating

Research from the University at Albany (Kaplan 2010) has revealed that about half of the people around the world utilize biomass such as wood, agricultural residues or coal to cook by and heat their homes with.

These fuels are not completely consumed by their ignition. They leave toxic residues in the form of carbon monoxide, arsenic and others that can significantly increase the body's burden of toxins when breathed in. This in turn increases the risk of damage to our mucosal membranes.

Volatile Organic Compounds (VOCs)

Researchers from the Texas Tech University Health Sciences Center (Arif and Shah 2007) studied the effects of volatile organic compounds (VOCs). They collected data on ten VOCs and 550 adults. Aromatic compounds and chlorinated hydrocarbons were specifically categorized. Exposure to aromatic compounds increased the incidence of asthma by 63%. In addition, exposure to aromatic compounds increased wheezing incidence from the previous year by 68%, and chlorinated hydrocarbon exposure increased wheezing incidence from the previous year by 50%.

Exposures to VOCs ranged from 0.03 micrograms per cubic meter for trichloroethene up to 14 microg/m3 for toluene. In other words, the higher the level of toxic inhalation, the higher the incidence of respiratory disorders. This is because VOCs present toxins that are quickly absorbed into the bloodstream through the airways. Once in the bloodstream, the body launches an inflammatory response to remove them.

First-, Second- and Third-Hand Smoke

Tobacco smoke is also a dangerous source of indoor pollution that can damage the mucosal membranes whether coming from first, second or third-hand smoke.

Recent research has indicated that not only is second-hand smoke dangerous to non-smokers, but second-hand smoke has more than *twice* the amount of tar, nicotine and other toxins than the smoker inhales. While the smoker will inhale the smoke through the filtering mechanism provided by the packed tobacco inside the cigarette paper—and many cigarettes also have additional filters to screen out toxins—the second-hand smoker will breathe all the smoke.

Second-hand smoke contains five times the amount of carbon monoxide—the lethal gas that de-oxygenates the blood—than the smoker inhales.

Second-hand smoke also contains higher levels of ammonia and cadmium. Its nitrogen dioxide levels are fifty times higher than levels considered harmful, and the concentration of hydrogen cyanide approaches toxic levels. Constant exposure to second-hand smoke increases the risk of lung disease by 25%, and increases the risk of heart disease by 10%.

Second-hand smoke exposure has also been irrefutably linked to emphysema, chronic bronchitis, asthma and other ailments, including GERD.

Synthetic Fragrances

Various scents and fragrances used in deodorizers, decorations, soaps, and furniture can be downright toxic. While a fragrance might smell like flowers or delicious foods, the typical commercial fragrance contains at least ninety-five percent synthetic chemicals. A single perfume may contain more than 500 different chemicals. Benzene derivatives, aldehydes, toluene, and petroleum-derived chemicals are just a few synthetics used in commercial fragrances. Toluene alone, for example, has been linked to respiratory disorders among previously healthy people.

For this reason, we should carefully consider any product with an ingredient called "fragrances." This includes laundry detergents, dishwashing and other soaps, shampoos and other types of hair products, disinfectants, shaving creams, fabric softeners, fragrant candles, air fresheners, and of course perfumes and colognes. Discernment also should also be given to the word "unscented," as this still may have some of the same synthetics, used instead as fragrance masking elements.

In one study (Anderson and Anderson 1997), mice were submitted to breathing with a commercial air freshener for one hour at different concentrations. A number of concentrations, including levels typically used by humans in everyday use, caused sensory and pulmonary irritation, decreased breathing velocity, and functional behavior abnormalities.

Another study, performed by the same researchers (Anderson and Anderson 1998) and published a year later, revealed that mice who were subjected to five commercial colognes or toilet water for an hour suffered various combinations of negative effects, including sensory irritation, pulmonary irritation, decreased airflow expiration, neurotoxicity and gastrointestinal issues.

Other Toxins

Offgassing from beds and other furniture can irritate the mucosal membranes. So can fabric softener emission. Several known irritants and toxins are typically found in fabric softeners, including styrene, isopropylbenzene, thymol, trimethylbenzene and phenols.

Another potential indoor trigger category is propellants. Propellants are used in sprays and pump bottles to disperse fluids. While chlorofluorocarbons (CFCs) have been practically eliminated from aerosols, today's aerosols and pump sprays often involves the use of volatile organic compounds (VOCs). Noxious propellants such as isobutane, butane and propane will typically linger in the air for several minutes after spraying. They can be quite toxic.

Formaldehyde has been shown to be a significant and prevalent toxin. Today so many building materials and furniture are built using formaldehyde. These include pressed wood, draperies, glues, resins, shelving, flooring, and so many other materials. The greatest source of formaldehyde appears to be those materials made using *urea-formaldehyde* resins. These include particleboard, plywood paneling, and medium density fiberboard.

There are many other toxins in our building materials—including many yet to be discovered. Certainly, we can safely say that any kind of building or decomposition of a modern building will likely impart various hazardous chemicals, including but not exclusively asbestos and formaldehyde.

Polybrominated diphenyl ethers or PBDEs provide one example. PBDEs is an organobromine used as a fire retardant. It is used to make automobiles, polyurethane foams, furniture, electronic goods, textiles, airplanes and of course, building materials.

This means that the air during any kind of sanding, crushing, fire or demolition should be treated with extreme caution. Using a particle or gas mask is more than a good idea under these circumstances, though it should be noted that most particle masks do not form a tight enough bond with the face to filter much at all. Best is to use a gas filter or a mask with a rubber barrier that fits tightly onto the face.

With regard to off-gassing, prior to bringing in any type of new furniture or wood into the house, it is best to off-gas the product by setting it in the sunshine for a couple of days or at least for a full day. As the sun's resonating waves connect with the material, many of its toxins are disassociated and released. Not such a good thing for the environment, but at least it will disburse outside of our immediate breathing environment. Off-gassing can help us avoid more than a potent toxin.

Fresh paint can also be toxic. This is because paint typically contains VOCs.

Many other indoor pollutants exist, depending upon the structure and condition of the environment. For example, automobiles, trains, planes, or buses can provide a whole range of triggers, from carbon monoxide to lead, formaldehyde and plasticizers—which can off-gas (also called *outgassing*), especially when the weather gets warmer.

This is especially the case for new cars. That 'new car smell' is the toxic off-gassing of a mixture of plasticizers, formaldehyde and other synthetics. In the case of older cars, air vents may be clogged with a number of molds, dust and bacteria, which may spray out whenever the "air" is turned on.

It might help to periodically clean out the filters of any car—especially older ones. In the case of a newer car, we might also consider leaving the windows cracked while parking in sunny locations between drives for a few weeks, to let the various materials outgas.

Our mucous membranes can become damaged by any number of toxins. Nausea and digestive discomfort are thus frequent symptoms of those subjected to toxic exposures. Here is a small list of occupations and their toxins, and following that, a partial list of mucosal irritants:

Occupation	Exposures
Agricultural workers	Pesticides, herbicides
Plastics manufacturers	Plasticizers, VOCs, polymers
Painters	Paints/thinners (VOCs)
Drivers	Carbon, soot, formaldehyde, micro
Metal workers	Metallic dusts, heavy metals
Saw millers	Wood dust, preservatives
Janitorial and housekeepers	VOCs, cleaning chemicals
Bakers and food workers	Airborne food particles
Home builders	VOCs, formaldehyde, asbestos
Health workers	SBS, microorganisms, chemicals

And finally, here is a listing of the toxins that irritate and damage our mucosal membranes around the body:

Some Mucosal Irritants and their Sources

Source	Toxins
Air pollutants	Lead, mercury, carbon monoxide, sulfur, arsenic, nitrogen dioxide, ozone…
Carpets, rugs	Molds, dander, lice, PC-4, latex
Cigarette/Cigar/Pipe Smoke	Carbon monoxide, nicotine, aldehydes, ketones, soot, formaldehyde, others
Cosmetics	Aluminum, phosphates and chemicals
Spray cans	Propellants, other chemicals
Foods/Additives	Food colors, preservatives, trans fats, pesticides, arachidonic acids, acrylamide, phytanic acid, artificial flavors, refined sugars and much, much more
House	Radon, formaldehyde, pollen, dust, mold, dander, pesticides, cleaning products, asbestos, lead, paint, endotoxins
Household chemicals	Cleaners, pesticides, herbicides, paints
Insects	Endotoxins from dust mites, cockroaches and other insects
Laundry soaps	Fragrances, detergents, surfactants
Microorganisms	Mold, bacteria, viruses, parasites
Mattresses/pillows	Endotoxins, molds, formaldehyde
Paints	Lead, arsenic, VOCs, adhesives
Pets	Dander, up to 240 infectious diseases & parasites (65 from dogs/39 from cats)
Pharmaceuticals	Many-see short list on pages 112-113
Water	Chorine byproducts, pesticides, pharmaceuticals, many others
Pools and spas	Chlorine byproducts such as trihalomethanes (THMs), various carbonates
Soaps and Shampoos	Fragrances, detergents, surfactants
Stoves, Fireplaces	Carbon monoxide, NO_2, arsenic, soot
Work and school environments	SBS, practically all of the above

The bottom line is the mucosal membranes of our esophagus epithelia, sphincters and stomach walls can become damaged by what we eat, what we breathe and what pharmaceuticals we take. These can either directly effect the mucosal membranes of our mouth and esophagus, or effects us after consuming them. They can inhibit the activities of our submucosal glands from within, and dry out and thin our mucous on contact by contributing free radicals. This of course results in not enough membrane to protect our epithelial cells from exposure to stomach acids, toxins and food acids.

This means that there is an accumulative effect to toxin exposure. Should a healthy person just take some aspirin for a headache now and then, there typically is not a big heartburn response.

But should the person be otherwise burdened by toxicity from another source—such as what we are eating, drinking or breathing—this can produce a significant accumulative effect upon the mucosal membranes and underlying epithelia of the esophagus and stomach wall.

Chapter Five

GERD Strategies

Anti-GERD Herbs

Herbs versus Meds

Traditional medicines of the world have been treating gastrointestinal conditions and digestive discomfort with success for thousands of years. While GERD has not been a condition of epidemic proportions as it is today, it is an ailment that traditional medicine has experience treating successfully over thousands of years.

While specific herbal treatments differ around the world, many independently utilized the same herbs—often with different names and different formulations.

Herbs work completely differently than do pharmaceuticals. While pharmaceuticals typically contain one or two synthesized active ingredients that can cause serious side effects, herbs typically contain tens if not hundreds of active constituents that each balance and buffer each other. As a result, many herbs will accomplish multiple effects at the same time. In the case of some of the herbs we'll discuss here, we find that many reduce inflammation and render pain relief, while stimulating healthy mucosal membrane secretions at the same time.

Herbal medicine has successfully treated billions of people over the centuries, and this clinical experience has been handed down through thousands of generations. Unlike modern conventional medicine, there has been no financial conflict of interest incumbent in the research and study of traditional herbs. Since they grow freely, there has been no competition or need to patent. Herbal medicine has remained an honorable institution of devoted individuals.

In comparison, there is a huge conflict of interest in the study of pharmaceuticals—as pharmaceutical companies can spend billions of dollars on the development of a single drug. Once a pharmaceutical company has designed a new drug, it can receive patent protection for that chemical combination, giving it up to twenty years of potential exclusivity for selling that drug—at least where patent laws exist. This means a guarantee of profits as long as doctors prescribe that drug. With a patent, there is protection from competition, guaranteeing salaries and profits for many years.

This means that the relationship between the doctor and patient has changed. Without the doctor prescribing the medication, there is no continual use. Thus, market control must include both patent and doctor. For this reason, pharmaceutical giants focus their attention on a combination of drug research, patent protection, regulation, and marketing to physicians and patients.

In our modern medical institutions, pathology instruction relating to diagnosis also accompanies the use of specific pharmaceutical drugs. Western medical institutions synchronize with the pharmaceutical industry due to financial relationships between pharmaceutical companies, medical schools, medical licensure and pathology documentation. Drug research by doctors—many of whom are also medical school professors—is often funded by pharmaceutical manufacturers. This means that the incentives become financial rather than based upon the health of each individual patient.

This has been illustrated among several investigative reports over the past couple of years showing that doctors have fudged research papers and not disclosed information about certain drugs due to their financial relationship with pharmaceutical companies. When financial incentives become a primary concern among medical institutions, the patient's well being gets marginalized.

This has become evident from the massive side effects of pharmaceutical medicines.

The *Journal of the American Medical Association* (Lazarou *et al.* 1998) reported that in 1994, 2,216,000 Americans were hospitalized, permanently disabled, or died as a result of pharmaceutical use. This is over 2.2 million Americans annually with *reported* injury from pharmaceuticals. The study, done at the University of Toronto, also showed that approximately 106,000 people die each year from taking *correctly prescribed* FDA-approved pharmaceuticals. This does not include the number of deaths resulting by misuse, overdose or addiction to these same drugs.

Furthermore, the U.S. FDA was sent 258,000 adverse drug events in 1999. Harvard researcher and associate professor of medicine Dr. David Bates told the *Los Angeles Times* in 2001 "...*these*

146

numbers translate to 36 million adverse drug events per year" (Rappoport 2006).

The plausibility of this huge number was confirmed in another study published in the *Journal of the American Medical Association* in 1995 (Bates *et al.*). This revealed that over a six month study period, 12% of 4031 adult hospital admissions had either a confirmed adverse drug event or a potentially adverse drug event.

In addition to these facts, estimates from several sources have confirmed that about 16,000 deaths occur and about 100,000 people are hospitalized from NSAID use alone. This computes to 50 NSAID-related deaths and 300 hospitalizations every day as a result from NSAID use. About 100 million prescriptions of NSAIDs are written in addition to millions of over the counter purchases.

The damage to Americans by pharmaceutical medication does not stop there. *The Nutrition Institute of America* has reported that over 20 million unnecessary antibiotic prescriptions are written by doctors per year. Over seven million medical and surgical procedures a year are unnecessary. Over eight million people are hospitalized without need. Our medical institution is quite simply suffocating in its own mismanagement.

According to a nationwide poll conducted by Louis Harris and Associates released in 1997 by the *National Patient Safety Foundation* and the *American Medical Association,* an estimated 100 million Americans experienced a medical mistake: 42% of those randomly surveyed. Misdiagnosis and wrong treatments accounted for 40% of those mistakes. Medical medication errors accounted for 28%, while medical procedure errors accounted for 22% of these medical mistakes (NPSF 1997).

In a study of four Boston adult primary care practices involving 1202 outpatients, 27% of responders experienced adverse drug events (Gandhi *et al.* 2003).

In a 2004 interview with Dr. Lucian Leape, a physician, medicine professor, expert in patient safety, and author of numerous studies, reported that over the past ten years since the 1997 NPSF studies were performed, improvements in our medical system have been inadequate. Barriers to improvement cited physician denial, hospital environment, lack of leadership and little system review (Leape 2004).

Indeed, over the past few decades, our medical industry has become the leading cause of death and injury in the United States. Carolyn Dean, M.D., N.D., in her book *Death By Medicine* (2005), found that over 105,000 deaths occurred from medications in 2005. Another 98,000 died from medical errors and 199,000 died from outpatient adverse reactions. In total, her study found that over 783,000 deaths were caused by conventional medical treatments in 2005.

This accounting of deaths out-numbers both U.S. heart disease death rates and cancer death rates. In 2002 for example, 450,637 people died of heart disease and 476,009 died of cancer.

Even if a pharmaceutical results in an improved condition for a particular ailment, there are often dangerous side effects. Some of these can be worse than the original ailment. In addition, most medications stress the liver and kidneys in one respect or another— shortening the lifespan of these critical organs.

Some medications, like aminoglycoside antibiotics streptomycin, kanamycin, garamicin and others have been shown to cause kidney damage in as many as 15 percent of patients. Others, such as acetaminophen, carbamazepine, atenolol, cimetidine, phenylbutazone, acebutolol, piroxicam, mianserin, naproxen, sulindac, ranitidine, enflurane, halothane, valproic acid, phenobarbital, isoniazid and ketoconazole can cause acute dose-dependent liver damage. This is because the liver and the kidneys work together to process most chemicals out of the body.

Together these organs must break down and excrete the chemical byproducts of medications, resulting in their hopeful elimination from the body. During their journey out, these derivatives can damage the body's cells and tissue systems.

The P450 liver enzyme process moves chemicals through the extraction pathway in many cases. This enzyme is effective in most healthy bodies for a few chemicals at a time. Yet multiple drugs can overwhelm and deplete this pathway. With the P450 pathway overloaded by various chemicals, additional drugs can damage tissues incrementally. For this reason, a higher number of liver enzymes in a blood analysis is seen by doctors as a dangerous sign indicating an overload of pharmaceuticals.

This means that like most toxic chemicals, many pharmaceuticals put a burden on the liver. This is because the liver must work harder to filter and break down the chemicals—before sending them out through the kidneys, colon, lungs and/or sweat glands. This of course, directly affects mucosal membrane health.

The central issue related to the burdening of liver is the fact that synthetic chemicals are foreign to the body.

Most botanicals are quite the opposite. Botanicals are highly recognized by the body, simply because humans have been consuming these and similar plant products for thousands of years. Thus, the body processes the constituents of a plant compound amicably and without duress.

In fact, many medicinal herbs provide a broad spectrum of healthy effects, which work together to heal concurrent issues. These effects include antioxidant activity and immune stimulation. Some are also antiseptic and antibiotic as well. Some increase detoxification, stimulate the liver, increase kidney efficiency and stimulate the adrenal glands all at the same time.

While pharmaceuticals are isolated chemicals with often one central mechanism of action within the body, most botanicals have many—some even hundreds—of pharmacological constituents and complementary actions. For example, according to research by James Duke, Ph.D. of the U.S. Department of Agriculture and Norman Farnsworth, Ph.D., a research professor at the University of Illinois, ginger contains at least 477 active constituents (Schulick 1996). While botanicals produce active biochemicals that act in a healing manner, they also produce active multiple constituents that buffer and balance each other.

Separately, one of ginger's active constituents might produce side effects along with its actions. The other constituents balance these mechanisms, however. Together the many constituents in ginger make it one of the most active and effective medicinal botanicals for many ailments. Many herbal medicine experts consider it one of the best anti-inflammatory botanicals.

Like a number of other anti-inflammatory herbs, ginger has been shown to suppress the expression of both cyclooxygenase-1 and cyclooxygenase-2; yet without slowing down the production and secretion of mucosal membranes around the body.

As a result, whole ginger has been shown to slow leukotriene production through the blocking of the 5-lipooxygenase enzyme (Grzanna *et al.* 2005) without adverse side effects. This slows inflammation and pain without sacrificing the health of the mucosal membranes. In fact, ginger has been shown to actually stimulate mucosal membrane health. For this reason, ginger is one of the best herbal strategies to employ for those with GERD or gastritis, as we'll illustrate later.

Ginger is not alone in its broad swath of medicinal constituents. As mentioned above, research has confirmed that many other botanicals also have dozens if not hundreds of constituents.

Unlike the parade of adverse side effect-ridden COX inhibiting non-steroidal anti-inflammatory drugs introduced by the pharmaceutical industry over the past half century, anti-inflammatory botanicals provide a level of safety and a myriad of benefits to our mucosal membranes and esophageal epithelia.

We might add that most pharmaceuticals—some of which have been pulled from the market because they have injured hundreds of thousands of people—require billions of dollars of taxpayer investment in regulation and oversight.

The complexity of these drugs is met with a double-whammy of risk. If even a small amount of this wasted effort could be diverted to the growing and production of the anti-inflammatory botanicals discussed here, we could be saving billions of taxpayer dollars, not to speak of the damage to the environment from the dumping of toxic synthetics and the deaths of hundreds of thousands of people each year.

The central issue modern medicine has with herbal medicine is the speed in which its therapeutic effects can be seen. This is also its benefit, however. While pharmaceuticals are fast acting, they also create imbalances within the body, and require the body to work harder to detoxify the drug.

Most medicinal botanicals have no toxicity when dosed correctly, but their effects are typically more gradual. This forces the patient to be disciplined, and well, *patient*. It is because natural herbal medicines are complex and balanced that they tend to act more deeply. They also produce a result that is longer-lasting, working with the body to strengthen its immunity and ability to resist the problem in the future.

Rather than causing negative side effects by blocking the immune system, anti-inflammatory botanicals produce *positive* side effects. While gradually reducing pain, fever and inflammation, many modulate eicanosoids and boost mucosal membrane secretions.

Many also stimulate detoxification; increase healthy appetite; reduce nausea; protect against ulcers; increase liver vitality; stimulate circulation; calm nerves; balance endocrine function; encourage bone healing; improve lung and gum health; and neutralize oxidative (free) radicals.

Many are also antiseptic, anesthetic, and antiemetic. Such are a few of the many "side effects" of medicinal herbs. Laboratory studies have also shown many of these to be protective against cancer (LaValle, 2001; Shukla and Singh 2007; Schulick 1996).

There are a number of excellent pain-relieving botanicals that physicians can consider before resorting to the array of increasingly toxic pharmaceutical analgesics. Botanicals such as white willow tree bark and meadowsweet are good examples. White willow tree bark and meadowsweet both contain a constituent called salicin. This of course is the natural version of the synthetic *acetyl-salicylic acid* we discussed in the last chapter, known by its expired patented trademark name of *aspirin.*

As discussed previously, acetyl-salicylic acid and its non-acetylated, isolated *salicylic acid* both come with a number of adverse side effects, including internal bleeding and gastro-intestinal upset sometimes leading to ulceration, GERD and stomach bleeding.

Far from its natural origins, today's aspirin is usually manufactured from phenol, which can be derived from coal or isolated from other materials. The phenol is treated with sodium and then carbon dioxide under pressure, rendering salicylate.

After acidification into salicylic acid, it is acetylated with acetic anhydride to yield the final product. The manufacturing facility hosting these reactions produces pollutants to yield the synthetic result. Though it successfully relieves pain, aspirin also creates adverse side effects as we have discussed.

We've discussed how NSAIDs disrupt the cyclooxygenation (COX) process, which oxidizes arachidonic acid utilizing the en-

151

zyme called cyclooxygenase. By blocking COX, the production of prostaglandins and prostanoids such as thromboxane is interfered with.

This also interferes with sub-mucosal gland production, and the secretion of mucosal membranes. This is the relationship between these NSAID and selective COX-inhibitors and their various GI side effects. When the stomach and intestinal mucosal membranes are not secreted, intruders and even the stomach's own acids can damage the epithelial cells of the stomach wall and the intestinal walls.

What we may not realize is that the original botanical sources of *salicylic acid*—white willow bark and meadowsweet flowers—also perform this same inhibition of COX. The difference, however, is that these botanicals also balance the actions of its salicins by activating other physiological mechanisms, which increase the secretion of mucosal membranes. This is an example of the incredible balancing effect of the many constituents within nature's herbal medicines.

Many herbs also increase the body's detoxification process concurrently to their other actions. This in turn speeds healing and promotes healthy mucosal membranes, leading to better protection for the esophagus and stomach wall.

Aspirin's disruptive mechanisms are illustrated in its effective depletion of a number of nutrients from the body. These include iron, potassium, folic acid, and vitamin C. According to Kauffman (2000), death rates among populations of aspirin users are significantly higher than non-aspirin populations.

In contrast, the botanical versions *supply* many of these nutrients. Botanicals not only relieve pain and boost the immune system. They also supply nutrients to balance the system.

In other words, white willow bark and meadowsweet—by nature's design—contain a biomolecular version of salicin, moderated by a variety of constituents to balance its effects. Subsequently, whole-plant salicin botanicals do not have a history of the negative side effects. Their molecular arrangements are synergistically oriented with a balance of constituents, which resonate with and stimulate our body's immune system while slowing the conversion of prostaglandins and leucotrienes to gradually ease inflammation.

Unlike aspirin, willow and meadowsweet actually *promote* a healthy stomach lining while reducing inflammation and pain, rather than causing gastrointestinal problems. For this reason, traditional herbalists often recommend meadowsweet specifically for acid reflux, gastritis and ulcerative conditions.

Botanical pain relievers have the ability to gradually modulate the eicanosoid response in order to ease inflammation and pain. They also stimulate the body's own healing mechanisms to help solve the root problem.

Many herbal medicines also strengthen and unburden the liver. Nearly every medicinal botanical contains constituents that provide antioxidant and blood-purifying effects. They will thus neutralize toxic free radicals and stimulate glutathione scavenging. They will stimulate the immune system to respond more efficiently.

In addition, many botanicals stimulate more efficient filtration and excretion among the kidneys, colon, liver, sweat glands and lungs to speed the removal of waste products from the blood and tissues.

In contrast, pharmaceutical chemicals typically burden the liver and bloodstream with toxicity. Their foreign molecules must be broken down by liver enzymes, which is why liver enzymes tend to increase amongst patients who take multiple medications.

This all means, frankly, that herbs are simply not comparable to pharmaceutical drugs. They are entirely different creatures. It would be like comparing a rocking chair to a helicopter. Herbs produce multiple health effects, while most pharmaceuticals halt or engage one type of process, unbalancing others.

This is critical in a multi-functional machine like the body. You can't just change one process without other processes being altered. The body is finely tuned in health. When we start tinkering with some processes, others are affected. This is what causes side effects.

The incredible thing about herbs is that while they change some processes, they also buffer and alter others so that the body trends toward *more* balance.

Just as botanicals affect the body vastly different from pharmaceuticals, traditional health practitioners look at pain much differently than do medical doctors. Traditional health practitioners such as herbalists, naturopaths and acupuncturists are not focused upon naming the illness (diagnosis). They are focused upon the root cause of the imbalances that exist within the body, and thus seek to find those natural elements that help to rebalance the body's metabolism so that it will heal itself. This in turn should remove the cause of the pain.

We must remember that plants are living organisms. They have their own immune systems. They produce an array of biochemicals that protect them and keep them balanced. These same biochemicals become available to humans when we consume their leaves, bark and roots.

Because plants are stationary, they must protect themselves with their various biochemicals. This means the biochemicals they produce interact with environmental threats in the same way those biochemicals will interact with environmental threats within the human body.

One might wonder why there is not more information being made available about the many positive effects of botanical foods and medicines. There is one large glaring reason for the lack of rigorous clinical studies for many botanical products: Botanical medicine is simply not profitable enough for the financial appetites of most large scientific institutions. Researchers have to be paid, and the pharmaceutical giants are very generous with their support for research, so long as that research supports something the pharmaceutical company can patent.

The other reason relates to the media. A reasonable survey of mass media advertising illustrates the financial power pharmaceutical giants now wield over our media. Should a network or media outlet attempt to broadcast objective information about botanical medicines, they will likely be reined in pretty quickly, because the salaries of those executives are also derived from the ability of pharmaceutical companies to sell their patented medicines.

At least for now, natural botanical plants cannot be patented. (Genetically engineered plants can, however. We should be leery of this, because this offers to those companies who provide genetically engineered seeds the ability to control our food production.)

If we consider that hundreds of thousands of people die each year from medications, while very few if any die of herbal supplement use, the numbers do not imply any safety issue with botanicals. Yet every day research institutions are warning people about the dangers of using herbal medications. Ironically, much of these warnings are about problems caused by the *interactions* between herbs and pharmaceuticals.

Let's look at a few key examples of pain-relieving and inflammation-reducing herbs that actually promote mucosal membrane health. For the first few, we'll show some of their pain-relieving properties along with digestive comfort effects. We'll also list some of the active constituents within the herb to illustrate our point about herbs having many biochemicals that balance and buffer each other.

This presentation of the science and traditional use of medical herbs is not simply the personal opinion of the author. Rather, this discussion utilizes the documentation and research of numerous researchers, scientists and physicians trained in herbal medicines. Here traditional clinical uses of herbal medicine have been derived from a number of *Materia Medica* texts from various traditions, as well as from documented histories of using these herbs upon significant populations over centuries—some even over thousands of years. Unless otherwise noted in the text, this information utilizes the following reference materials (see reference section for complete citation):

Bensky *et al.* 1986; Bisset 1994; Blumenthal 1998; Blumenthal and Brinckmann 2000; Bruneton 1995; Chevallier 1996; Chopra *et al.* 1956; Christopher 1976; Clement *et al.* 2005; Duke 1989; Ellingwood 1983; Fecka 2009; Foster and Hobbs 2002; Frawley and Lad 1988; Gray-Davidson 2002; Griffith 2000; Gundermann and Müller 2007; Halpern and Miller 2002; Hobbs 2003; 1997; Hoffmann 2002; Hope *et al.* 1993; Jensen 2001; Kokwaro 1976; Lad 1984; LaValle 2001; Lininger *et al.* 1999; Mabey 1988; Mehra 1969; Mindell and Hopkins 1998; Murray and Pizzorno 1998; Nadkarni and Nadkarni 1908/1975; Newall *et al.* 1996; Newmark and Schulick 1997; O'Connor and Bensky 1981; Potterton 1983; Schulick 1996; Schauenberg and Paris 1977; Schulz *et al.* 1998; Shi *et al.* 2008; Shishodia *et al.* 2008; Tierra 1992; Tierra 1990; Tiwari 1995; Tisserand 1979; Tonkal and Morsy 2008; Weiner 1969; Weiss 1988; Williard 1992; Williard and Jones 1990; White and Foster 2000; Wood 1997.

Aloe vera

Aloe has been used traditionally for inflammation, constipation, wound healing, skin issues, ulcers and intestinal issues for at least five thousand years. Aloe's constituents include anthraquinones, barbaloins and mucopolysaccharides, which help replenish the mucosal membranes.

Bittersweet - *Solanum dulcamara*

This creeping shrub that grows along streams and bogs has been used extensively in traditional Western herbal medicine for all varieties of allergic epithelial issues and inflammatory conditions. It has been used for rheumatism and circulatory problems. The alkaloid solamine and the glucoside dulcamarin have been recognized as its active constituents, solasodine appears to be intricately involved in stimulating corticoid production, and the production of mucosal membranes.

Perhaps it is for this reason that many traditional herbalists have recommended bittersweet in cases of allergic skin conditions and mucous membrane issues. We should note that another constituent, solanine, can be poisonous in significant amounts. Therefore, as in all herbal products, consultation with a health professional is suggested before use.

Black Pepper - *Piper nigrum*

While *Piper nigrum* is considered Ayurvedic, it is probably one of the most common spices used in Western foods. In fact, the world probably owes its use of Black pepper in foods to Ayurveda.

Black pepper is used in a variety of Ayurvedic formulations because of its anti-inflammatory action. Ayurvedic doctors describe Black pepper as a stimulant, expectorant, carminative (expulsing gas), anti-inflammatory and analgesic. It has been used traditionally for heartburn, rheumatism, bronchitis, coughs, asthma, sinusitis, gastritis and other histamine-related conditions. It is also thought to stimulate a healthy mucosal membrane among the stomach and intestines.

Black pepper used as a spice to increase taste is certainly not unhealthy, but it takes a significantly greater and consistent dose to produce its anti-inflammatory effects.

A traditional Ayurvedic prescription for gastroesophageal reflux or GERD, for example, is to take Black pepper in a warm glass of water on an empty stomach first thing in the morning over a period of time. This dose of Black pepper, according to Ayurveda, stimulates mucosal secretion, and purifies the mucosal membranes of the stomach and intestines.

Researchers from South Korea's Wonkwang University (Bae *et al.* 2010) found that the *Piper nigrum* extract piperine significantly inhibited inflammatory responses, including leukocytes and TNF-alpha.

Boswellia (Frankincense)

The medicinal Boswellia species include *Boswellia serratta, Boswellia thurifera,* and *Boswellia spp.* (other species). Boswellia contains a variety of active constituents, including a number of boswellic acids, diterpenes, ocimene, caryophyllene, incensole acetate, limonene and lupeolic acids.

The genus of *Boswellia* includes a group of trees known for their fragrant sap resin that grow in Africa and Asia. Frankincense was extensively used in ancient Egypt, India, Arabia and Mesopotamia thousands of years ago, as an elixir that relaxed and healed the body's aches and pains. The gum from the resin was applied as an ointment for rheumatic ailments, urinary tract disorders, and on the chest for bronchitis and general breathing problems. It is classified in Ayurveda as bitter and pungent.

Over the centuries, boswellia has been used as an internal treatment for a wide variety of ailments, including ulcers, heartburn, bronchitis, asthma, arthritis, rheumatism, anemia, allergies and a variety of infections. Its properties are described as stimulant, diaphoretic, anti-rheumatic, tonic, analgesic, antiseptic, diuretic, demulcent, astringent, expectorant, and antispasmodic.

Boswellia has also shown to be beneficial for esophagitis and GERD.

In two studies, boswellic acids extracted from Boswellia were found to have significant anti-inflammatory action. The trials revealed that Boswellia inhibited the inflammation-stimulating LOX enzyme (5-lipoxygenase) and thus significantly reduced the production of inflammatory leukotrienes (Singh *et al.* 2008; Ammon 2006).

Another study (Takada *et al.* 2006) showed that boswellic acids inhibited cytokines and suppressed cell invasion through NF-kappaB inhibition.

Indian researchers found that Boswellia successfully treated ulcerative colitis in rats (Singh *et al.* 2008) in rats.

Boswellia also inhibits inflammation. In an *in vitro* study also from the University of Maryland's School of Medicine (Chevrier *et al.* 2005), boswellia extract proved to modulate the balance between Th1 and Th2 cytokines. This illustrated Boswellia's ability to strengthen the immune system and increase tolerance.

A similar-acting Ayurvedic herb is Guggul. Guggul is another gum derived from the resin of a tree—*Commiphora mukul.*

Bupleurum - *Bupleurum chinense; Bupleurum falcatum*

Bupleurum has also been called Hare's Ear, Saiko and Thorowax. Bupleurum belongs in the Umbelliferae family, and thus is related to fennel, dill, cumin, coriander and others—and exerts similar medicinal effects.

The root is typically used, and its constituents include triterpenoid saponins called saikosides, flavonoids such as rutin, and sterols such as bupleurumol, furfurol and stigmasterol. The saikosides in Bupleurum have been known to boost liver function and reduce liver toxicity, as well as strength the mucosal membrane integrity.

This last effect appears to be the result of a special class of constituents called saikosaponins. Like other saponins, these have a balancing and protective effect upon the epithelial membranes and sphincters of the esophagus.

GERD is often described in Chinese traditional medicine as related to spleen weakness. Bupleurum was studied by researchers at the Beijing University of Traditional Chinese Medicine (Chen *et al.* 2005) on 58 patients with spleen deficiency. After one month of treatment, tests showed that levels of epinephrine and dopamine were decreased and beta-endorphin levels had increased substantially among the Bupleurum-treated group. They concluded that Bupleurum significantly *"regulates nervous and endocrine systems."* As we've discussed, this directly affects sphincter tone and efficiency.

Calendula (marigold) - *Calendula officinalis*

Marigold flowers, as beautiful as they are, provide potent antiseptic and antibacterial properties according to research and clinical application. It is also been used for ulcers and heartburn, due both to its soothing effects and antibacterial properties.

Calendula contains a variety of flavonoids, saponins, mucilage and bitter compounds. It has been used traditional herbalists for healing wounds, and ulcerative conditions. Its antimicrobial effects have been shown to inhibit Candida species as well.

Cayenne *Capiscium frutescens or Capiscium annum*

This red pepper contains the alkaloid capsaicin—known to reduce the amount of substance P in nerves, thereby reducing pain transmission. Cayenne also has the distinction of stimulating the production of mucosal membranes among the esophagus and digestive tract. It also stimulates the production of gastric acids at the same time—increasing digestion.

Capiscium contains capsaicinoids; various carotenoids such as zeaxanthin, beta-cryptoxanthin, and beta-carotene; steroid glycosides, vitamins A & C and volatile oils; and at least twenty-three flavonoids including quercetin, luteolin and chysoeriol. These constituents work together to provide a number of anti-inflammatory benefits.

Researchers from Singapore's National University Hospital found that those who ate the most foods containing chili powder also contained the least incidence of ulcers.

Cayenne is known to increase circulation; increase detoxification; stimulate appetite; increase liver and heart function; stimulate the immune system and increase metabolic function. It is also a recognized antibacterial and antiviral agent. Some research has compared cayenne's antiseptic abilities to that of an antibiotic. Its actions have also been described as carminative, alterative, hemostatic, anthelmintic, stimulant, expectorant, antiseptic and diaphoric.

Comfrey - *Symphtum officinale*

Comfrey has been a favorite among traditional European herbalists for thousands of years. It contains mucilate (mucilage), allontoin, glycosides, saponins, triterpenoids, tannins, alkaloids and many other components.

159

Because of its saponin and mucilage content, comfrey is considered strengthening for mucous membranes throughout the body, including the esophagus and stomach wall. It is used as a poultice for healing skin wounds, and it is steeped into a tea infusion for digestive conditions.

Comfrey has been shown to inhibit prostaglandins and slow pain, while helping to rebuild the mucosal membranes. For this reason, Comfrey has been recommended for gastritis, ulcers and heartburn for many centuries, and has a long history of success with no side effects.

Chamomile - *Matricaria recutita*

Chamomile has been shown to effectively relieve inflamed and irritated mucosal membranes, especially those within the esophagus, stomach and intestines. Chamomile is also anti-inflammatory and has been found to benefit digestion in general.

Chamomile contains alpha-biasabolol, matricin, apingenin, luteolin, quercetin, azulene and others.

Some of these effects seem to come from the azulene—found to relax the smooth muscles around the intestines. Azulene also relaxes the smooth muscles around the airways as well.

Chamomile has also been used to soothe anxiety with success.

Chinese Licorice and Common Licorice

Glycyrrhiza uralensis is also called Chinese Licorice. It is not the common Licorice (*Glycyrrhiza glabra*) known in Western and Ayurvedic herbalism. However, the two plants have nearly identical uses and constituents. So this discussion also serves *Glycyrrhiza glabra*.

Chinese licorice is known in Chinese medicine as giving moisture and balancing heat to mucosal membranes of the airways and esophagus. It is also soothing to the throat and eases muscle spasms. The root is described as antispasmodic.

A Bulgarian study (Korlarski *et al.* 1987) gave deglycyrrhized licorice extract to 80 patients, and found that 75% experienced relief from GERD symptoms.

Due to adrenal effects, many natural physicians have suggested that the deglycyrrhized form of licorice extract is better suited for GERD sufferers.

160

Researchers from New York's Mount Sinai School of Medicine (Jayaprakasam *et al.* 2009) extensively investigated the anti-asthmatic properties of *Glycyrrhiza uralensis*. They found that *G. uralensis* had five major flavonoids: liquiritin, liquiritigenin, isoliquiritigenin, dihydroxyflavone, and isoononin. Liquiritigenin, isoliquiritigenin, and dihydroxyflavone were found to suppress airway inflammation via inhibiting eotaxin. Eotaxin stimulates the release of eosinophils to asthmatic airways during inflammation.

Licorice also contains glactomannan, triterpene saponins, glycerol, glycyrrhisoflavone, glycybenzofuran, cyclolicocoumarone, glycybenzofuran, cyclolicocoumarone, licocoumarone, glisoflavone, cycloglycyrrhisoflavone, licoflavone, apigenin, isokaempferide, glycycoumarin, isoglycycoumarin, glycyrrhizin and glycyrrhetinic acid (Li *et al.* 2010; Huang *et al.* 2010).

One of its main active constituents, isoliquiritigenin, has been shown to be a H2 histamine antagonist (Stahl 2008). Chinese Licorice has been shown to prevent the IgE binding that signals the release of histamine. This essentially disrupts the histamine inflammatory process while modulating immune system responses (Kim *et al.* 2006).

Another important constituent, glycyrrhizin, is a potent anti-inflammatory biochemical. It has also been shown to halt the breakdown of cortisol produced by the body. Let's consider this carefully. Like cortisone, cortisol inhibits the inflammatory process by interrupting interleukin cytokine transmission. If cortisol is prevented from breaking down, more remains available in the bloodstream to keep a lid on inflammation.

This combination of constituents gives Licorice aldosterone-like effects. This means that the root balances the production and maintenance of steroidal corticoids. A recent study by University of Edinburgh researchers (Al-Dujaili *et al.* 2012) found, for example, that licorice ingestion reduced cortisone levels in saliva.

Glycyrrhizin and other constituents in licorice (such as licochalcone A) have also been found to alter inflammatory cytokines such as IL-6, which in turn moderate inflammation and pain (Honda *et al.* 2012).

These effects in turn stimulate the secretion of healthy of mucosal membranes. This is confirmed by animal research that has

161

confirmed that Licorice is anti-allergic, and decreases anaphylactic response, and balances electrolytes and inflammatory edema (Lee *et al.* 2010; Gao *et al.* 2009).

Cinnamon - *Cinnamomum cassia*

Cinnamon is also referred to as *Ramulus cinnamomi cassiae* in traditional Chinese medicine. It is commonly called cinnamon—a delicious culinary spice present in most kitchens.

Cinnamon is used in just about every traditional medicine. The bark is often used, although the twigs are also utilized. Its constituents include limonene, camphor, cineole, cinnamic aldehyde, gums, mannitol, safrole, tannins and oils.

According to Western herbalism, Ayurvedic medicine and traditional Chinese medicine, it is useful for colds, sinusitis, bronchitis, dyspepsia, asthma, muscle tension, toothaches, the heart, the kidneys, and digestion. It is also thought to strengthen circulation in general. Its properties are described as expectorant, diuretic, stimulating, analgesic and alterative. In other words, it is an immune-system modulator. It is also described as dilating to the blood vessels and warming to the body according to some traditional disciplines.

Cumin Seed - *Cuminum cyminum*

Cuminum cyminum has a long history of use among European and Asian herbalists. It is described as antispasmodic and carminative, so it tends to soothe inflammatory responses. Cumin has been used traditionally to ease abdominal cramping and gas.

Cumin seed contains mucilage, gums and resins. Traditional herbalists consider these constituents primarily responsible for Cumin's ability to help strengthen the mucosal membranes. This makes Cumin part of a strategy to rebuild the mucosal membranes of the esophagus and digestive tract.

Dandelion - *Taraxum officinale, Taraxum mongolicum, Taraxum spp.*

Dandelion has hundreds of active constituents, including aesculetin, aesculin, arabinopyranosides, arnidiol, artemetin, B vitamins, benzyl glucoside, beta amyrin, beta-carboline, alkaloids, beta-sitosterol, bitter principle, boron, caffeic acid, caffeic acid ethyl, various esters, calcium, chicoric acid, chlorogenic acid, chlorophylls, choline, cichorin, coumaric acid, coumarin, deacetylmatricarin, di-glucopyranoside, dihydroconiferin, dihydrosyringin, dihydroxylben-zoic, acid, esculetin, eudesmanolides, faradiol, four steroids, furulic acid, gallic acid, gallicin, genkwanin-lutinoside, germacranolide ac-ids, glucopyranosides, glucopyranosyl-arabinopyranoside, glu-copyranosyl-glucopyranoside, glucopyranosyl-xyloypyranoside, guai-anolide, hesperetin, hesperidin, indole alkaloids, inulin, ionone, iron, isodonsesquitin A, isoetin, isoetin-glucopyranosyl, lactupicrine, lu-penol acetate, lutein, luteolin, luteolin-7-O-, gluccoside, magnesium, mannans, mongolicumin A, mongolicumin B, monocaffeyltartaric, acid, monoterpenoid, myristic acid, pyridine derivative, palmitic acid, pectin, phi-taraxasteryl acetate, phosphorus, p-hydroxybenzoic acid, p-hydroxyphenylacetic, acid, polyphenoloxidase, polysaccha-rides, potassium, quercetins, rufescidride, scopoletin, sesquiterpene, sesquiterpene ketolac-, tone, sesquiterpene lactones, seventeen anti-oxidants, several caffeoylquinic , acids, several luteolins, silicon, so-dium, sonchuside A, steroid complexes, stigmasterol, syringic acid, syringin, tannins, taraxacin, taraxacoside, taraxafolide, taraxafolin-B, taraxasterol, taraxasteryl acetate, taraxerol, taraxinic acid beta-, glu-copyranosyl, taraxinic acid, derivatives, taraxol, thirteen benzenoids, trime-thyl ether, triterpenoids, violaxanthin, vit. A (7000 IU/oz), vitamin C, vitamin D, vitamin K, xyloypyranosides, and zinc.

As such, it is no surprise that dandelion has the ability to strengthen the immune system and the mucosal membranes.

It has also been used to treat stomach problems, and is thought to reduce blood pressure. In Chinese medicine, dandelion is known to clear heat, more specifically in the liver, kidney and skin. Dande-lion has been used to increase urine excretion, and reduce pain and inflammation. Yet it also contains an abundance of potassium—which balances its diuretic effect (as potassium is lost during heavy urination). It has been documented as a blood and digestive tonic, laxative, stomachic, alterative, cholagogue, diuretic, choleretic, anti-inflammatory, antioxidant, anti-carcinogenic, analgesic, anti-hyperglycemic, anti-coagulation and prebiotic.

In a 2007 study from researchers at the College of Pharmacy at the Sookmyung Women's University in Korea (Jeon *et al.* 2008), dandelion was found to reduce inflammation, leukocytes, vascular permeability, abdominal cramping, pain and COX levels among exudates and *in vivo*.

Dandelion was found to stimulate fourteen different strains of probiotic bifidobacteria—important components of the immune system that inhibit pathogenic bacteria (Trojanova *et al.* 2004).

Other studies have illustrated that dandelion inhibits both inter-leukin IL-6 and TNF-alpha—both inflammatory cytokines (Seo *et al.* 2005).

Dandelion was shown to stimulate the liver's production of glutathione (GST)—an important component of mucosal membranes (Petlevski *et al.* 2003).

Another study by University of British Columbia researchers showed that dandelion extract was capable of reducing copper radicals—showing its ability to reduce heavy metals in the body (Hu and Kitts 2003).

Dandelion increased the liver's production of superoxide dismutase and catalase, increasing the liver's ability to purify the blood of toxins (Cho *et al.* 2001).

Dandelion illustrated the ability to inhibit IL-1 and inflammation in Kim *et al.* (2000) and Takasaki *et al.* (1999).

In a study of 24 patients with chronic colitis, pains in the large intestine vanished in 96% of the patients by the 15th day after being given a blend of herbs including Dandelion (Chakŭrski *et al.* 1981).

Both the leaves and the root of Dandelion have been used to reduce heartburn among some traditional medicines.

Evening Primrose - *Oenothera spp.*

Another herb known by traditional herbalists to be beneficial for allergic or inflamed epithelial issues. The seeds are rich in gamma-linolenic acid (GLA)—a fatty acid known to slow inflammatory responses of prostaglandins, especially those relating to epithelial hypersensitivity. The oil from Evening primrose can be taken internally in capsules or as oil. Herbalists give it credit for being helpful for epithelial permeability issues.

Fennel - *Foeniculum vulgare*

Foeniculum vulgare contains anetholes, caffeoyl quinic acids, carotenoids, vitamin C, iron, B vitamins, and rutins. Ayurvedic and traditional herbalists from many cultures have used Fennel to relieve digestive discomfort, gastritis, gas, abdominal cramping, bloating and irritable bowels; and to treat asthmatic hypersensitivities. Fennel stimulates bile production. Bile digests fats and other nutrients, increasing their bioavailability.

One of Fennel's constituents, called anethole, is known to suppress pro-inflammatory tumor necrosis factor alpha (TNF-a). This inhibition slows excessive immune response. The combination of anethole and antioxidant nutrients such as rutin and carotenoids in Fennel also strengthen immune response while increasing tolerance.

Fennel is not appropriate for pregnant moms, because it has been known to promote uterine contractions. As with any herbal supplement, Fennel should be used under the supervision of a health professional. Those with birch allergies should also be aware that they may also be sensitive to Fennel. (The same goes for Cumin, Caraway, Carrot seed and a few others).

Gentian - *Gentiana lutea*

This traditional herb is also known as bitter root, and has been referred to by traditional herbalists as a "bitter."

Typically the root is used, which contains various glycosides, including amarogentin, gentiopicrin, sweitiamarin and others, as well as alkaloids like gentianine and gentialutine, triterpenes, and several xanthones.

Root bitters have been used to increase appetite, stimulate bile secretions and stimulate mucosal secretions. It has been shown in research to be anti-inflammatory and used to stem fevers.

Ginger *Zingiber officinalis*

Ginger is one of the most powerful natural digestive aids, with thousands of years of use in Ayurveda and Chinese Medicine. In Ayurveda—the oldest medical practice still in use—ginger is the most recommended botanical medicine. As such, ginger is referred to as *vishwabhesaj*—meaning "universal medicine"—by Ayurvedic physicians. As mentioned earlier, an accumulation of studies and chemical analyses in 2000 determined that ginger has at least 477 active constituents.

As in all botanicals, each constituent will stimulate a slightly different mechanism—often moderating the mechanisms of other constituents. Many of ginger's active constituents have anti-inflammatory and/or pain-reducing effects. Research has illustrated that ginger inhibits COX and LOX enzymes in a balanced manner (Grzanna *et al.* 2005; Schulick 1996; and others). This allows for a gradual reduction of inflammation and pain without the negative GI side effects that accompany NSAIDs. Ginger also stimulates circulation, inhibits various infections, and strengthens the liver. It also stimulates the submucosal glands to produce healthy mucous membranes.

Ginger has therefore been used as a treatment for gastritis, GERD, rheumatoid arthritis, respiratory ailments, fevers, nausea, colds, flu, hepatitis, liver disease, headaches and many digestive ailments to name a few. Herbalists classify ginger as analgesic, tonic, expectorant, carminative, antiemetic, stimulant, anti-inflammatory, and antimicrobial.

Whole ginger is clinically proven to reduce nausea, stomachache, ulcers and many other gastrointestinal problems. These effects combine with its inflammation-reduction effects.

Many remedies use ginger extract. Through extraction, many constituents are often lost. Some are sensitive to heat and light. Others are sensitive to ethanol or methanol extraction methods. Therefore, during the pulverization, dehydration and refining process used to make ginger extract, there is a great likelihood that many constituents will not remain in the extract.

In other words, it is suggested that ginger be consumed only in its raw form. Fresh ginger root can be purchased at practically any grocery or health food store. It then can be washed like any other fresh food, and then grated onto a salad or other dish. If it is put onto a cooked dish, it is recommended that it be put in after the cooking. Just grate onto the food before serving. Ginger root can also be bitten into and chewed raw, and it can also make a nice tea—not steeped too long of course.

Goldenseal - *Hydrastis canadensis*
Goldenseal is also called yellow root and Indian turmeric. Typically the root is used. Goldenseal contains a number of alkaloids, one of the most effective being berberine. It also contains hydrastine, resins and various volatile oils.

Goldenseal is well-known among North American Indians and early Americans, who used it for curing peptic ulcers, heartburn, digestive conditions, fevers, infections and inflammation. It is considered to have a rejuvenative effect upon mucosal membranes and those supporting glands and tissue systems.

Berberine has been found in a number of studies to be antibiotic and anti-inflammatory. Its antibiotic effect may well be one reason for its usefulness with peptic ulcers, as it combats *H. pylori* growth.

Goldenseal is very potent, and most herbalists advise that it be used no more than five days in a row before taking a break. It can then be resumed. Berberine has also been advised not to use during pregnancy.

Herbs that have similar activity as goldenseal include **Barberry, Oregon Grape** and to some extent, **Yarrow.**

Gold Thread - *Coptis chinnensis*

Gold thread is often referred to as *Rhizoma coptidis* in Chinese medicine. Its common names include Gold thread or Golden thread. In Ayurveda, other species of *Coptis* spp. are also considered Gold thread.

Materia Medica of traditional Chinese medicine have documented that Gold thread removes heat associated with histamine responses affecting the eyes, throat and skin. It has also proved helpful for digestion. Applied topically, it has been used to calm skin rash, and has been used to treat boils and abscesses.

In Ayurveda, Gold thread is considered a bitter and tonic herb that reduces fever (antipyretic). It is also reputed to belong in the same category as Goldenseal.

Grapple Plant - *Harpagophytum procumbens, Harpagophytum spp.*

Harpagophytum contains a number of constituents, including acetylacteoside, acteoside, aucubinine B, beatrine A, beatrine B, beta-sitosterol, caffeic acid, cannamic acid, chlorogenic acid, cinnamic acid, cinnamoylmyoporoside, coumaroylharpagide, coumaroylharpagide, coumaroyl-procumbide, diacetylacteoside, feruloylharpagide, galactopyranosylharpagoside, harpagide, harpagoside, harprocumbide A, harprocumbide B, iridoid glycosides, isoacteoside, other phenolic glycosides, pagoside, p-coumaroylharpagide, procumbide, pyridine monoterpene, alkaloid (PMTA), stigmasterol, triterpenes and verbascoside.

The grapple plant has been studied extensively in Europe, with great success among pain patients, especially those with arthritis and heartburn.

It is native to Africa, and is rare in any other part of the world. This often makes the herb rather expensive and not readily obtainable. Indigenous peoples of South Africa have used the dried roots of harpagophytum in decoctions for a variety of ailments, particularly rheumatic conditions and gastrointestinal problems. G. H. Mehnert, a German farmer in South Africa, noticed these qualities and introduced the herb into the medical institutions of Europe.

It is considered a bitter—with a bitter value of about 6,000—matching that of gentian root. Over time, European herbalists came to use grapple for gastrointestinal upset, rheumatoid arthritis, osteoarthritis, backache, gallbladder disorders, diabetes, lumbago, headaches, backaches, gout and menstruation pain.

Several herbalists have noted its ability to clear the bloodstream, and it has also been known to clear up skin ulcers with external use. Others have noted its ability to strengthen the liver and gall bladder.

Interestingly—and quite opposite to the effects of NSAIDs—harpagophytum has been used for pain as well as in the treatment of ulcers, heartburn and gastritis.

In a study from France's Saint-Jacques Hospital (Moussard et al. 1992), harpagophytum was given to 25 healthy human volunteers for 21 days. Blood levels of PGE2, thromboxane, PGF-1 and leukotriene were tested before and after the dosage. None of the levels changed significantly, as other studies have indicated takes place among typical COX-inhibiting NSAIDs. Therefore, the researchers concluded that harpagophytum does not have the familiar mechanisms for reducing inflammation observed for other arthritic herbs and drugs.

Another study on the mechanisms for harpagophytum (Huang et al. 2006) illustrated that harpagoside blocked the movement of NF-kappaB, which would inhibit the COX-2 enzyme with nitric oxide, "thereby inhibiting downstream inflammation and subsequent pain events," the researchers explained. In the situation where there is no critical process of pain occurring, blocking the cascade at the NF-kappaB point would likely not occur. This again indicates a different mechanism for harpagophytum outside of direct COX inhibition.

Herbalist Richard Mabey (1988) commented that while harpogoside and beta sitosterol are known to have anti-inflammatory properties, the actions of harpagophytum are best with the whole plant—as they are with most medicinal herbs.

Jujube - *Ziziphus zizyphus*

The Jujube plant produces a delicious sweet date that tastes very much like a sweet apple. The fruit has many different properties in traditional medicine. It has been used to stimulate the immune system. It has been used to reduce stress, reduce inflammation, sooth indigestion, and repeal GERD.

Jujube contains a variety of constituents, including mucilage, ceanothic acid, alphitolic acid, zizyberanal acid, zizyberanalic acid, zizyberanone, epiceanothic acid, ceanothenic acid, betulinic acid, oleanolic acid, ursolic acid, zizyberenalic acid, maslinic acid, tetracosanoic acid, kaempferol, rutin, quercetin and others.

These constituents suggest the extensive support that this fruit can render for asthma sufferers with regard to rebuilding the mucosal membranes, reducing inflammation, relaxing the mind and nerves, and soothing the stomach and esophagus.

Long Pepper - *Piper longum*

The related Ayurvedic herb, *Piper longum,* has similar properties and constituents as Black pepper. It is used to inhibit the inflammation and histamine activity that results in lung and sinus congestion. Like Black pepper, Long pepper is also known to strengthen digestion by stimulating the secretion of the mucosal membranes within the stomach and intestines. It is also said to stimulate enzyme activity and bile production.

One study by researchers from India's Markandeshwar University (Kumar *et al.* 2009) found that the oil of Long pepper fruit significantly reduced inflammation.

Mallow - *Malva silvestris*

Malva silvestris grows throughout Europe and has enjoyed an extensive and popular reputation among Western and Middle Eastern traditional medicines as a demulcent herb: It soothes irritated tissues. Mallow contains polysaccharides, asparagine and mucilage—which stimulates a balance and coating among the body's mucosal membranes. The leaves are typically used.

The mucilage is primarily composed by polysaccharides. These include beta-D-galactosyl, beta-D-glucose, and beta-D-galactoses.

Mallow has been clinically used for sore throats, heartburn, dry sinuses, and irritable bowels.

This herb has also been used in decoctions by European herbalists for allergic skin responses and eczema. For this reason, Swiss doctors during the World Wars would apply mallow compresses onto skin rashes with good success.

Mallow's leaves, flowers and roots are all used. It is an emollient and demulcent, rendering the ability to soften and coat, while stimulating healthy mucous among the airways.

Mallow has been documented among traditional medicines to successfully treat GERD, sinusitis and asthma.

Marsh Mallow - *Althaea officinalis*

Marsh mallow—also called marshmallow—has similar properties and constituents as the *Malva verticillata* L (Mallow). It belongs in the same family, Malvaceaea, and has similar constituents.

Marsh mallow has also been reputed among traditional medicines around the world. This is because it contains mucilage, which supports and stimulates a healthy mucosal membrane.

For this reason, Marsh mallow is considered a demulcent: its leaves soothe irritated sore throats, heartburn, dry sinuses, and irritable bowels.

The leaves, flowers and roots are all used in healing. Marsh mallow is known to be emollient, which gives it properties that soften and coat practically any membrane within the body, including the sinuses, throat, stomach, intestines, urinary tract and of course, the esophagus.

The root of the Marsh mallow will contain up to 35% mucilage. It also contains a variety of long-chain polysaccharides. Extracts use cold water, so they dissolve the mucilage without the starches. For this reason, tea infusions for drinking and gargling using Marsh mallow often use cold water overnight, although it can also be steeped for 15-20 minutes using hot water.

Meadowsweet - *Spiraea ulmaria, Filipendula ulmaria, Spiraea betulifolia, Filipendula glaberrima, Filipendula vulgaris*

Also sometimes called *Queen of the Meadow*, this perennial bush grows throughout Europe and North America in damp grasslands and by streams in the forests.

Meadowsweet also contains numerous constituents, including multiple types of salicins, avicularin, coumarin, ellagitannins, volatile oils, eugenol, gallic acid, gaultherin, hydrolysable rugosin, hyperoside, meth-oxybenzaldehyde, monotropitin, mucilage, opiraein, phenolic glycodides, phenylcarboxylic acids, pireine, quercetin, rugosins, rutin, spiraein, spiraeoside, tannins and many others.

It has small, sweet-smelling white flowers that bloom in the summer. Its flowers, leaves and root extracts have been used to reduce digestive discomfort, fevers, aches, pains and inflammation for thousands of years. The Egyptians, Greeks, Romans and Northern Europeans were known to have utilized meadowsweet extracts for the treatment of rheumatism, infection of the urinary tract and abdominal discomfort. North American Indians used meadowsweet for bleeding, kidney issues, gastritis, colds and menstrual pain. Traditional herbalist Dr. Nicholas Culpeper wrote that meadowsweet "helps in the speedy recovery from cholic disorders and removes the instability and constant change in the stomach." [Cholic refers to increased bile acids.]

It is meadowsweet's soothing mucilage effects that provide much of its benefit in gastritis, esophagitis and GERD. The mucilage adds tone and thickness to our mucosal membranes, providing protection for our cells.

According to herbalist Richard Mabey, the tannin and mucilage content in meadowsweet moderate the adverse gastrointestinal side effects of isolated salicylates. For this reason, it is often used for heartburn, hyperacidity, acid reflux, gastritis and ulcers.

A purified version of salicin was isolated from meadowsweet in 1830 by Swiss Johann Pagenstecher. This led to the production of acetylsalicylic acid by the Bayer Company, now known by its common name of aspirin. The root of the word aspirin, "spirin" is derived from meadowsweet's genus name *Spiraea*.

The tannins within meadowsweet have been documented to have beneficial effects upon digestion as well. Thus, meadowsweet is often recommended for digestive disorders such as gastritis, GERD, indigestion, diarrhea and colitis. Meadowsweet is also often recommended for the removal of excess uric acid because of its diuretic and detoxifying effects. It has been used for kidney stones as well.

Herbalist David Hoffman documents its ability to reduce excess acidity in the stomach and ease nausea. Meadowsweet has been described as astringent, aromatic, antacidic, cholagogue (increasing bile flow), demulcent (soothing and providing mucilage), stomachic (tonic to digestive tract), and analgesic. The German Commission E monograph suggests the flower and herb for pain relief.

Unlike its pharmaceutical alternatives, meadowsweet flower extracts exhibit liver-protective effects against toxic hepatitis. Meadowsweet has been found to stimulate a normalization of liver enzymes, liver antioxidant effects. It also proved to normalize lipid peroxidation (cholesterol production) within the liver (Shilova *et al.* 2008).

Meadowsweet's phenolic extracts were found to have significant antioxidant and free radical scavenging potential (Sroka *et al.* 2005; Calliste *et al.* 2001).

Meadowsweet extract decreased inflammation, which included suppressing proinflammatory cytokines, decreasing IL-2 synthesis, and eliminating hypersensitivity *in vivo* (Churin *et al.* 2008).

Meadowsweet's antioxidant capacity was one of the highest levels in one test of 92 different phenolic plant extracts (Heinonen 1999).

Meadowsweet showed significant inhibition of several bacteria (Rauha *et al.* 2000). It was also shown to be antimicrobial by Radulović *et al.* (2007). This makes it applicable to *H. pylori* overgrowths.

Meadowsweet extract also exhibited the ability to reduce blood clotting. During *in vivo* and *in vitro* research (Liapina and Koval'chuk 1993), meadowsweet was determined to have anticoagulant (reducing clotting) and fibrinolytic (breaking down fibrin) properties, making it useful for speeding tissue healing.

Meadowsweet's anticoagulant and fibrinolytic properties were considered similar to heparin in another study (Kudriasho *et al.* 1990).

Contrasting with NSAIDs, meadowsweet was also found to be curative and preventative for acetylsalicylic acid-induced ulcers in rats (Barnaulov and Denisenko 1980).

Furthermore, meadowsweet has been found to inhibit the growth of *H. pylori*—the microorganism thought to cause or contribute to the majority of gastritis cases as well as GERD conditions (Cwikla *et al.* 2009).

Mullein - *Verbascum theapsiforme*

The leaves, flowers and herbs of *Verbascum theapsiforme* and *V. philomoides olanum* have been part of the traditional herbalist repertory for thousands of years. It is classified as a demulcent and expectorant, because it is known to soothe irritations among the airways and esophagus, and help clear thickened mucous.

Mullein's soothing and demulcent properties are due primarily to its mucilage content, which can be as high as 3%. Other constituents include saponins, which are believed to produce the expectorant properties of this herb.

Mullein has thus been used for centuries for hypersensitivity among the mucosal membranes, including coughing and bronchialspasm, skin irritations and throat infections. In all these cases, its effects have been considered soothing to epithelial cells.

Mucilage Seeds

A number of seeds are helpful for calming and settling the airways, including seeds such as Flax, Safflower, Rapeseed, Caraway, Anise, Fennel, Licorice seed, Black seed and others. Seeds contain basic compounds that offer mucilage, saponins and other polysaccharides that contribute to the health of the mucous membranes.

Not surprisingly, combinations or single versions of these seeds have been used in traditional medicine for centuries.

Pharmacology researchers from Cairo's Helwan University (Haggag *et al.* 2003) treated allergic asthmatic patients with an herbal blend containing of Anise, Fennel, Caraway, Licorice, Black seed and Chamomile—all known for their mucosal-rebuilding effects. They found that the extract significantly decreased cough frequency and intensity. It also increased lung function, with higher FEV1/FVC percentages among the asthmatic patients, as compared to those who consumed a placebo tea.

Panex Ginseng

Panex ginseng is a traditional remedy for allergies and hypersensitivity with thousands of years of use. Panax ginseng will come in white forms and red forms. The color depends upon the aging or drying technique used.

The Ginseng in the FAHF formula is termed *Radix* Ginseng or Ren shen but it is *Panex ginseng*. Depending upon how the Ginseng is cured, there are several types of Ren shen.

When Ginseng is cultivated and steamed, it is called 'red root' or Hong Shen. Ginseng root will turn red when it is oxidized or processed with steaming. Some feel that red root is better than white, but this really depends upon its intended use, the age of the root, and how it was processed. Soaking Ginseng in rock candy produces a white Ginseng that is called Bai shen. This soaking seems odd, but this has been known to increase some of its constituent levels such as superoxide and nitric oxide. When the root is simply dried, it is called 'dry root' or Sheng shaii shen. Korean Red Ginseng is soaked in a special herbal broth and then dried.

There are a number of species within the *Panax* genus, most of which also contain most of the same adaptogens, referred to as gensenosides. Most notable in the *Panex* genus is American Ginseng, *Panax quinquefolius*.

Ginseng contains camphor, mucilage, panaxosides, resins, saponins, gensenosides, arabinose and polysaccharides, among others.

Eleutherococcus senticosus, often called Siberian Ginseng, is actually not Ginseng. While it also contains adaptogens (eleutherosides), these are not the gensenoside adaptogens within Ginseng that have been observed for their ability to relieve hypersensitivity.

Researchers from Italy's Ambientale Medical Institute (Caruso *et al.* 2008) tested an herbal extract formula consisting of *Capparis spinosa, Olea europaea, Panax ginseng* and *Ribes nigrum* (Pantescal) on allergic patients. They found that allergic biomarkers, including basophil degranulation CD63 and sulphidoleukotriene (SLT) levels

174

were significantly lower after 10 days. They theorized that these bio-markers explain the herbal formulation's *"protective effects."*

Ginseng has been found to stimulate circulation and improve appetite, and as a mild stimulant and potent antioxidant.

Pine Bark Extract

Traditional herbalists have used pine bark extracts for respiratory conditions and other mucosal-related conditions for centuries. The process of extraction is complex, however. Pine bark contains numerous constituents that yield health benefits, but also contains a high-density tannin complex requiring careful purification.

Today's standard for pine bark extracts is an extract of French Maritime Pine (*Pinus pinaster*) called Pycnogenol®. This extract is produced using a process patented by the Swiss company Horphag Research, Ltd. The process renders a number of bioavailable pro-cyanidolic oligomers (PCOs), including catechin and taxifolin, as well as several phenolic acids.

Pycnogenol® has undergone extensive clinical study and laboratory research. Today, Pycnogenol® has been the subject of nearly 100 human clinical studies, testing over 7,000 patients with a variety of conditions. This extract's unique layered proanthocyanidin content has been shown, among other things, to significantly reduce systemic inflammation.

Meanwhile, German researchers (Rohdewald *et al.* 2008) found in a laboratory that Pycnogenol significantly inhibited the growth of *H. pylori* bacteria that are at the root of many GERD conditions.

Pycnogenol also strengthens our mucosal membranes. In a study of allergic rhinitis to birch pollen, for example, 39 allergic patients were given Pycnogenol® several weeks before the start of the 2009 birch allergy season. The treatment reduced allergic eye symptoms by 35% and sinus symptoms by 20%, compared to the placebo group. Better results were found among those who took Pycnogenol® seven to eight weeks before the birch pollen season began (Wilson *et al.* 2010).

We've discussed the relationship between GERD and inflammation. Pycnogenol® reduces a number of pro-inflammatory mediators.

Reishi - *Ganoderma lucidum*

This a popular medicinal mushroom. Reishi has been shown in numerous studies to significantly moderate inflammation, stimulate the mucosal membranes and aid digestion.

Reishi contains many constituents, including steroids, triterpenes, lipids, alkaloids, glucosides, coumarin glycoside, choline, betaine, tetracosanoic acid, stearic acid, palmitic acid, nonadecanoic acid, behenic acid, tetracosane, hentriacontane, ergosterol, sitosterol, ganoderenic acids, ganolucidic acids, lucidenic acids, lucidone and many more.

Ling Zhi strengthens immunity and modulates the body's tolerance and responses to allergens. Reishi has been shown to increase production of IL-1, IL-2 and natural killer cell activity. A number of studies have shown that Reishi can significantly lower IgE levels specific to allergens, and reduce inflammatory histamine levels. It has also been shown to improve lung function and has been used traditionally for bronchitis and asthma.

Recently, researchers from Japan's University of Toyama (Andoh *et al.* 2010) found that Reishi also relieves skin itching and rash *in vivo*.

Slippery Elm - *Ulmus fulva*

Slippery elm has long been used to soothe irritated throats and esophagi. It contains high mucilage and mucopolysaccharide content, along with tannins, starches and others. It is considered a demulcent, and used by Northern American Indians and European herbalists for ulcers, heartburn and general stomach upset. The inner bark is typically used and has the highest mucilage content, as it adds lubrication to the mucosal membranes, giving credence to its namesake, "slippery." It is also mildly astringent, which helps stimulate digestion.

Triphala

Triphala means *"three fruits."* Triphala is a combination of three botanicals: *Terminalia chebula, Terminalia bellirica* and *Emblica officinalis.* They are also termed Haritaki, Bibhitaki and Amalaki, respectively. This combination has been utilized for thousands of years to rejuvenate the intestines, regulate digestion and balance the mucosal membranes of within the digestive tract.

The 'three fruits' also are said to produce a balance among the three doshas of *vata, pitta* and *kapha*. Each herb, in fact, relates to a particular *dosha:* Haritaki relates to *vata*, Amalaki relates to *pitta* and Bibhitaki relates to *kapha*. The three taken together comprise the most-prescribed herbal formulation given by Ayurvedic doctors for digestive issues.

This use has been justified by preliminary research. For example, in a study by pharmacology researchers from India's Gujarat University (Nariya *et al.* 2003), triphala was found to significantly reverse intestinal damage and intestinal permeability *in vivo*.

The traditional texts and the clinical use of triphala today in Ayurveda have confirmed these types of intestinal effects in humans.

We might want to elaborate a little further on Haritaki in particular. *Terminalia chebula* has been used by Ayurvedic practitioners specifically for conditions related to asthma, coughs, hoarseness, abdominal issues, skin eruptions, itchiness, and inflammation. It is also called He-Zi in traditional Chinese medicine.

Research has found that Haritaki contains a large number of polyphenols, including ellagic acids, which have significant antioxidant and anti-inflammatory properties (Pfundstein *et al.* 2010).

Turmeric - *Curcuma longa*

Turmeric can also either be considered a medicinal herb or a food-spice. It is a root (or rhizome) and a relative of ginger in the *Zingiberaceae* family. Just as we might expect from a botanical, turmeric has a large number of active constituents. The most well known of these are the curcuminoids. These include curcumin (diferuloylmethane), demethoxycurcumin and bisdemethoxycurcumin. Others include volatile oils such as tumerone, atlantone, and zingiberone, polysaccharides, proteins, and a number of resins.

These work together to stimulate the immune system along with mucosal secretions. For these reasons, turmeric is known for its anti-inflammation effects.

As stated in a recent review from the Cytokine Research Laboratory at the University of Texas (Anand 2008), studies have linked turmeric with "suppression of inflammation; angiogenesis; tumor genesis; diabetes; diseases of the cardiovascular, pulmonary, and neurological systems, of skin, and of liver; loss of bone and muscle; depression; chronic fatigue; and neuropathic pain."

Indeed, turmeric has been used for centuries for gastritis, heartburn, inflammation, gallbladder problems, diabetes, wound-healing, liver issues, hepatitis, menstrual pain, anemia, and gout. It is considered alterative, antibacterial, carminative and stimulant.

In a study on 45 patients with peptic ulcers (Prucksunand 2001), ulcers were completely resolved and absent in 76% of the group taking turmeric powder in capsules.

Other studies have also shown similar positive gastrointestinal effects of turmeric. We can conclude that not only is turmeric a known anti-inflammatory, but its *positive* gastrointestinal side effects greatly contrast the negative GI side effects of NSAIDs.

Turmeric can certainly be taken in a capsule as the above studies mention. However, because turmeric is readily available as a delicious spice, there is every reason to conclude that adding it (along with ginger) to our daily meal-plans in its raw or powdered form. This said, some herbalists, such as James LaValle, R.Ph, N.M.D., suggest that for best results turmeric should also be taken as a supplement.

Willow Bark - *Salix alba, Salix spp.*

The willow tree can grow to 75 feet tall, but many species are smaller trees and even shrubs. It has rough bark with narrow, glandular, pointed leaves and small yellow flowers. It grows along streams and fields—and often in neighborhood yards. There are some 450 species of the genus *Salix,* and most contain similar constituents. Willow species grow practically all over the world.

Willow contains numerous medicinal constituents, including various types of salicins, catechins, procyanidins, flavones, various tannins, helicon, isoquercitrin, isosalipurposide, leonuriside, luteolins, naringenin, naringin, picein, piceoside, populin, and salidroside, sisymbrifolin, tremulacin and many others.

Along with decreasing pain, Willow has been used to soothe irritated throats and digestive tracts for thousands of years by traditional herbalists from around the world. This comes from willow's mucilage effects, and the ability to add tone to our esophageal sphincters.

178

Anti-GERD Formulation:

Rikkunshi-to / Liu Jun Zi Tang

This is an ancient formula used in Chinese Traditional Medicine and Japanese Kampo Medicine. It has been used for digestive issues, swelling, edema and others. The formula, however, has been the subject of considerable research, after it was established that it reversed GERD, gastritis and heartburn conditions. Let's look at some of the research and then we'll take a look at what the formula contains:

Researchers from the Osaka Medical Center and Research Institute for Maternal and Child Health (Kawahara *et al.* 2007) gave eight children suffering from GERD—six severely—0.3 grams of rikkunshito (TJ-43) per kilogram of body weight per day to the children for seven days.

After the seven days, emesis symptoms decreased among three of the children. Among the other patients, other symptoms were significantly decreased, including nausea, hematemesis (vomiting blood), and wheezing.

The researchers also used a pH electrodes to gauge the esophageal pH and the time that the pH was less than 4.0. They found that the average reflux pH decreased significantly.

The researchers concluded that, "The short-term administration of TJ-43 relieved symptoms and reduced the distal esophageal acid exposure through improved esophageal acid clearance."

The last part is key to the mechanism: "esophageal acid clearance." What is "esophageal acid clearance?"

This is the removal and neutralizing of acids through the mucosal membrane chemistry and current. One of the activities of the mucosal membranes, remember, is to flush out toxins and constantly cycle out old mucous, so the mucosal glands—where ever located—can continue to produce mucous. And remember, that it is this mucous that provides the barrier and protectant to the cells of the esophagus, stomach lining and other epithelial membranes covered with mucosal membranes.

In other words, this herbal combination stimulates the natural function of the mucosal membranes.

Gastroenterology researchers from Japan's Osaka City University Graduate School of Medicine (Tominaga *et al.* 2011) compared Rikkunshi-to to the GERD medication rabeprazole with 104 GERD patients. After four weeks of treatment, the patients using Rikkunshi-to had success rates that were comparative to a double-dose of the pharmaceutical medication.

Researchers from Japan's Gunma University Graduate School of Medicine (Mochiki *et al.* 2010), reviewed the research related to the use of Rikkunshi-to. They found that Rikkunshito stimulates metabolic activity along the digestive tract (also referred to as motility).

The formula has also been shown to increase ghrelin secretion. Ghrelin is a hormone secreted in the stomach and intestines, as well as the pancreas. Ghrelin is integral in increasing appetite, which means increasing enzyme and bile acid production, as well as stimulating submucosal gland production of protective mucous.

The researchers concluded that: "Rikkunshito is effective for improving the symptoms of functional dyspepsia, gastroesophageal reflux disease, and cisplatin-induced anorexia and vomiting."

The Rikkunshito formula contains eight herbs:
- ➤ Ginseng (Ren shen)
- ➤ Atractylodes Rhizome (Bai zhu)
- ➤ Hoelen mushroom (Fu ling)
- ➤ Pinellia Tuber (Ban xia)
- ➤ Tangerine Peel (Chen pi)
- ➤ Jujube (Da zao)
- ➤ Licorice (Gan cao)
- ➤ Ginger (Sheng jiang)

Modern TCM and Kampo formulations will typically be standardized to the constituents Hesperidin (contained in the tangerine peel and likely also jujube fruit) and Glycyrrhizin (contained in the licorice). While a number of the above herbs are mentioned above, a few are not, as these would be considered supporting herbs to the formula.

Others Herbs to Consider

In addition to these herbs, several others have also been used in traditional medicine to help heartburn:

➤ Anise (*Pimpinella anisum*): Some similarities with licorice, stimulates mucosal integrity.

➤ Barberry (*Berberis vulgaris*): A bitter, with significant berberine content, which repels *H. pylori*.

➤ Borage (*Borago officinalis*): Relative of Chamomile, stimulates mucosal membrane integrity.

➤ Chaparral (*Larrea tridentata*): Stimulates wound healing, reduces irritation.

➤ Cinnamon (*Cinnamomum zeylanicum*): Inhibits *H. pylori* and Candida.

➤ Horehound (*Marrubium vulgare*): Stimulates gastric secretions and saliva secretions.

➤ Lavender (*Lavandula augustifolia*): Relaxes nerves and reduces stress. Also inhibits *H. pylori*.

➤ Lemon Balm (*Melissa officinalis*): Sedative and soothing to the digestive tract.

➤ Oregon Grape (*Berberis aquifolium*): Contains berberine, which inhibits *H. pylori*. Also has bitter principle, which stimulates digestion.

➤ Yarrow (*Achillea millefolium*): Used traditionally by North American Indians and others for heartburn.

➤ Yellow Dock (*Rumex crispus*): Bitter principle stimulates secretion of gastric acids and enzymes, speeding stomach emptying.

Herbal Techniques

We've discussed a long list of herbs that can provide numerous benefits and healing properties to an irritated esophagus and sphincters. Choosing the right herb and/or formula for a particular case can thus be a little tricky. For this reason, a seasoned expert in herbal formulations can offer specific suggestions relating to ones constitution and precise level of sensitivities.

This said, not all traditional health practitioners approach GERD the same. Still, a western herbalist and a Chinese medicine herbalist may both recommend the same kind of herbs for GERD. The Chinese and Kampo medicine practitioner views the condition related to a balanced meridian flow and heat present in that part of the body.

For example, Traditional Chinese Medicine often refers to the presence of symptoms that resemble GERD as "disharmony of stomach." To test whether this diagnosis is correct, Chinese researchers (Chen *et al.* 2010) analyzed the contents of the sputum of patients with the "disharmony of stomach" diagnosis. They discovered that the sputum revealed increased levels of by eosinophils—immune cells that indicate an inflammatory condition.

They followed by treating the patients with Chinese herbs used for "disharmony of the stomach" and then retested the sputum of the patients.

They found that the sputum indicated the Chinese herbs reduced the eosinophil count down to normal, healthy levels—indicating that the Chinese herbs helped relieve GERD symptoms that extended into the esophagus and airways. So the language may be different, the remedies are often similar.

The choice of application will likely depend also upon the part of the body affected. While most of these medicinal herbs help stimulate mucosal membrane health in general, some benefit particular tissue systems better than others. Some, like mullein, will benefit the lungs, while ginger will benefit the digestive tract. Still, mullein will benefit the GI tract and ginger will benefit the lungs as well. So these kinds of crossovers occur, but at the same time, ginger is better for digestive issues than it is for lung issues.

Another example might be that Marsh mallow, Mallow and Mullein might be recommended in a case of GERD along with asthmatic symptoms, because GERD illustrates a weakness in the mucosal membranes.

Or perhaps, for issues where sinusitis presents along with asthmatic hyperreactivity, the herbalist may recommend the use of ventilation or ointment of camphor, menthol and eucalyptus along with anti-asthma herbs to clear the sinus passageways, speed the removal of mucous from the nasal region, and exert some antimicrobial effects that these bring.

Dosages and Methods

We have not detailed precise dosages in this section because there are many considerations when determining dosages. These include age, physical health, constitution, unique weaknesses, diet, lifestyle and other factors. Herbs should also be carefully matched, and some herbs and formulations have been known to interact with certain medications.

Therefore, it is suggested that herbs are chosen, formulated and dosed by an experienced herbalist. If there are any medications being used, the prescribing physician should be consulted.

This said, most of the herbs mentioned above, with the exception of essential oils, are safest when used as *infusions*. An infusion is simply the steeping of the fresh or dried root, bark, leaf, seed, stem or fruit in water.

In the case of most herb leaves and stems, the water is brought to a boil, and the herb can be steeped for 5-10 minutes using a strainer or tea-ball.

In the case of most roots, seeds and barks, the root can be steeped a little longer, for 10-20 minutes, depending on the herb. In some cases a seed, root or bark is better when it is soaked overnight in room temperature water.

Another strategy is to simply ingest a capsule or pressed tablet of a powdered version of the herb or herbal formulation. Liquid extracts are also available from many reputable herbal suppliers. In these cases, the literature accompanying these products should be closely examined for dosages and possible interactions. Be wary that extracts may not have the same effects as the raw or infused herb.

A number of the formulations (or their derivatives) mentioned in this section are available as encapsulated, pressed tablets or liquid extracts, together with dosage suggestions. Before using this strategy, care should be taken to assure that the herbal formulation has been ultimately designed by a reputable herbalist. Most of the popular commercial brands of herbal formulations employ professional herbalists to design their formulations. Many will also name the herbalist on the marketing material or label of the product. These should be considered more trustworthy formulations.

By far the best approach is to have an herbalist formulate and recommend herbs specific to ones constitution, symptom severity, medication and lifestyle. In the alternative, a commercial formula (such as ones discussed in this chapter) blended or overseen by a reputable herbalist, together with instructions on the packaging, can be used.

Remember, if taking pharmaceutical medications, the prescribing physician should be consulted to avoid possible interactions. Also, very small doses, gradually building up to the suggested dose, are usually recommended in the beginning to test tolerances.

Anti-reflux Nutrition Strategies

Most GERD sufferers will experience heartburn after eating certain foods. The strange thing is that while many react to the same types of foods—such as fatty foods—some react to foods that others with GERD don't. Why is this?

It is a combined effect. It has to do with the condition of our mucosal membranes, and the type of damage our epithelial tissues within the esophagus, sphincter and stomach wall have suffered. It depends upon our digestive tract's ability to produce enzymes. It can also depend upon our body's sensitivities—if any—to certain types of foods.

As mentioned previously, research illustrates that GERD sufferers can have a wide range of pH within the esophagus and stomach. It is not a one-size-fits-all proposition.

What is common among most with GERD is the damage to our mucosal membranes, allowing acids and toxins to penetrate and harm the underlying epithelial cells.

The actual damage to the membranes can vary, from simply being thinned from lack of hydration or stress to a thickening of mucous within the membranes in the regions of the esophagus, sphincter and stomach wall.

This mucosal thickness can be due to an viral infection or increased amount of toxins in the area, producing inflammation. It may also be caused by repeated exposures to a particular toxin. Or it may also be related to an infection of microorganisms that are damaging the tissues of the region.

For others, damage to the sphincter from a hiatal hernia or chronic overeating may be at issue with GERD. In this case, the weakened lower esophageal sphincter is allowing too many gastric acids into the esophagus, which may overwhelm mucous membranes over time. This mechanical issue, as mentioned earlier, is also connected to other related causes (damage to mucosal membranes) because only a small percentage (approaching 5%) of hiatal hernia patients have GERD.

Regardless of the particular issue, we illustrated research in the last chapter that showed that diets high in plant-based fiber and nutrients typically help our mucosal membranes and damaged epithelial surfaces—inclusive of the sphincters.

And fattier meals—especially animal fats—tend to slow the rate of stomach emptying and release reactive oxidative species (ROS); and as a result stimulate high acidity within the esophagus. This was shown by research from Wake Forest's School of Medicine, which found that meals containing more fat resulted in a lower pH (more acid) within the esophagus than less fatty foods.

Plant-based foods provide numerous compounds that promote this reviving of these tissues and mucosal membranes. Before we get into the specifics of these, let's look at how plant foods prevent many mucosal membrane-related conditions, including those related to the health of the airways, esophagus and stomach, including some of the studies we reviewed earlier for clarity:

Remember the review of research from Mount Sinai School of Medicine (Friedman 1989) finding that heartburn from gastroesophageal reflux can be reduced by eliminating fatty foods, alcohol, and chocolate from the diet.

Remember the research from the Chinese Academy of Medical Sciences (Chen *et al.* 2011), which compared the diets of 751 esophageal cancer cases with 2,253 healthy persons. They found that the cancer patients were more than three times more likely to eat fried foods, 40% less likely to eat fresh vegetables daily, and more likely to have an inconsistent diet. They characterized eating daily fresh vegetables were "protective."

Remember the research from India's Seth G S Medical College and The Indian Society of Gastroenterology (Bhatia *et al.* 2011). In a study of 3,224 people, the strongest determinant of GERD was eating more fried foods and more meats. GERD incidence was also associated with carbonated sodas, black tea and coffee.

And remember the research from New Jersey's Montclair State University (Navarro *et al*. 2011) that utilized a large population-based study conducted in the states of Connecticut, New Jersey, and Washington. They found six patterns among those with esophageal cancers, which included eating more red meats, more fried foods and less fruits and vegetables. In addition, those who drank more alcohol and smoked more likely suffered from GERD.

In addition, we've shown other research showing that chocolate, peppermint, and sugary carbonated beverages can encourage sphincter weakness and GERD symptoms.

These findings are not isolated, as most are confirmed by multiple studies. We also find that many are common among other mucosal membrane conditions such as wheeze, asthma, allergies and sinus issues. This indicates that not only are certain foods disruptive to our mucosal membrane health in general, but certain diets promote the health of our mucosal membranes:

A study that on mucosal-membrane related disorders conducted among eight Pacific countries included subjects from Samoa, Fiji, Tokelau, French Polynesia and New Caledonia. The research found that the risk factors for increased rhinoconjunctivitis included the regular consumption of meat products, butter and margarine; along with regular television viewing, acetaminophen use and second-hand smoke.

Allergic eczema was also associated with regular meat consumption and butter consumption; along with regular television viewing, acetaminophen use and second hand smoke. Major predicating factors for asthma and wheeze were regular margarine consumption, electric cooking, and maternal smoking.

The researchers concluded that: "*Regular meat and margarine consumption, paracetamol [acetaminophen] use, electric cooking and passive smoking are risk factors for symptoms of asthma, rhinoconjunctivitis and eczema in the Pacific.*"

In a study of 460 children and their mothers on Menorca—a Mediterranean island—medical researchers from Greece's Department of Social Medicine and the University of Crete (Chatzi *et al*. 2008) found that children of mothers eating primarily a Mediterranean diet (a predominantly plant-based diet) produced significantly lower rates of asthma among the children.

They found that mothers with a high Mediterranean Diet Score during pregnancy reduced the incidence of persistent wheeze among their children by 78%. Their children also had 70% lower incidence of allergic wheezing; and a 45% reduction in allergies among their children at age six (after removing other possible variables).

The research from Sweden's Uppsala University discussed earlier (Uddenfeldt *et al.* 2010) studied the lifestyle and diets in 12,560 adolescents, adults and elderly adults with a follow-up period of 13 years, between 1990 and 2003. The researchers found that those eating a diet heavy with fruit and fish significantly reduced rates of asthma. In elderly persons, the rates were reduced by nearly 50%.

Medical researchers from Britain's University of Nottingham (McKeever *et al.* 2010) researched the relationship between diet and respiratory symptoms, including forced expiratory volumes. Their data was derived from 12,648 adults from the Monitoring Project on Risk Factors and Chronic Diseases in The Netherlands. They also included dietary patterns and lung function decline over a five-year basis.

They found that diets with higher intakes of meat and potatoes, and lower levels of soy and cereals, was linked to reduced lung function and lower expiratory levels (FEV1) levels. They also found that the heavy meat-and-potatoes diet produced higher levels of chronic obstructive pulmonary disease. They also found that a "cosmopolitan diet" with heavier intakes of fish and chicken (both of which are commonly fried) produced higher levels of wheeze and asthma.

Remember the research from the University of Athens (Bacopoulou *et al.* 2009). Here 2,133 children at ages seven and eighteen were studied. The daily consumption of fruit and vegetables significantly reduced the risk of asthma symptoms through age 18.

Researchers from the Johns Hopkins School of Medicine (Matsui and Matsui 2009) studied 8,083 people over two years old using data from the National Health and Nutrition Examination Survey (2005-2006). They found that among patients diagnosed by a doctor as having asthma and/or wheeze in the last year, higher blood levels of folate was linked to lower total IgE levels—a sign of reduced allergy and hypersensitivity (atopy). They also found a dose-dependent relationship between higher folate levels and doctor-diagnosed wheeze and/or asthma.

Good sources of folate include lettuce, spinach, lentils, beans, asparagus and other plant-based foods.

Researchers from Mexico's Institute of National Public Health (Romieu *et al.* 2009) followed 158 asthmatic children and 50 healthy children from Mexico City for 22 weeks. Diet, lung function testing and sinus mucous analysis was done every two weeks. Diets with greater amounts of fruits and vegetables resulted in lower levels of pro-inflammatory IL-8 cytokines. A diet that most closely trended towards the Mediterranean diet (index) resulted in better lung function tests. Children with the higher Mediterranean diet index scores also scored the highest in forced expiratory volume (FEV1) testing. The researchers concluded: *"Our results suggest that fruit and vegetable intake and close adherence to the Mediterranean diet have a beneficial effect on inflammatory response and lung function in asthmatic children living in Mexico City."*

Another study by researchers from the University of Crete's Faculty of Medicine (Chatzi *et al.* 2007) surveyed the parents of 690 children ages seven through 18 years old in the rural areas of Crete. The children were also tested with skin prick tests for 10 common allergens. This research found that consuming a Mediterranean diet reduced the risk of allergic rhinitis by over 65%. The risk of skin allergies and respiratory conditions (such as wheezing) was also reduced, but by smaller amounts. They also found that greater consumption of nuts among the children cut wheezing rates in half, while consuming margarine more than doubled the incidence of both wheezing and allergic rhinitis.

Nutrition researchers from Italy's D'Annunzio University (Riccioni *et al.* 2007) also studied the relationships between nutrition and bronchial asthma. They found significant evidence that inflammatory activity associated with the asthmatic hyperresponse relates directly to the production of reactive oxygen species. Furthermore, they determined that the damage done by these free radicals produces *"specific inflammatory abnormalities"* within the airways of asthmatics.

188

A related study by these researchers (Riccioni *et al.* 2007) tested 96 people—which included 40 asthmatics and 56 healthy control subjects—for blood levels of vitamin A and lycopene. They found that lycopene and vitamin A levels were significantly lower among the asthmatic patients versus the healthy controls.

As part of the International Study on Allergies and Asthma in Childhood (ISAAC), a contingent of researchers from around the world (Nagel *et al.* 2010) convened to analyze studies on asthma and diet conducted between 1995 and 2005 among 29 research facilities in 20 different countries. In all, the dietary habits of 50,004 children ages eight through twelve years old were analyzed.

This study revealed that those with diets containing large fruit portions had significantly lower rates of asthma. This link occurred among both affluent and non-affluent countries. Fish consumption in affluent countries (where vegetable intake is less) and green vegetable consumption among non-affluent countries were also associated with reduced asthma. In general, the consumption of fruit, vegetables and fish was linked with less lifetime asthma incidence among the entire population. Frequent consumption of beef burgers, on the other hand, was linked with greater incidence of lifetime asthma.

Researchers from the Harvard School of Public Health (Varraso et a. 2007) studied the effects of nitrites in the diet and the lungs. They analyzed 111 diagnosed cases of COPD between 1986 and 1998 among 42,915 men that participated in the Health Professionals Follow-up Study. The average consumption of high-nitrite meats (processed meats, bacon, hot dogs) was calculated from surveys conducted in 1986, 1990, and 1994. They found that consuming these meats at least once a day increased the risk of contracting COPD by more than 2-1/2 times over those who almost never ate high-nitrite meats. (Remember other research illustrating that high nitrite meals were also associated with GERD symptoms.)

These same Harvard researchers (Varraso et a. 2007) used a similar analysis of 42,917 men, but with more dietary parameters. The analysis found that the "Western" diet consisting of refined grains, cured and red meats, desserts and French fries increased the risk of COPD by more than four times, while a "prudent" diet, rich in fruits, vegetables and fish halved the risk of COPD.

The same researchers from the Harvard School of Public Health (Varraso *et al.* 2007) studied lung function and chronic obstructive pulmonary disease (COPD) and diet among 72,043 women between 1984 and 2000 in the Nurses' Health Study. Diets that had more fruit, vegetables, fish and whole-grain products reduced the risk of COPD by 25%, while a diet heavy in refined grains, cured and red meats, desserts and French fries increased the risk of COPD by 31%.

Researchers from Spain's University of Murcia (Garcia-Marcos *et al.* 2007) examined the effects of diet on asthma in 106 six and seven year-old children. Utilizing a Mediterranean diet score along with a survey of symptoms, they found that eating a predominantly Mediterranean diet decreased severe asthma symptoms among the girls. Diets high in cereal grains produced 46% lower incidence of severe asthma. Frequent fruit eating decreased rhinoconjunctivitis incidence by 24%. In contrast, diets higher in fast foods produced 64% greater incidence of severe asthma.

Meanwhile, research from the National Center for Chronic Disease and Prevention (Cory *et al.* 2010) indicated that only 11-30% of adult Americans eat the recommended amounts of fruits and vegetables—some of the lowest levels in the world.

Nutrition scientists from Korea's Kyung Hee University (Oh *et al.* 2010) studied the relationship between allergies, asthma and antioxidants. They found by testing 180 allergic and 242 non-allergic Korean children that higher serum levels of beta-carotene, dietary vitamin E, iron and folic acid were associated with lower incidence of atopic reactions among the children. These antioxidant nutrients are derived primarily from plant-based foods.

Many other studies have shown these associations between diet and asthma. Researchers from the Allergy and Respiratory Research Group Center for Population Health Sciences at the University of Edinburgh's Medical School (Nurmatov *et al.* 2010) analyzed 62 international asthma studies for control protocols and study design. They found that 17 of 22 well-designed studies that compared dietary fruit and vegetable intake with asthma showed that higher fruit and vegetables in the diet lowered asthma incidence.

Their analyses found that asthmatic children had significantly lower levels of vitamin A; and that greater levels of vitamin D, vitamin E and zinc was *"protective for the development of wheezing outcomes."*

The researchers concluded that adequate intake of antioxidant vitamins including vitamins A, C, and E were critical to reducing free radicals and inflammatory abnormalities. They also determined that antioxidants are able to reduce damage from incoming bacteria, viruses, toxins and xenobiotics (pollutants to the body). The researchers referenced a number of other studies that successfully associated oxidative stress with bronchial inflammation and subsequent asthma development.

Researchers from Italy's University G. D'Annunzio Chieti (Riccioni and D'Orazio 2005) discovered in their research that persistent asthma is linked to an increase in reactive oxygen species. Their research also found that antioxidant nutrients such as selenium, zinc and other antioxidant vitamins have the potential to help reduce asthma symptoms and severity.

Yes, many of these studies focused on asthma, allergies and other airway issues. But as we illustrated earlier, GERD and asthma are specifically linked in the research. People with asthma more likely have GERD and vice versa.

We also showed other research that found fatty diets were linked with GERD. Since fatty diets are linked with both GERD and asthma, and GERD is associated with asthma, these studies confirm over and over the link between certain diets and GERD.

We can also conclude from this research that consuming a predominantly plant-based diet (such as the Mediterranean diet), has clear results: It is linked with reduced incidence of GERD, allergies and other airway conditions. All of these conditions are connected to healthy mucosal membranes, because the airways, sinuses and esophagus are all similarly protected by mucosal secretions.

Anti-GERD Diet Strategies

Noting this research, we can see that a diet with plenty of plant-based foods, whether it be the Mediterranean diet, a vegetarian diet, vegan diet, a raw food diet or simply a diet with more fresh fruits, vegetables, seeds and nuts will help promote healthy mucosal secretions. In addition to this, foods that add to our body's probiotic colonies and/or nourish those probiotics (probiotics) within our digestive tracts will also help our mucosal health.

Foods to consider along these lines would be:

✓ Whole grain pastas, rice, potatoes and other complex carbohydrates (have been shown to reduce acidity and increase stomach emptying)

✓ Plant-based proteins such as nuts, beans, greens and (cultured only) dairy

✓ Unrefined oils with a healthy balance of omega-3 fats (see below)

✓ Foods cultured or fermented with probiotic microorganisms, whether with probiotic yeasts or probiotic bacteria

✓ Sprouted grains or beans

✓ Plant-based foods harvested whole and prepared as whole foods, with minimal cooking and processing

✓ Fresh fruits, especially those with seeds and peels.

On the last point, citrus peels have been shown to stimulate mucosal membrane health. Peels of citrus can be eaten by shaving the outer peel but leaving the bulk of the inner peel intact.

The Role of Fats, Calories and Volume

Remember the significant research mentioned earlier that illustrated that eating high fat meals—especially fried foods—dramatically increased the risk of GERD. This must also mean that we'll immediately feel better when we cut back on the fats in our meals, right? Not so fast.

Medical researchers from Italy's University of Milan (Colombo *et al.* 2002) compared the effects of high calorie diets versus high fat diets on reflux symptoms.

They tested thirteen young healthy adults with pH monitoring for three hours after meals. On separate days, they gave the subjects a meal with high fat content (56% fat), "balanced" fat content (23% fat) or a "balanced" low calorie meal with 25% fat.

They found that the pH in the esophagus was significantly lower after the low calorie meal as compared with the fatty meals. But they found little different in stomach pH levels and the acid clearance between the high fat meals and the low fat meals. They concluded that, "advice on dietary habits in patients with gastroesophageal reflux disease should be concentrated on decreasing the caloric load of meals rather than their fat content."

German researchers (Pehl *et al.* 1999) at Munich's Academic Teaching Hospital confirmed this in a study of 12 GERD sufferers, showing that reducing fats in a meal did little to curb immediate GERD symptoms.

It must be noted that the protocols of these studies did not go beyond the three hour period following each meal. There were no long term parameters gauged whatsoever.

These studies might sound contradictory with the previous research clearly showing that diets high in fats and fried foods increased GERD incidence. As anyone who does not suffer from GERD knows, a few fatty meals won't cause GERD, and not eating a fatty meal will necessarily relieve their GERD symptoms. In other words, the process is more gradual, and a specific meal will not make a radical difference one way or another.

We might compare it to rocky cliffs that sit on the ocean's edge. As we watch the waves hitting a big rock, we get the feeling that the waves do not affect the rock. A wave hits the rock, and splashes far and wide. The rock, meanwhile, stands its ground solidly with no apparent change.

Yet over time, as waves continuously hit the rock over period of years, we find the rock will be bent and slimmed towards the direction of the waves over time.

In the same way, it took a lot of fatty, fried meals and other bad habits to wear away at our mucosal membranes. This process may have been helped by other factors, including COX-inhibiting pharmaceutical use, stress, dehydration and other things that helped thin our esophageal mucosal membranes. But even with these factors, the process is typically gradual and cumulative.

We say cumulative because this also depends upon the quantity of the exposure. In the rock and water example, we might suggest that if the water was filled with shards of metal, the wearing away of the rock will occur faster than with simple salt water. In the same way, GERD can erupt sooner when a combination of risk factors are "thrown" at it.

This works both ways. If the water that hits the rock not impact it with much force, the rock will change little, even over time. In the same way, if a person were to have a more lightweight penchant for eating fatty foods or other GERD risk factors, then they likely would either have very occasional heartburn or none at all.

Eating volume may stimulate GERD symptoms more immediately, however. This is simply because of the relationship between mechanical pressure on the lower sphincter and the amount of food in our meals.

Illustrating this, some of the same German researchers (Pehl *et al.* 2001) gave twelve healthy young adults solid and liquid meals with higher and lower calories, and tested the response on their esophageal pH and sphincter pressure.

They found that the calorie levels made little difference in sphincter pressure. They concluded that, "gastroesophageal reflux induced by ingestion of a meal seems to depend on the volume but not on the caloric density of a meal."

Fiber and Gastric Emptying

While fiber is essential to maintaining normal digestion and cholesterol levels, acute GERD symptoms can be worsened by eating certain types of fibers, such as guar gum (Harju and Larmi 1985). At the same time, fibers like pectin and cereal grains are important because they help balance the pH of our digestive tract as a whole. And research has found that fibers like pectin increases the emptying rate.

Researchers from Japan's Gunma University Medical School (Shimoyama *et al.* 2007) confirmed this in a study that tested 11 healthy volunteers after eating meals with high pectin levels. The researchers found that the stomach emptied faster after the pectin meal when compared to other meals. They concluded: "In healthy individuals, pectin increased the viscosity of enteral nutrition and accelerated gastric emptying."

This said, high-fiber meals sometimes will cause a GERD sufferer discomfort. The reason that high-fiber foods can exacerbate GERD symptoms is that some GERD sufferers do not produce enough enzymes, and this results in a slower emptying rate.

On the other hand, if enzymes are not the problem, then fiber—especially pectin—is critical to keeping the digestive system running well and maintained. If fiber is a problem, enzyme levels (see below) and slower eating should be looked at. We should also consider whether the fiber is being eaten with fatty foods—which together will slow digestion down.

We should remember that the stomach's emptying rate is also connected with the emptying rate of the intestines, and that is connected with movement through the colon. When the colon and intestines are moving slowly, the rate of emptying through the pyloric sphincter will slow stomach emptying.

The consumption of fiber directly effects the rate of intestinal and colon movement. This is why many people become constipated: Their intake of fiber is deficient. Fiber accelerates intestinal and colon movement.

Fiber is either soluble or insoluble. Both soluble and insoluble fibers are not assimilated. They both move through out intestinal tract, escorting waste, facilitating digestion, and balancing nutrient absorption. They eventually facilitate our bowel movements.

While soluble fiber becomes gelatinous in the presence of liquids, insoluble fiber passes through our small and large intestines without much change. Soluble fiber will bind with fats in the stomach, slowing down the process of absorption. This delays glucose absorption into the bloodstream, which means that it provides an evenly balanced stream of energy to the cells. For this reason, soluble fiber is good for regulating blood sugar in those who have blood sugar issues—either diabetic (hyper-) or hypoglycemic problems.

Soluble fiber also lowers levels of the "bad" forms of LDL cholesterol by rendering LDL particle size at more optimal levels. Soluble fiber is plentiful in oats, flax, vegetables, psyllium husk, and various other nuts, beans and grains. Apples are a great source as well.

Insoluble fiber facilitates the easier movement of food through our intestines. This means that insoluble fiber helps prevent constipation and helps eliminate toxicity in the colon due to its aiding regular, rhythmic bowel movements. It is like an escort service.

Insoluble fiber also helps balance the pH of the intestinal tract. This of course assists the survival and viability of the important probiotic colonies so important to the immune system. Sources of insoluble fiber include various whole wheats, whole oats, corn, green leafy vegetables (cellulose is an insoluble fiber), and various nuts, seeds, green beans and green peas. Apples are also a great source of insoluble fiber.

A typical adult should have at least 30-40 grams of total fiber per day, with about 75% of that fiber being insoluble. By focusing our eating on whole natural foods, we will likely get enough of both fibers. However, should our diet contain a sizeable portion of processed or convenient foods, we might consider measuring our fiber consumption periodically. If we have constipation, irritable bowels, or just a lack of regular bowel movements, a lack of insoluble fiber is probably a contributing factor.

Fiber is composed of a number of polysaccharides and oligosaccharides. These are utilized by plants for stability with some flexibility, allowing for circulation and the ability to stand tall against the elements. Plants also use dextrins, inulins, lignans, pectins, chitins, waxy substances, and beta-glucans to create their root, leave and stem structures. All of these bind to toxins in the intestines and lower low density lipoproteins.

The health of the colon is a critical part of the health of the entire body. The colon provides the body with the ability to eliminate waste products. Without good elimination, waste products will putrefy, possibly finding their way back into the bloodstream.

Lack of fiber in the diet also causes a build up of thickened plaque around the walls of the intestine and colon. There are a number of ailments that have been associated with this build up of plaque. Constipation is obvious, as the opening (or *lumen*) becomes constricted. Other issues not so obvious are sinusitis; allergies; GERD; asthma; bronchitis; back pain; liver and gall bladder problems; skin issues like psoriasis and eczema; chronic fatigue and food sensitivities. Other disorders are worsened by or connected to this build up of mucoid plaque in the colon.

GERD-Friendly Fats

The types of fats we eat directly nourish our mucosal membranes and the cell membranes of our cells—including those cells that make up our epithelial layers and sphincters. The types of fats we eat also either increase or decrease our body's tendency for inflammation.

The fat balance of our diet is critical to our cell membranes and our mucosal systems because our these membranes are made of different lipids and lipid-derivatives like phospholipids and glycolipids.

An imbalanced fat diet therefore can lead to weak cell membranes. The cell membrane in a poor fat diet is more susceptible to oxidative radicals.

Good fats impact our mucosal membranes because they bond easily with phosphates and glycogen molecules to form durable phospholipids and glycolipids, creating more stability amongst our mucosal membranes.

This stability relates to the molecular bonds within the fat molecule—whether the bonds between the carbons and hydrogens are saturated or unsaturated.

Researchers from Germany's University of Regensburg (Schmitz and Ecker 2008) studied the relationship between polyunsaturated fatty acids and the body's mucous membranes. They concluded that both omega-6s and omega-3s stimulate receptors and signalling molecules at the genetic level, which influence inflammation. However, the omega-6s stimulate pro-inflammatory effects and omega-3s stimulate anti-inflammatory effects.

When these two fats—omega-3s and omega-6s—maintain a particular proportion, the create equilibrium amongst the body's membranes. When the omega-6s dominate, the mucous membranes are more sensitive, and more easily triggered. The predominant n-6 fatty acid is arachidonic acid, which is converted to prostaglandins, leukotrienes and other lipoxygenase or cyclooxygenase products."

Their research went on to classify the pro-inflammatory mediators that are stimulated by the over-availability of omega-6 fatty acids. These include NFkappaB, PPAR and SREBP-1c. These three regulate inflammation and fat metabolism within the cells and the mucosal membranes. They added that the balance of omega fatty acids also dictates the longevity and health of each cell.

Here is a quick review of the major fatty acids and the foods they come from:

Major Omega-3 Fatty Acids (EFAs)

Acronym	Fatty Acid Name	Major Dietary Sources
ALA	Alpha-linolenic acid	Walnuts, soybeans, flax, canola, pumpkin seeds, chia seeds
SDA	Stearidonic acid	hemp, spirulina, blackcurrant
DHA	Docosahexaenoic acid	Body converts from ALA; also obtained from certain algae, krill and fish oils
EPA	Eicosapentaenoic acid	Converts in the body from DHA

Major Omega-6 Fatty Acids (EFAs)

Acronym	Fatty Acid Name	Major Dietary Sources
LA	Linoleic acid	Many plants, safflower, sunflower, sesame, soy, almond especially
ARA	Arachidonic acid	Meats, salmon
PA	Palmitoleic acid	Macadamia, palm kernel, coconut
GLA	Gamma-linolenic acid	Borage, primrose oil, spirulina

Major Omega-9 Fatty Acids

Acronym	Fatty Acid Name	Major Dietary Sources
EA	Eucic acid	Canola, mustard seed, wallflower
OA	Oleic acid	Sunflower, olive, safflower
PA	Palmitoleic acid	Macadamia, palm kernel, coconut

Major Saturated Fatty Acids

Acronym	Fatty Acid Name	Major Dietary Sources
Lauric	Lauric acid	Coconut, dairy, nuts
Myristic	Myristic acid	Coconut, butter
Palmitic	Palmitic acid	Macadamia, palm kernel, coconut, butter, beef, eggs
Stearic	Stearic acid	Macadamia, palm kernel, coconut, eggs

Essential fatty acids (EFAs) are fats the body does not form. Eaten in the right proportion, they can also lower inflammation and speed healing. EFAs include the long-chain polyunsaturated fatty acids—and the shorter chain linolenic, linoleic and oleic polyunsaturates. EFAs include omega-3s and omega-6s. The omega-3s include alpha linolenic acid (ALA), docosahexaenoic acid (DHA) and eicosapentaenoic acid (EPA). EPA and DHA are found in algae, mackerel, salmon, herring, sardines, sablefish (black cod). The omega-6s include linoleic acid, (LA), palmitoleic acid (PA), gamma-linoleic acid (GLA) and arachidonic acid (ARA). The term *essential* was originally given with the assumption that these types of fats could not be assembled or produced by the body—they must be taken directly from our food supply.

This assumption, however, is not fully correct. While it is true that we need *some* of these from our diet, our bodies can readily convert LA to ARA, and ALA to DHA and EPA as needed. Therefore, these fats can be considered essential in the sense that they are not generated by the body, but we do not necessarily have to consume each one of them.

Monounsaturated fats are high in omega-9 fatty acids like oleic acid. A monounsaturated fatty acid has one double carbon-hydrogen bonding chain. Oils from seeds, nuts and other plant-based sources have the largest quantities of monounsaturates. Oils that have large proportions of monounsaturates such as olive oil are known to lower inflammation when replacing high saturated fat in diets. Monounsaturates also aid in skin cell health and reduce atopic skin responses.

Monounsaturated fatty acids like oleic acid have been shown in studies to lower heart attack risk, aid blood vessel health, and offer anti-carcinogenic potential. They are typical among Mediterranean diets, which have been shown to reduce heart disease risk and cancer risk—related to their lower levels of lipid peroxidative radicals. The best sources of omega-9s are olives, sesame seeds, avocados, almonds, peanuts, pecans, pistachio nuts, cashews, hazelnuts, macadamia nuts, several other nuts and their respective oils.

Polyunsaturated fats have at least two double carbon-hydrogen bonds. They come from a variety of plant and marine sources. Omega-3s ALA, DHA and EPA simply have longer chains with more double carbon-hydrogen bonds. ALA, DHA and EPA are known to lower inflammation and increase artery-wall health. These *long-chain* omega-3 polyunsaturates are also considered critical for intestinal health.

The omega-6 fatty acids are the most available form of fat in the plant kingdom. Linoleic acid is the primary omega-6 fatty acid and it is found in most grains and seeds.

Saturated fats have multiple fatty acids without double bonds (the hydrogens "saturate" the carbons). They are found among animal fats, and tropical oils such as coconut and palm. Milk products such as butter and whole milk contain saturated fats, along with a special type of healthy linoleic fatty acid called CLA or *conjugated linoleic acid*.

The saturated fats from coconuts and palm differ from animal saturates in that they have shorter chains. This actually gives them—unlike animal saturates—an antimicrobial quality.

Medium chain fatty acids like coconut and palm oils have been shown in human studies to lower lipoprotein-A concentrations in the blood while having fibrinolytic (plaque and clot reduction) effects (Muller *et al.* 2003).

Trans fats are oils that either have been overheated or have undergone hydrogenation. Hydrogenation is produced by heating while bubbling hydrogen ions through the oil. This adds hydrogen and repositions some of the bonds. The "trans" refers to the positioning of part of the molecule in reverse—as opposed to "cis" positioning. The cis positioning is the bonding orientation the body's cell membranes work best with. Trans fats have been known to be a cause for increased radical species in the system; damaging artery walls; contributing to inflammation, heart disease, high LDL levels, liver damage, diabetes, and other metabolic dysfunction (Mozaffarian *et al.* 2009). Trans fat overconsumption slows the conversion of LA to GLA.

Conjugated linolenic acid (CLA) is a healthy fat that comes from primarily from dairy products. CLA is also a trans fat, but this is a trans fat the body works well with—it is considered a healthy trans fat.

Researchers from St Paul's Hospital and the University of British Columbia (MacRedmond *et al.* 2010) gave 28 overweight adults 4.5 g/day of CLA or a placebo for 12 weeks in addition to their medications. After the twelve weeks, those in the CLA group experienced significantly better lung function compared to the placebo group. The CLA group also experienced a significant reduction of weight and BMI compared with the control group. The CLA group also had lower leptin/adiponectin ratios—associated with balanced metabolism.

Other research has also found that CLA can to reduce lipid peroxidation and provide better balance among lipids (Noone *et al.* 2002).

Arachidonic acid (ARA): ARA is considered an essential fatty acid, and research has shown that it is vital for infants while they are building their intestinal barriers. However, ARA is pro-inflammatory and stimulates pro-inflammatory mediators like leukotrienes. Too much of it as we age thus burdens our immune systems, pushing our bodies towards systemic inflammation and slower detoxification.

Red meats provide the highest levels of arachidonic acid. Because arachidonic acid stimulates the production of pro-inflammatory prostaglandins and leucotrienes in an enzyme conversion process, too much ARA leads to a greater level of toxicity, producing more inflammation.

Interestingly, carnivorous animals cannot or do not readily convert linoleic acid (found in many common plants) to arachidonic acid, but herbivore animals do convert linoleic acid to arachidonic acid, as do humans. This conversion—on top of a red meat-heavy diet—produces high arachidonic acid levels. In contrast, a diet that is balanced between plant-based monounsaturates, polyunsaturates and some saturates (such as the Mediterranean diet) will balance arachidonic acids with the other fatty acids.

Gamma linoleic acid (GLA): A wealth of studies have confirmed that GLA reduces or inhibits the inflammatory response. Leukotrienes produced by arachidonic acid stimulate inflammation, while leukotrienes produced by GLA block the conversion of polyunsaturated fatty acids to arachidonic acid. This means that GLA lowers inflammation, and promotes a healthy immune system.

A healthy body will convert linoleic acid into GLA readily, utilizing the same delta-6 desaturase enzyme used for ALA to DHA conversion. From GLA, the body produces *dihomo-gamma linoleic acid,* which cycles through the body as an eicosinoid. This aids in skin health, healthy mucosal membranes, and down-regulates inflammatory hypersensitivity.

In addition to conversion from LA, GLA can also be obtained from the oils of borage seeds, evening primrose seed, hemp seed, and from spirulina. Excellent food sources of LA include chia seeds, seed, hempseed, grapeseed, pumpkin seeds, sunflower seeds, safflower seeds, soybeans, olives, pine nuts, pistachio nuts, peanuts, almonds, cashews, chestnuts, and their respective oils.

The conversion of LA to GLA (and ALA to DHA) is reduced by trans fat consumption, smoking, pollution, stress, infections, and various chemicals that affect the liver.

Docosahexaenoic acid (DHA) obtained from algae, fish and krill, has significant therapeutic and anti-inflammatory effects according to the research. DHA is also associated with stronger cell membranes, and lower levels of lipid peroxidation.

It appears that the anti-inflammatory effects of DHA in particular relate to a modulation of a gene factor called NF-kappaB. The NF-kappaB is involved in signaling among cytokine receptors. With more DHA consumption, the transcription of the NF-kappaB gene sequence is reduced. This appears to reduce inflammatory signaling (Singer *et al.* 2008).

DHA readily converts to EPA by the body. EPA degrades quickly if unused in the body. It is easily converted from DHA as needed. Our bodies store DHA and not EPA.

Because much of the early research on the link between fatty acids and inflammatory disease was performed using fish oil, it was assumed that both EPA and DHA fatty acids reduced inflammation. Recent research from the University of Texas' Department of Medicine/Division of Clinical Immunology and Rheumatology (Rahman *et al.* 2008) has clarified that DHA is primarily implicated in reducing inflammation. DHA was shown to inhibit RANKL-induced pro-inflammatory cytokines, and a number of inflammation steps, while EPA did not.

The process of converting ALA to DHA and other omega-3s requires an enzyme produced in the liver called delta-6 desaturase. Some people—especially those who have a poor diet, are immune-suppressed, or burdened with toxicity such as cigarette smoke—may not produce this enzyme very well. As a result, they may not convert as much ALA to DHA and EPA.

For those with low levels of DHA—or for those with problems converting ALA and DHA—low-environmental impact and low toxin content DHA from microalgae can be supplemented. Certain algae produce significant amounts of DHA. They are the foundation for the DHA molecule all the way up the food chain, including fish. This is how fish get their DHA, in other words. Three algae species—*Crypthecodinium cohnii*, *Nitzschia laevis* and *Schizochytrium spp.*—are in commercial production and available in oil and capsule form.

Microalgae-derived DHA is preferable to fish or fish oils because fish oils typically contain saturated fats and may also—depending upon their origin—contain toxins such as mercury and PCBs (though to their credit, many producers also carefully distill their fish oil). However, we should note that salmon contain a considerable amount of arachidonic acid as well (Chilton 2006).

Thus, the DHA derived from fish sources, because it requires increased levels of filtering and processing to remove PCBs and mercury, would not be considered a living source of DHA, as it is too far removed from the living source. Algae-derived DHA is a wholesome source, as it is derived directly from living algae. Algae-derived DHA also does not strain sensitive fishery populations.

Algal-DHA also decreases pro-inflammatory arachidonic acid levels. One study (Arterburn *et al*. 2007) measured pro-inflammatory arachidonic acid levels within the body before and after supplementation with algal DHA. It was found that arachidonic acid levels decreased by 20% following just one dose of 100 milligrams of algal DHA.

For those who consider fish the superior source of DHA: In a study by researchers from The Netherlands' Wageningen University Toxicology Research Center (van Beelen *et al*. 2007), all three species of commercially produced algal oil showed equivalency with fish oil in their inhibition of cancer cell growth. Another study (Lloyd-Still *et al*. 2007) of twenty cystic fibrosis patients concluded that 50 milligrams of algal DHA was readily absorbed, maintained DHA bioavailability immediately, and increased circulating DHA levels by four to five times.

In terms of DHA availability, algal-DHA is just as good as fish. In a randomized open-label study (Arterburn *et al*. 2008), researchers gave 32 healthy men and women either algal DHA oil or cooked salmon for two weeks. After the two weeks, plasma levels of circulating DHA were bioequivalent.

Alpha-linolenic acid (ALA) is the primary omega-3 fatty acid the body can most easily assimilate. Once assimilated, the healthy body will convert ALA to omega-3s, primarily DHA, at a range of about 7-40%, depending upon the health of the liver. One study of six women performed at England's University of Southampton (Burdge *et al*. 2002) showed a conversion rate of 36% from ALA to

203

DHA and other omega-3s. A follow-up study of men showed ALA conversion to the omega-3s occurred at an average of 16%.

We should include that ALA, which comes from plants, has been shown to halt or slow inflammation processes, similar to DHA. In studies at Wake Forest University (Chilton *et al.* 2008), for example, flaxseed oil produced anti-inflammatory effects, along with borage oil and echium oil (the latter two also containing GLA).

Furthermore, flaxseed has been recommended specifically for toxicity and inflammation for centuries. This is not only because of its omega-3 levels: it is also because flaxseed contains mucilage, which helps strengthen our mucosal membranes. An infusion (tea) made of flaxseed has thus been recommended with great success by numerous traditional physicians over the centuries.

The healthy fat balance: In a meta-study by researchers from the University of Crete's School of Medicine (Margioris 2009), numerous studies showed that long-chain polyunsaturated omega-3s tend to be anti-inflammatory while omega-6 oils tend to be pro-inflammatory.

This simplifies the equation too much. Most fat research has also shown that most omega-6s are healthy oils. Balance is the key.

Research has illustrated that reducing animal-derived saturated fats reduces inflammation, cardiovascular disease, high cholesterol and diabetes (Ros and Mataix 2008). All of these relate to toxicity, because as we've discussed, lipid peroxidation lies at the root of these conditions.

The relationships became clearer from a study performed at Sydney's Heart Research Institute (Nicholls *et al.* 2008). Here fourteen adults consumed meals either rich in saturated fats or omega-6 polyunsaturated fats. They were tested following each meal for various inflammation and cholesterol markers. The results showed that the high saturated fat meals increased inflammatory activities and decreased the liver's production of HDL cholesterol; whereas (good) HDL levels and the liver's anti-inflammatory capacity were increased after the omega-6 meals.

What this tells us is that the omega-3/omega-6 story is complicated by the saturated fat content of the diet and subsequent liver function. High saturated fat diets increase (bad) LDL (lipid peroxidation) content and reduce the anti-inflammatory and antioxidant capacities of the liver. Diets lower in saturated fat and higher in omega-6 and omega-3 fats encourage antioxidant and anti-inflammatory activity.

We also know that diets high in monounsaturated fats—such as the Mediterranean diet—are also associated with significant anti-inflammatory effects. Mediterranean diets contain higher levels of monounsaturated fats like oleic acids (omega-9) from foods like olives and avocados (and their oils); as well as higher proportions of fruits and vegetables, and lower proportions of saturated fats.

High saturated fat diets are also associated with increased obesity, and a number of studies have shown that obesity is directly related to inflammatory diseases—including allergies as we've discussed. High saturated fat diets and diets high in trans fatty acids have also been clearly shown to accompany higher levels of inflammation—illustrated by increases in inflammatory factors such as IL-6 and CRP (Basu *et al.* 2006).

To maximize anti-inflammatory factors, the ideal proportion of omega-6s to omega-3s is recommended at about two to one (2:1). The western diet has been estimated by researchers to up to thirty to one (30:1) of omega-6s to omega-3s. This large imbalance (of too much omega-6s and too little omega-3s) has also been associated with inflammatory diseases, including asthma, arthritis, heart disease, ulcerative colitis, Crohn's disease, and others. When fat consumption is out of balance, the body's metabolism will trend towards inflammation. This is because in the absence of omega-3s and GLA, omega-6 oils convert more easily to arachidonic acid. And remember, ARA is pro-inflammatory (Simopoulos 1999).

Noting the research showing the relationships between the different fatty acids and inflammation, and the condition of the liver (which can be burdened by too much saturated fat), scientists have logically arrived at a model for dietary fat consumption for a person who is either dealing with or wants to prevent inflammation-oriented conditions and toxicity:

Omega-3	20%-25% of dietary fats
Omega-6+Omega-9	40%-50% of dietary fats
Saturated	5%-10% of dietary fats
GLA	10%-20% of dietary fats
Trans fats	0% of dietary fats

Nuts, seeds, grains, beans, olives and avocados can provide the bulk of these healthy fats in balanced combinations. Walnuts, pumpkin seeds, flax, chia, soy, canola and algal-DHA can fill in the omega 3s. Healthy saturated fats can be found in coconuts, palm and dairy products. These foods are typical of the Mediterranean diet.

Cabbage

Cabbage has been used for centuries among traditional medicines to curb stomach upset, ulcers and reflux symptoms. Cabbage contains a unique constituent, s-methylmethionine, also referred to as vitamin U. Through a pathway utilizing one of the body's natural enzymes, called Bhmt2, s-methylmethionine is converted to methionine and then to glutathione in several steps.

In this form, glutathione has been shown to stimulate the repair of the mucosal membranes within the stomach, intestines and airways. Glutathione has also been shown to increase the health and productivity of the liver.

Raw cabbage or cabbage juice has been used as a healing agent for ulcers and intestinal issues for thousands of years among traditional medicines, including those of Egyptian, Ayurvedic and Greek systems. The Western world became aware of raw cabbage juice in the 1950s, when Garnett Cheney, M.D. conducted several studies showing that methylmethionine-rich cabbage juice concentrate was able to reduce the pain and bleeding associated with ulcers.

In one of Dr. Cheney's studies, 37 ulcer patients were treated with either cabbage juice concentrate or a placebo. Of the 26-patient cabbage juice group, 24 patients were considered "successes"—achieving an astounding 92% success rate.

Medical researchers from Iraq's University Department of Surgery (Salim 1993) conducted a double-blind study of 172 patients who suffered from gastric bleeding caused by nonsteroidal anti-inflammatory drugs (NSAIDs). They gave the patients either cysteine, methylmethionine sulfonium chloride (MMSC) or a placebo. Those receiving either the cysteine or the MMSC stopped bleeding. Their conditions became *"stable"* as compared with many in the control group, who continued to bleed.

Plants use s-methylmethionine to help heal cell membrane damage among their leaves and stems. This is reminiscent of antioxidants: Plants produce antioxidants to help to protect them from damage from the sun, insects and diseases. In other words, the very same biochemicals that protect plants also help heal our bodies.

Note that MMSC or cabbage juice does not inhibit the flow of gastric juices in the stomach to produce these effects as do acid blocking medications. Rather, they stimulate the body's natural production of mucous membranes, which serve to protect the esophagus epithelia from the effects of acids, toxins and microorganisms.

Raw Vinegars

Vinegars are quite acidic, so they can be extremely helpful to someone with low stomach acidity, or non-acid reflux. For someone with high acidity GERD, vinegar should be used with caution, and combined with alkaline foods.

Remember that if we have low stomach acidity, our GERD may be the result of our stomach emptying rate being so slow that food is backing up into our esophagus—likely made worse by a problematic lower sphincter.

There are a variety of different types of vinegars, depending upon the raw material used. In all cases, the raw material of a healthy vinegar will be a plant source, fermented by a healthy yeast culture. The yeast culture will convert the sugars of the plant source (and added sugars if used) to alcohol. As the alcohol is fermented further, it is oxidized by the zymase enzymes in the yeast, which convert to alcohol to carboxylic acetic acids. These acetic acids are the main constituent of vinegar, and what gives vinegar its tartness.

To speed up the process, alcohols are often used commercially to make vinegars. These include cheaper or turned wines, distilled alcohol (from wood or grain) and other spirits. The conversion of alcohol to vinegar is much quicker because the first step (sugar to alcohol) has already been made.

Raw vinegar made from apples, grapes or other fruits is suggested, as they will contain a variety of antioxidants, as well as acetic acid, which helps stimulate a good environment for our body's own probiotics, and one that repels pathogenic microorganisms.

207

Vinegar can also encourage our parietal cells to produce normal levels of acidity, assuming our acid levels are low—which is the case for many GERD sufferers as we've discussed. If a little vinegar with a meal increase GERD symptoms, then it should be avoided. But if it helps, we should consider adding more to our meals, up to two or three tablespoons.

Vinegar can be used in salads, for pickling vegetables and other creative recipes. It can also simply be taken by the teaspoon but this is to be avoided by acidic reflux sufferers. Raw apple cider vinegar is considered by many as the most healthy vinegar currently available.

Bananas

Several studies have shown that bananas are helpful for both ulcer sufferers and GERD sufferers. Some have called banana a natural antacid—yet its effects are much more complex than that.

Banana contains a number of important minerals, including potassium. Potassium is an electrolyte that is important to the health of our mucosal membranes. Bananas also contain protease inhibitors, which apparently inhibit *H. pylori* and other bacteria growth in the gut. In addition, bananas contain sitoindoside-IV, which stimulates mucosal membrane health.

In addition, bananas contain the prebiotic FOS, which feeds our probiotic populations. As these feed and grow, they inhibit *H. pylori* and others, as we've shown earlier.

While ripe bananas have these effects, unripe bananas and unripe plantains seem to have more of these compounds at their peak availability.

(Goel *et al.* 2001; Prabha *et al.* 2011; Sumona *et al.* 2009; Agarwal *et al.* 2009; Lewis *et al.* 1999)

Anti-GERD Recipes:

Here are several general recipes to help heal the esophageal sphincters and epithelial walls of the esophagus:

> ➢ *Smoothies:* Drinking our fruits and even vegetables, together with kefir or yogurt takes pressure off the sphincters because the food is already masticated, and thus more readily digested. Fruits and berries with seeds such as strawberries and raspberries, along with bananas, are wonderful smoothie ingredients.

➢ *Raw vegetable juices:* Juiced endive, celery and carrots. These feed us with readily-available nutrients that stimulate our immune system and alkalize our blood. Cucumbers are particularly good for the mucosal membranes. Remember, though, that much of the good fiber is left behind in juicing. Blending our vegetables into a smoothie is a better method.

➢ *Super soup:* Barley, lentils celery, carrots, beets and ginger. These also provide significant pH balancing effects. Lentils are a traditional favorite to help soothe heartburn.

➢ *Miso soup:* Miso provides a fermented form of soybeans that soothes and helps clear our mucous membranes. This remedy has been a long-time favorite among Asian countries.

➢ *Turmeric curry dishes:* Ayurvedic cooking provides many traditional dishes steeped in spices that stimulate the immune system and provide antioxidants. Some may be too spicy for comfort. Turmeric is likely an exception, because of its ability to stimulate the submucosal glands.

➢ *Salsa with chilies:* Conventional medicine assumed that chilies were too spicy for GERD sufferers. This has proved quite the opposite. Chilies increase mucosal integrity and help remove *H. pylori* and other infections. A healthy chili salsa can include both green and red chilies. Don't forget the cilantro—a great blood purifier.

➢ *Yogurt with every dish:* Fresh yogurt is an excellent ingredient that can replace mayonnaise, butter, cream, milk and other dairy products that can slow down stomach emptying. To the contrary, live yogurt contains probiotics that speed along gastric emptying. They also nurture the esophagus epithelia and mucosal membranes. Yogurt is great on salads and as a side to practically any meal.

How Raw, Fresh Foods help GERD

One of the most important losses from food pasteurization is its enzyme content. Most foods contain a variety of enzymes that aid in the assimilation or catalyzing of nutrients and antioxidants.

These include xanthenes, lysozymes, lipases, oxidases, amylases, lactoferrins and many others contained in raw foods. The body uses food enzymes in various ways. Some enzymes, such as papain from papaya and bromelain from pineapples, aid digestion, speed gastric emptying, and even dissolve artery plaque and reduce inflammation.

While the body makes many of its own enzymes, it also absorbs many food enzymes or uses their components to make new ones. We'll discuss enzymes in more detail later.

Pasteurization also typically leaves the food or beverage with a residual caramelized flavor due to the conversation of the enzymes, flavonoids and sugars to denatured compounds. These can slow digestion, as they are more difficult for the body to break down. In milk, for example, there is a substantial conversion from lactose to lactulose (and caramelization) after UHT pasteurization. Lactulose can cause intestinal cramping, nausea and vomiting.

In the case of pasteurized juices, pasteurization can leave the beverage in a highly acidic state, which can irritate our mucous membranes, epithelial cells and sphincters, and in general increase the acid level of these regions.

As for irradiation, there is little research on the resulting nutrient content outside of a few microwave studies (which showed decreased nutrient content and the formation of undesirable metabolites). There is good reason to believe that irradiation may denature some nutrients.

Whole foods in nature's packages are significantly different from pasteurized processed foods. Fresh whole foods produced by plants contain various antioxidants and enzymes that reduce the ability of microorganisms to grow. The Creator also provided whole foods with peels and shells that protect nutrients and keep most microorganisms out. Microorganisms may invade the outer shell or peel somewhat, but the peel's pH, dryness and density—together with the pH of the inner fruit—provide extremely effective barriers to microorganisms and oxidation.

For this reason, most fruits and nuts can be easily stored for days and even weeks without having significant nutrient reduction. Once the peel or shell is removed, the inner fruit, juice or nut must be consumed to prevent oxidation and contamination—depending upon its pH and sugar content.

Whole natural foods also contain polysaccharides and oligosaccharides that combine nutrients and sugar within complex fibers. Fiber is important for gastric emptying. These combinations also help prevent oxidation and pathogenic bacteria colonization.

With heat processing, the complex sugars of natural foods are broken down into more simplified, refined form, which promotes *H. pylori* and *Candida* growth. Why? Because simple sugars provide convenient energy sources for these aggressive bacteria and fungi colonies. By contrast, our probiotics are used to eating the complexed oligosaccharides in fibrous foods. In other words, heat-processing produces the perfect foods for increased pathogenic microorganism colonization.

Anti-GERD Nutrients

Most of the research points to a diet of whole foods and nutrients. However, two studies have shown that a few key nutrients seem to greatly benefit GERD sufferers.

In the first, pharmacy research from Brazil's Estadual da Paraíba University (Pereira 2006) gave 176 patients with GERD a regimen of supplements; and they treated another matched group of 177 GERD patients with 20 milligrams per day of the pharmaceutical omeprazole.

The supplement blend included:

- **melatonin**
- **tryptophan**
- **vitamin B6**
- **folic acid**
- **vitamin B12**
- **methionine**
- **betaine**

After forty days of treatment, every patient in the group given the supplement regimen (that is, 100%) reported that their reflux symptoms were gone. Meanwhile 115 patients (out of 177) of the omeprazole group reported their symptoms were gone after 40 days of treatment. This means the supplements had 100% success versus 66% treatment success of omeprazole. The supplement group reported no side effects from the supplement treatment (refer to first chapter for omeprazole's known side effects.)

In a clinical application, leading nutrition researcher and physician Melvyn Werbach, M.D., treated a patient with chronic GERD who was taking PPIs and wanted off the meds. The patient was given the following cocktail of nutrients:

- melatonin 6 mg
- 5-hydroxytryptophan 100 mg
- D,L-methionine 500 mg
- betaine 100 mg
- L-taurine 50 mg
- riboflavin 1.7 mg
- vitamin B6 0.8 mg
- folic acid 400 micrograms
- calcium 50 mg

After 40 days on the supplements, the PPIs were able to be withdrawn, and the patient's GERD symptoms completely subsided.

During a ten month follow-up, Dr. Werbach was able to gradually reduce all the nutrients, except for melatonin, which could not be reduced below 3 milligrams without symptoms. This is primarily because endogenous melatonin production can slow down when it is supplemented over a long periods.

The patient continued to show no GERD symptoms throughout the withdrawal (Werbach 2008).

While Dr. Werbach's treatment followed only one case, the supplement list mirrored the supplements in the Brazilian study, which showed effectiveness among 176 GERD patients. And the follow up by Dr. Werbach illustrates that these nutrients have more than simply a treatment effect: They also have a therapeutic effect upon the GERD sufferer.

The Brazilian research was also confirmed by previous studies—which found that melatonin has a dual effect: 1) It moderates acidic pH and; 2) stimulates the formation of nitric oxide. Nitric oxide relaxes the lower esophageal sphincter, allowing it to function more mechanically correct.

Additional research has also found that melatonin helps protect against damage to the esophageal region, and is a primary ingredient within the digestive mucosal membranes. This means that its effects do not slow important gastric secretions as much as it helps promote mucosal secretions.

The Brazilian researchers characterized the other supplements given as having "anti-inflammatory and analgesic effects." They concluded that the "formulation promotes regression of GERD symptoms with no significant side effects."

While most of these nutrients are available from a diet rich in plant-based foods, melatonin is only available in a few foods, including dark sweet cherries.

However, we also know the body will produce more of its natural melatonin when the body is exposed to significant sunlight during the day, balanced by a gradual darkening of lights into the later evening, and of course, a good night's sleep. The body produces significant melatonin as we fall asleep, as melatonin slows down the body's metabolism.

This relates specifically, by the way, to stress—which has also been linked to GERD as we've discussed. When a person is stressed, they will produce less melatonin.

Melatonin is important to the health of the digestive tract in general. Without it, the intestinal cells become irritated and damaged.

In addition to these, there are nutrients that have been shown to directly or indirectly reduce inflammation and increase the integrity of the esophageal sphincters. Most of these are also available from whole foods:

Vitamin C is considered by researchers as one of the "first line of defense" antioxidants, because it is readily available to neutralize free radicals in mucosal membranes and tissue fluids. A number of studies have shown that vitamin C can reduce inflammation.

Vitamin C supplement doses aimed at reducing inflammation typically range from one to three grams per day. As mentioned, chelated versions and versions with bioflavonoids help the potency of vitamin C. Some health researchers have also noted that vitamin C and quercetin tend to work well together. This is why apples and onions are so healthy. Fruits and many vegetables offer readily-assimilable doses of vitamin C with bioflavonoids. Vitamin C drink powders with chelated ascorbates also provide a good way to supplement extra vitamin C.

Lycopene: This phytonutrient, usually isolated from tomatoes, has been shown in some research to reduce inflammation. Best approach here is to consume tomatoes, which have been found to contain about 10,000 different nutrients.

Beta-carotene and other Carotenoids: These vitamin A precursors are essential antioxidants often lacking in many diets. Some research has shown that carotenoids can reduce radical damage to the eyes and other organs. Carrots, tomatoes, and other orange- or red-colored foods contain carotenoids.

Vitamin E: Most people consider vitamin E a single nutrient. But there are actually at least eight forms of vitamin E. Four of them are tocopherols, which include alpha-tocopherol, beta-tocopherol, gamma-tocopherol, and delta-tocopherol. There are also four tocotrienol forms of vitamin E. This includes alpha-tocotrienol, beta-tocotrienol, gamma-tocotrienol, and delta-tocotrienol. The primary vitamin E form in most supplements is alpha-tocopherol.

Most of the research on vitamin E has utilized only alpha-tocopherols. Ongoing research has established that alpha-tocopherols do provide some benefits, but a mix of tocotrienols provide more benefit—especially with regard to cardiovascular health.

Diets can vary in terms of their vitamin E forms. Western diets are typically restricted to alpha-tocopherols and gamma-tocopherols. However, a mixed plant-based diet that includes coconut and palm foods, whole grain rice and other whole grains will render more of the tocotrienol forms.

The bottom line is that the E vitamins are essential antioxidants that help prevent lipid peroxidation—as discussed earlier.

Quercetin: This flavonoid inhibits histamine and leukotrienes—inflammatory mediators—in the body. High-quercetin foods include apples, onions, garlic and many herbs—although onions have been known to worsen GERD symptoms for some.

Vitamin Bs: All the vitamin Bs are important to the body's mucosal systems. They are most known for donating methyl groups, used by the liver and glutathione to scavenge free radicals. We should also note that toxins and pharmaceuticals will reduce our stores of Bs. Also, many people lack the intrinsic factor that allows for B vitamin—especially B12—assimilation. For these people, many doctors have advised B12 shots.

For those questioning their B12 intake, many probiotics produce B12 or useful B12 analogs. Spirulina also contains B12, as does yogurt, kefir and other fermented dairy products.

As far as supplementing goes, research has recently illustrated, however, that sublingual (under the tongue) B12 is absorbed just as readily into the blood as a B12 shot. There are several sublingual B vitamin supplements on the market today.

Hydrocloric Acid

The supplementation of hydrochloric acid (HCl) has been recommended by numerous natural physicians for well over a century. This is specifically suggested for those with hypochlorhydria, or low stomach acidity.

As we've discussed, low stomach acidity is often a result of infection by *H. pylori*. It can also be caused by a slowing metabolism, obesity, antacids and other possibilities.

The point of supplementing HCl is to encourage the acidic balance of the gut, which may or may not stimulate normal gastric secretion over time. Most clinicians who have prescribed this method have found that the parietal cells indeed do resume their production of gastric acids to normal levels with HCl supplementation.

To determine whether HCl is advisable, a pH test or Heidelberg gastric analysis can be performed. The Heidelberg analysis uses a capsule on a string as we described earlier.

Another possible test is to take a small amount of vinegar during a meal. If the vinegar eases the symptoms then low acidity should be considered. If the vinegar increases the burning sensation, this is likely too much acidity.

Assuming low acidity, the procedure is typically to start with one HCl dose of 300-600 milligrams (capsule) with a meal. If the symptoms increase or a warming of the gut is felt, then this dose is too high. If the symptoms decrease, then at the next meal, two capsules can be taken. This can be repeated to the next meal until the warming of the gut is felt. If the warming is felt in the gut, the dose is too much. The next meal can go back to the last dose assuming symptoms have decreased with the HCl.

Over time, the parietal cells may increase their acidic production and whatever dose we're at may cause the warming in the gut. The dose should be gradually decreased with the warming.

Minerals

Minerals are critical to our detoxification and cleansing processes because they donate ions that neutralize radicals, and are part of key enzymes. Without enough of these important minerals, the body's metabolic systems slow down, due to the lack of enzymes and ion donators.

Magnesium deficiency has been found to be at the root of a number of conditions, especially those related to anxiety, spasms and muscle cramping. Not surprisingly, inflammation can be significantly reduced with magnesium supplementation.

Magnesium, along with calcium, is critical for smooth muscle tone and nerve conduction. Magnesium is part of the calcium ion channel system. Magnesium regulates calcium infusion into the nerves, which helps keep them stabilized and balanced. This is why magnesium deficiencies within the calcium ion channel system causes overstrain among muscles. This translates to spasms, cramping and muscle fatigue.

If magnesium levels are low, the ion channels will be unstable, stimulating nerve hyperactivity. This nerve hyperactivity can cause changes in the flow of nutrients into cells and toxins out of cells. In other words, magnesium deficiency can result in toxemia.

Magnesium is also a critical element used by the immune system. A body deficient in magnesium will likely be immunosuppressed. Animal studies have illustrated that magnesium deficiency leads to increased IgE counts, and increased levels of inflammation-specific cytokines. Magnesium deficiency is also associated with increased degranulation among mast/basophil/neutrophil cells, which stimulates the allergic response.

Dr. Jabar from the State University of New York Hospital and Medical Center, notes the blood magnesium levels can help determine if magnesium supplements can help. Magnesium levels among red blood cells indicate whether magnesium will likely have any effects.

It is no surprise that magnesium has also been shown to benefit anxiety, as it helps balance nerve firing. For those of us with high levels of stress in our modern lives, magnesium can help neutralize our body's over-response to stress.

Magnesium has also been shown to have anti-inflammatory effects when combined with dosing with larger (one gram or more) doses of vitamin C.

Foods high in magnesium include soybeans, kidney beans, lima beans, bananas, broccoli, Brussels sprouts, carrots, cauliflower, celery, cherries, corn, dates, bran, blackberries, green beans, pumpkin seeds, spinach, chard, tofu, sunflower seeds, sesame seeds, black beans and navy beans, mineral water and beets.

Calcium, is also critical for the functioning of nerves and muscles. Every cell utilizes calcium, evidenced by calcium ion channels present in every cell membrane. Therefore, calcium is necessary for a healthy esophagus and mucosal membranes.

Muscle cramping and airway constriction can result from calcium deficiency. Low calcium levels also result in deranged nerve firing, which can accelerate anxiety and depression. Supplementing calcium should also be accompanied by magnesium supplementing. For example, a supplement with 1,000 mg of calcium can be balanced by 600 mg of magnesium along with trace minerals.

Foods provide the most assimilable forms of calcium. Good calcium foods include carrots, probiotic dairy, bok choy, collards, okra, soy, beans, broccoli, kale, mustard greens and others.

Zinc is another important mineral for toxemia. Researchers from Italy's INRAN National Research Institute on Food and Nutrition (Devirgiliis *et al.* 2007) have investigated the relationship between zinc and chronic diseases. Their research determined that an "imbalance in zinc homeostasis" can impair protein synthesis, cell membrane transport and gene expression. These factors, they explained, stimulate imbalances among hormones and tissue systems, producing inappropriate inflammation.

As zinc ions pass through the cell membrane, they assist the cell in the uptake of nutrients. Zinc transporters interact with genes to regulate the transmission of nutrients within the cell, and the pathways in and out of the cell. Zinc concentration within the cell is balanced by proteins called metallothioneins. These proteins require copper and selenium in addition to zinc.

Metallothioneins are critical to the cell's ability to scavenge various radicals and heavy metals that can damage the cells. Deficiencies in metallothioneins have been seen among chronic inflammatory conditions, and even fatal diseases such as cancer.

Not surprisingly, research has also shown that zinc modulates T-cell activities (Hönscheid *et al.* 2009).

It is likely for these reasons that zinc has been used clinically with success to help soothe sore throats.

Good zinc foods include cowpeas, beans, lima beans, milk, brown rice, yogurt, oats, cottage cheese, bran, lentils, wheat and others.

Selenium: Research has shown that greater levels of lipid peroxidation (due to greater consumption of poor fats and fatty foods) decrease our body's levels of selenium. This is because selenium is a critical component of glutathione peroxidase—which reduces lipid peroxidation.

Those with higher levels of lipid peroxidation tend to require more selenium because they exhaust this nutrient more readily. This has the indirect effect of reducing the strength of our mucosal membranes. While selenium supplements might offer generous amounts of selenium, one brazil nut will supply about 120 micrograms of selenium. This is 170% of the recommended daily value.

Sulfur: Research has confirmed that dietary sulfur can significantly relieve inflammation and hypersensitivity. In a multi-center open label study by researchers from Washington state (Barrager *et al.* 2002), 55 patients with allergic rhinitis were given 2,600 mg of methylsulfonylmethane (MSM)—a significant source of sulfur derived from plants—for 30 days. Weekly reviews of the patients reported significant improvements in allergic respiratory symptoms, along with increased energy. Other research has suggested that sulfur blocks the binding of histamine among receptors.

Supplemental MSM is typically derived from plant sources. Good food sources of sulfur include avocado, asparagus, barley, beans, broccoli, cabbage, carob, carrots, Brussels sprouts, chives, coconuts, corn, garlic, leafy green vegetables, leeks, lentils, onions, parsley, peas, radishes, red peppers, soybeans, shallots, Swiss chard and watercress.

Potassium content within the mucosal membranes is specifically reduced by many pharmaceutical medications, as well as toxins and sweating. Low potassium levels will contribute to imbalances within the mucosal membranes, and will reduce these membranes' ability to clear toxins and protect our cells.

Good potassium foods include bananas, spinach, sunflower seeds, tomatoes, pomegranates, turnips, lima beans, navy beans, squash, broccoli and others.

Trace minerals: These should not be ignored in this discussion. Trace elements are important to nearly every enzymatic reaction in the body.

While minerals have been shown to provide therapeutic results, we must be careful about mineral supplements, especially those that provide single or a few minerals. Minerals co-exist in the body, and a dramatic increase in one can exhaust others as the body depletes the oversupply. Thus, an isolated macro-mineral supplement can easily produce a mineral imbalance in the body, which can produce a variety of hypersensitivity issues.

Better to utilize natural sources of minerals. These include, first and foremost, mineral-intensive vegetables. Nearly all vegetables contain generous mineral content in the combinations designed by nature. Best to eat a mixed combination of vegetables to achieve a healthy array of trace minerals.

Whole food mineral sources also contain many trace minerals in their more-digestible *chelated* forms. Chelation is when a mineral ion bonds with another nutrient, providing a ready ion as the body needs it.

Most organically-grown plant-based foods provide a rich supply of trace minerals, assuming we are eating enough of them. Other good sources of trace minerals include natural mineral water, whole (unprocessed) rock salt, coral calcium, spirulina, AFA, kelp and chlorella. These sources will typically have from 60 to 80 trace elements, all of which are necessary for the body's various enzymatic functions. See the author's book, *Pure Water*.

We should also note that research by David Brownstein, M.D. (2006) has illustrated that whole unprocessed salt does not affect the body with high blood pressure, cardiovascular disease, diabetes and so on, as refined salts (often called sodium but is actually purified sodium chloride) do.

Cooking with whole rock salts instead of refined salt is a great way to get numerous trace minerals.

Antioxidants

Remember that toxins provide one of the components that can damage the cells of our esophagus, sphincters and mucosal membranes. They accomplish this by releasing or becoming unbalanced radicals that "steal" atomic elements from our cell membranes or mucous membranes in order to become more balanced. This means that neutralizing toxins provides a strategy to help reduce GERD.

In addition, antioxidants reduce our total body toxin load, which serves to strengthen our body's immune system. This allows our body to better react to toxins without launching full-blown inflammation.

When we harvest a fresh plant-based food and eat it with minimal storage, processing and cooking, we are deriving significant benefits from the living organism that produced the food. Because living organisms defend themselves against toxins throughout their lives, by eating fresh whole foods or whole foods minimally cooked, our bodies can utilize the same elements the plant utilized to protect itself against toxins.

This in turn stimulates our immune systems, and also provides direct free radical protection. This is because antioxidants are designed to neutralize toxins.

As we've discussed, a plethora of research has confirmed that damage from free radicals is implicated in many health conditions. Free radicals from toxins damage cells, cell membranes, organs, blood vessel walls and airways—producing systemic inflammation—as the immune system responds to an overload of tissue damage.

Free radicals are produced by synthetic chemicals, pathogens, trans fats, fried foods, red meats, radiation, pollution and various intruders that destabilize within the body. Free radicals are molecules or ions that require stabilization. They reach stabilization by 'stealing' atoms from the cells or tissues of our body. This in turn destabilizes those cells and tissues—producing damage.

Antioxidants serve to stabilize free radicals before our cells and tissues are robbed—by donating their own atoms. A diet with plenty of fruits and vegetables supplies numerous antioxidants. Although antioxidants cannot be considered treatments for any disease, many studies have proved that increased antioxidant intake supports immune function and detoxification. These effects allow the immune system to respond with greater tolerance.

Antioxidant constituents in plant-based foods are known to significantly repeal free radicals, strengthen the immune system and help detoxify the system. These include *lecithin* and *octacosanol* from whole grains; *polyphenols* and *sterols* from vegetables; *lycopene* from tomatoes and watermelons; *quercetin* and *sulfur/allicin* from garlic, onions and peppers; *pectin* and *rutin* from apples and other fruits; *phytocyanidin flavonoids* such as *apigenin* and *luteolin* from various greenfoods; and *anthocyanins* from various fruits and oats.

Some sea-based botanicals like kelp also contain antioxidants as well. Consider a special polysaccharide compound from kelp called *fucoidan*. Fucoidan has been shown in animal studies to significantly reduce inflammation (Cardoso *et al.* 2009; Kuznetsova *et al.* 2004).

Procyanidins are found in apples, currants, cinnamon, bilberry and many other foods. The extract of *Vitis vinifera* seed (grapeseed) is one of the highest sources of bound antioxidant *proanthocyanidins* and *leucocyanidines* called *procyanidolic oligomers* or PCOs. Pycnogenol® also contains significant levels of these PCOs. Blueberries, parsley, green tea, black currant, some legumes and onions also contain PCOs and similar proanthocyanidins.

Research has demonstrated that PCOs have protective and strengthening effects on tissues by increasing enzyme conjugation (Seo *et al.* 2001). PCOs have also been shown to increase vascular wall strength (Robert *et al.* 2000).

Oxygenated carotenoids such as *lutein* and *astaxanthin* also have been shown to exhibit strong antioxidant activity. Astaxanthin is derived from the microalga *Haematococcus pluvialis*, and lutein is available from a number of foods, including spirulina.

Most of these phytonutrients specifically modulate the immune system. For example, the flavonoids *kaempferol* and *flavone* have been shown to block mast cell proliferation by over 80% (Alexandrakis *et al*. 2003). Sources of kaempferol include Brussels sprouts, broccoli, grapefruit and apples.

Furthermore, *resveratrol* from grapes and berries modulate nuclear factor-kappaB and transcription/Janus kinase pathways—which strengthens immunity. Good sources of resveratrol include peanuts, red grapes, cranberries and cocoa (wine is not advisable for cleansing as we'll discuss later).

Nearly every plant-food has some measure of phytonutrients discussed above and more. These phytonutrients alkalize the blood and increase the detoxification capabilities of the liver. They help clear the blood of toxins.

Foods that are particularly detoxifying and immunity-building include fresh pineapples, beets, cucumbers, apricots, apples, almonds, zucchini, artichokes, avocados, bananas, beans, collard greens, berries, casaba, celery, coconuts, cranberries, watercress, dandelion greens, grapes, raw honey, corn, kale, citrus fruits, watermelon, lettuce, mangoes, mushrooms, oats, broccoli, okra, onions, papayas, parsley, peas, whole grains, radishes, raisins, spinach, tomatoes, walnuts, and many others.

These plant-based foods are also our primary source of soluble and insoluble fiber. Diets with significant fiber help clear the blood and tissues of toxins, and lipid peroxidation-friendly LDL cholesterol. Fiber is also critical to a healthy digestive tract and intestinal barrier. Fiber in the diet should range from about 35 to 45 grams per day according to the recommendations of many diet experts. Six to ten servings of raw fruits and vegetables per day should accomplish this—which is even part of the USDA's recommendations. This means raw, fibrous foods should be present at every meal.

Good fibrous plant sources also contain healthy *lignans* and *phytoestrogens* that help balance hormone levels, and help the body make its own natural corticoids. Foods that contain these include peas, garbanzo beans, soybeans, kidney beans and lentils.

Plant-based foods provide these immune-stimulating factors because these vary same factors make up the plants' own immune systems. For example, the red, blue and green flavonoid pigments in plants and fruits help protect the plant from oxidative damage from radiation. The proanthocyanidins in grains like oats, for example, help protect the oat plant from crown rust caused by the *Puccinia coronata* fungus. So the same biochemicals that stimulate immunity in humans are part of plants' immune systems.

These same whole food phytonutrients also neutralize oxidative radicals in our bodies—the reason they are called antioxidants. How do we know this? Scientists can measure the ability of a particular food to neutralize free radicals with specific laboratory testing. One such test is called the *Oxygen Radical Absorbance Capacity Test* (ORAC). This technical laboratory study is performed by a number of scientific organizations that include the USDA, as well as specialized labs such as Brunswick Laboratories in Massachusetts.

Research from the USDA's Jean Mayer Human Nutrition Research Center on Aging at Tufts University has suggested that a diet high in ORAC value may protect blood vessels and tissues from free radical damage that can result in inflammation (Sofic *et al.* 2001; Cao *et al.* 1998). These tissues, of course, include the airways. Research has confirmed that consuming 3,000 to 5,000 ORAC units per day can have protective benefits.

ORAC Values (100 grams) of Selected (raw) Fruits (USDA, 2007-2008)

Fruit	Value		Fruit	Value
Cranberry	9,382		Pomegranate	2,860
Plum	7,581		Orange	1,819
Blueberry	6,552		Tangerine	1,620
Blackberry	5,347		Grape (red)	1,260
Raspberry	4,882		Mango	1,002
Apple (Granny)	3,898		Kiwi	882
Strawberry	3,577		Banana	879
Cherry (sweet)	3,365		Tomato (plum)	389
Gooseberry	3,277		Pineapple	385
Pear	2,941		Watermelon	142

There is tremendous attention these days on two unique fruits from the Amazon rain forest and China called *açaí* and *goji berry* (or wolfberry) respectively. A recent ORAC test documented by Schauss *et al.* (2006) gives açaí a score of 102,700 and tests documented by Dr. Paul Gross gives goji berries a total ORAC of 30,300. However, subsequent tests done by Brunswick Laboratories,

Inc. gave these two berries 53,600 (açaí) and 22,000 (goji) total-ORAC values.

In addition, we must remember that these are the dried berries being tested in the latter case, and a concentrate of acai being tested in the former case. The numbers in the chart above are for fresh fruits. Dried fruits will naturally have higher ORAC values, because the water is evaporated—giving more density and more antioxidants per 100 grams.

For example, in the USDA database, dried apples have a 6,681 total-ORAC value, while fresh apples range from 2,210 to 3,898 in total-ORAC value. This equates to a two-to-three times increase from fresh to dried. In another example, fresh red grapes have a 1,260 total-ORAC value, while raisins have a 3,037 total-ORAC value. This comes close to an increase of three times the ORAC value following dehydration.

Part of the equation, naturally, is cost. Dried fruit and concentrates are often more expensive than fresh fruit. High-ORAC dried fruits or concentrates from açaí or gogi will also be substantially more expensive than most fruits grown domestically (especially for Americans and Europeans). Our conclusion is that local or in-country grown fresh fruits with high total-ORAC values produce the best value. Local fresh fruit offers great free radical scavenging ability, support for local farmers, and pollen proteins we are most likely more tolerant to.

By comparison, spinach—an incredibly wholesome vegetable with a tremendous amount of nutrition—has a fraction of the ORAC content of some of these fruits, at 1,515 total ORAC. Spinach, of course, contains many other nutrients, including proteins lacking in many high-ORAC fruits.

Dehydrated spices can have incredibly high ORAC values. For example, USDA's database lists ground Turmeric's total ORAC value at 159,277 and oregano's at 200,129. However, while we might only consume a few hundred milligrams of a spice per day, we can eat many grams—if not pounds—of sweet colorful fruit every day.

Root Foods

It is no coincidence that many of the roots, such as ginger, turmeric, onions garlic, beets, carrots, turnips, parsnips and others, have a stabilizing effect upon the digestive tract. These root foods are known for their ability to alkalize the mucosal membranes and bloodstream. They are also known to help rejuvenate the liver and adrenal glands, which in turn nourish our mucosal membranes.

Beets, for example, contain, among other nutrients, betaine, betalains, betacyanin and betanin. Remember that betaine is one of the nutrients specifically found to reduce GERD symptoms and strengthen the sphincters. Beets are delicious foods that can be grated into salads, juiced, steamed, baked and simply eaten raw. Red beets are typically considered the healthiest, but pink and white beets also contain betaine.

We should note that while beets contain significant amounts of betaine, other betaine-rich foods include broccoli, spinach and some whole grains.

Root foods also contain generous portions of folate, iron and fiber. One of the primary fibers in beets is pectin, which is also found in apples. Pectin has a unique soluble and insoluble fiber content that maximizes the attachment of radical-producing LDL cholesterol in the intestines. Pectin also attaches to many other toxins, drawing them out of the body as well.

Each of the root foods listed above contain unique constituents that support liver health, detoxification and consequently, mucosal health.

Greenfoods

A greenfood is a category of foods considered nutritionally superior than many other foods. As a result, they are great strategies for increasing mucosal health. Greenfoods include the wheat grasses, sprouts, algae, and sea vegetables.

Greenfoods provide practically every nutrient imaginable, including enzymes, minerals, trace elements, essential and nonessential amino acids, vitamins, antioxidants and various phytonutrients. Many will provide over 1,000 nutrients.

A big benefit of greenfoods is their alkalinity. This gives them the ability to neutralize radicals and lipid peroxides, and help balance the pH of our various mucosal systems.

Much of this alkalinity comes from greenfoods' bioavailable mineral content. Many of these minerals are also are colloidal. They tend to be hydrophobic, and maintain a positive electrical charge—rendering them alkaline.

Cereal Grasses

Wheat grass is the young grass of the wheat species, *Triticum aestivum*. In addition to a plethora of vitamins, minerals, amino acids, phytonutrients, metabolic enzymes—including superoxide dismutase and cytochrome oxidase—wheat grass maintains up to 70% chlorophyll.

Early research by Dr. Charles Schnabel, Dr. George Kohler and Dr. A.I. Virtanen in the 1925-1950 era found that cereal grasses like wheatgrass achieved their highest nutrient content at around 18 days—right before the first jointing.

Wheat grass can increase blood hemoglobin levels. Wheat grass tablets decreased blood transfusion needs by 25% among 20 children requiring frequent blood transfusions in a recent study.

Barley grass maintains similar properties. Research has found that barley grass is a potent free radical scavenger; significantly reduces total cholesterol and LDL-cholesterol; and inhibits LDL oxidation. Barley grass juice powder can have 14 vitamins, 18 amino acids, 15 enzymes, 10 antioxidants, 18 minerals and 75 trace elements.

Another cereal grass is Kamut grass. The khorasan wheat has higher protein levels than most wheat varieties, and contains higher zinc, selenium and magnesium content. Selenium is known for stimulating glutathione activity as we've discussed.

Coriander/Cilantro/Parsley

Coriandrum sativum has documented throughout traditional medicines as an anti-allergy and antioxidant herb. The seeds are called Coriander, and the leaves are called Cilantro. Cilantro has been popularly used throughout Central America, Italy, and also Asia—where it is sometimes called Chinese parsley. Cilantro is the backbone ingredient—together with tomatoes and garlic—of salsa. It is related to Italian parsley, with many of the same constituents. Coriander is taken as fresh or juiced fresh, and it has been used by Ayurvedic practitioners primarily for allergic skin rashes and hay fever.

Fresh Italian parsley can readily be found in supermarkets and farmers' markets. While often used as a garnish (for looks and/or to clean the breath), a therapeutic quantity of parsley is about a *bunch*. A bunch of parsley is about two ounces or about ten stalks together with their branches and leaves. A *bunch* can be added to a salad or put into a soup. Parsley can be delicious with tomatoes, vinegar and olive oil. And of course, it can also freshen the breath.

Sprouts

Sprouts and their powders are nutritional powerhouses. They have exponential nutritional value, well above the nutrient content of their seeds or the fully-grown plants. This was confirmed in 1970s experiments by former Hippocrates Health Institute Director of Research, Viktoras Kulvinskas, M.S. Kulvinskas, who found that ascorbic acid levels in soybean sprouts increased from zero to 103 milligrams per 100 grams by day six—about the ascorbic acid content found in lime juice. These levels fall off significantly within days.

Each plant has a different nutrient peak. Ascorbic acid content in broad bean sprouts—used to cure scurvy during World War I—peaks in three days, after which the levels fall off.

Many believe that sprouts produce this greater antioxidant content to defend themselves against threats from the soil.

Great nutritional sprouts include wheat grass sprouts, barley, oats, beans, broccoli and cabbage. The latter two provide a class of nutrients called glucosinolates. These glucosinolates yield sulfur compounds and indole-3 carbinols. Both have shown to have significant anticarcinogenic and anti-inflammatory effects in the body.

Seed selection is critical. A good quality seed will germinate at least 50%. Heirloom seeds often germinate at much higher rates.

Sea Grasses

Kelps might be called seaweeds, but these phytonutrient powerhouses are anything but weeds. About 1,500 species of sea kelps flourish, many in the North Pacific and North Atlantic oceans.

Most kelps are stationary, and sustainably harvested in the wild. This means they must be allowed to regrow to guarantee future harvests. *Ascophyllum nodosum* kelp contains an impressive array of vitamins—more than many vegetables. They include over 60 essential minerals, amino acids and vitamins. They also contain growth promoters, according to kelp researchers.

Most kelps also contain fucoidan, a sulfated polysaccharide. Laboratory studies have indicated fucoidan has anti-tumor, antico-agulant and anti-angiogenic effects. It down-regulates Th2 (inhibiting allergic response), inhibits beta-amyloid formation (implicated in Alzheimer's), inhibits proteinuria in Heymann nephritis and decreases artery platelet deposits.

Other kelps include dulse, sargasso seaweed, *Undaria pinnatifida*, sea palm and others.

Spirulina

Spirulina use dates back to the Aztecs. A good source of carotenoids, vitamins (including vegan B12 according to independent laboratory tests) and minerals, spirulina contains all essential and most non-essential amino acids, with up to 65% protein by weight. It also contains antioxidant phytonutrients such as zeaxanthin, myxoxanthophyll and lutein. It also will contain antioxidant carotenoids, vitamins and minerals.

Spirulina also contains phycobiliprotein, a unique blue pigment anti-inflammatory and antioxidant. Research has showed that phycobiliproteins can protect the liver and kidney from toxins. They are also anti-viral, and stimulate the immune system.

In one study from the University of California-Davis, 12 weeks of 3000 milligrams of Hawaiian spirulina per day significantly increased hemoglobin concentration and mean corpuscular hemoglobin among 30 adults over the age of 50. IDO (indoleamine 2,3-dioxygenase) enzyme activity—a sign of increased immune function—was also higher among the subjects.

Chlorella

More than 800 published studies have verified the safety and efficacy of *Chlorella pyrenoidosa*. Chlorella's reputation of drawing out heavy metals and other toxins make it a favorite among health practitioners.

Chlorella maintains considerable vitamins minerals, and phytonutrients—including chlorella growth factor (CGF), known to stimulate cell growth. It is also a complete protein, with about 60% protein by weight and every essential and non-essential amino acid.

Clinical studies have shown that chlorella stimulates T-cell and B-cell activity and contributes to the improvement of fibromyalgia, ulcerative colitis and hypertension. Another study showed that chlorella increases IgA levels and lowers dioxin levels in breast milk.

Chlorella's tough cell wall must be broken down mechanically to allow these nutrients' bioavailability. Our digestive enzymes cannot digest these outer cell walls. For this reason, quality chlorella growers will pulverize this tough outer cell wall.

Haematococcus and Astaxanthin

Another greenfood algae is *Haematococcus pluvialis*, known for its high astaxanthin content. Astaxanthin is a strong carotenoid similar to beta-carotene. For this reason, astaxanthin is one of the most powerful natural antioxidants known. It also has anti-inflammatory effects, and has been used for eye health, joint healthy, muscle soreness, cardiovascular health, and skin health. It can also protect against damage from UV radiation.

Aloe Vera

While aloe has long been known for its skin irritation and wound healing abilities, science on its internal use is still emerging.

Aloe is now used for gastrointestinal health, immune support and cardiovascular health, as well as the health of the skin and mucosal membranes.

A study from London's Queen Mary School of Medicine on 44 active ulcerated colitis patients found that internal aloe use resulted in clinical improvement. And double-blind, randomized research using Aloecorp's Qmatrix processed aloe has shown that it reduces oxidative stress markers and stimulates the immune system.

Aloe can be taken as a juice or a gel.

The soothing mucopolysaccharides content of aloe can also be found among other cactus plants, including nopalea and others.

Raw Honey

Raw honey, especially the Manuka variety, can be extremely helpful for GERD sufferers. This is because raw honey contributes a number of key enzymes, as well as antibiotics produced by bees that apparently reduce *H. pylori* colonization.

Refined or heated honey will likely not contain these antibiotics and enzymes, as these are heat sensitive.

Some have advocated taking a teaspoon a day on an empty stomach.

Papaya

Papaya contains several protease enzymes such as papain, which help speed stomach emptying. Papain and other elements of papaya (such as a high carotenoid content) also help strengthen the mucosal membranes of the esophagus and stomach wall.

Probiotic and Prebiotic Strategies

As we've discussed, probiotics are key to mucosal membrane and digestive health. Probiotics help us digest food and they secrete beneficial nutritional products. Unbelievably, probiotics are a good source of a number of essential nutrients. They can manufacture biotin, thiamin (B1), riboflavin (B2), niacin (B3), pantothenic acid (B5), pyridoxine (B6), cobalamine (B12), folic acid, vitamin A and vitamin K. Their lactic acid secretions also increase the assimilation of minerals that require acid for absorption, such as copper, iron, magnesium, chromium, selenium and manganese among many others.

Probiotics are also critical to nutrient absorption. They break away amino acids from complex proteins, and mid-chain fatty acids from complex fats. They help break down bile acids. They help convert polyphenols from plant materials into assimilable biomolecules. They also aid in soluble fiber fermentation, yielding digestible fatty acids and sugars. Among many other nutritive tasks, they also help increase the bioavailability of calcium.

Probiotics also assist in peristalsis—the rhythmic motion of the digestive tract—by helping move intestinal contents through the system. They also produce antifungal substances such as acidophillin, bifidin and hydrogen peroxide, which counteract the growth of not-so-friendly yeasts. Probiotic hydrogen peroxide secretions are also oxygenating, providing free radical scavenging. In addition, they can manufacture some essential fatty acids, and are the source of 5-10% of all short-chained fatty acids essential for healthy immune system function.

An example of the extent of probiotics' ability to produce antimicrobials is the antibiotic streptomycin. This antibiotic, produced by the probiotic bacteria, *Streptomyces griseus* was discovered in 1943 by Selman Waksman.

Probiotics directly and indirectly break down toxins utilizing biochemical secretions and colonizing activities. Nutrients produced by probiotics have been found to have antitumor and anticancer effects within the body. Some probiotics can prevent assimilation of toxins like mercury and other heavy metals. Others will directly bind these toxins or will facilitate their binding to other molecules in order to remove them.

Probiotic nutrients are instrumental in slowing cellular degeneration and the diseases associated with it. Through their nutritive mechanisms, probiotics help normalize serum levels of cholesterol and triglycerides. Some probiotics even help break down and rebuild hormones.

Probiotic nutrients can also increase the productivity of the spleen and thymus—the key organs of the immune system.

Probiotics are necessary components to healthy digestion. Their populations dwell along and within the intestinal mucosal lining, providing a protective barrier to assist in the process of filtering and digesting toxins and other matter prior to these toxins encountering the intestinal wall cells. This mechanism helps maintain the brush barrier cells and keep the mucosal lining beginning from the esophagus down to the colon.

Probiotics will also compete with pathogenic organisms for nutrients. Assuming good numbers, this strategy can check pathobiotic growth substantially. Nutrients produced by probiotics will also help stimulate the immune cell production, and normalize their activity during inflammatory circumstances.

Probiotics are available from a variety of cultured foods. These fermented foods teeming with probiotic bacteria and yeasts include yogurt and kefir, raw cheeses, traditional cottage cheese, traditional sour cream, traditional buttermilk, traditional sauerkraut, lassi, amasake (Japanese sweet rice drink), traditional miso, traditional tempeh, traditional tamari, traditional soy sauce and traditional kombucha tea and others.

Other foods utilize probiotics in their preparation. Traditional sourdough bread and bauerbrot are good examples. Most bread, in fact, uses some sort of (often probiotic) yeast fermentation process to prepare the flour for baking. In these, however, the probiotics are likely all killed during baking.

Some of the foods mentioned here are preceded by the word "traditional" because sadly, many of today's versions are pasteurized or otherwise acidified enough to kill any viable probiotic colonies.

Both cottage cheese and butter were originally probiotic foods, for example, when we used to eat dairy products from our local dairies or own farms. Today, these two foods are produced commercially without probiotics. Ironically, even many commercial yogurts are unbelievably pasteurized prior to shipping—killing off most if not all of their viable colonies.

Another example is tamari and soy sauce. Today, most commercial versions are brewed with solvents. Probiotics are no longer part of these processes, as were the traditional versions.

For example, there is a lot that can be done with yogurt. We've all heard of frozen yogurt, and certainly that is one. But yogurt in some cultures, such as among Indians, is eaten with every meal. It is eaten with and in salads, and rice dishes. Yogurt is creamy and delicious, and can make for an excellent salad dressing with a little oil and vinegar and dill. It can also be added to nearly every sauce to make the sauce creamy and delicious.

Kefir and lassi cultures can be added to nearly every combination of beverage, including smoothies and shakes.

Just about every vegetable can be pickled. Pickles using brine with probiotics is delicious and healthy. We can pickle peppers, olives and so many other foods.

Fermented beverages are now the rage among healthy foods. There are now many fermented beverages, including kombucha and others.

Milk: Raw or Pasteurized?

This naturally brings us to the topic of milk, since there are many reports that indicate that dairy may not be so healthy—especially when it comes to GERD and GERD-related mucosal conditions.

As for raw milk, numerous experiments have shown that raw milk, and dairy containing probiotics such as yogurt is not only healthy, but stimulates the immune system and fights off disease.

First let's consider a study by researchers at Switzerland's University of Basel (Waser *et al.* 2007). The researchers studied 14,893 children between the ages of five and 13 from five different European countries, including 2,823 children from farms, and 4,606 children attending a Steiner School (known for its farm-based living and instruction). The researchers found that drinking farm milk was associated with decreased incidence of (mucosal membrane-oriented) allergies and asthma. Why?

Raw milk from the cow can contain a host of bacteria, including *Lactobacillus acidophilus, L. casei, L. bulgaricus* and many other healthy probiotics. Cows that feed from primarily grasses will have increased levels of these healthy probiotics.

This is because a grass diet provides prebiotics that promote the cow's own probiotic colonies. Should the cow be fed primarily dried grass and dried grains, probiotic counts will be reduced, replaced by more pathogenic bacteria. As a result, most non-grass fed herds must be given lots of antibiotics to help keep their bacteria counts low. Probiotics, on the other hand, naturally keep bacteria counts down.

As a result, the non-grass fed cow's milk will have higher pathogenic bacteria counts than grass-fed cows. This means that the milk itself will also have high counts. When the non-grass-fed cow's milk is pasteurized, the heat kills most of these bacteria. The result is a milk containing dead pathogenic bacteria parts. These are primarily proteins and peptides, which get mixed with the milk and are eventually consumed with the milk.

In other words, pasteurization may kill the living pathogenic bacteria, but it does not get rid of the bacteria proteins. This might be compared to cooking an insect: If an insect landed in our soup, we could surely cook it until it died. But the soup would still contain the insect parts—and proteins.

Now the immune system of most people, and especially infants with their hypersensitive immune system, is trained to attack and discard pathogenic bacteria. And how does the body identify pathogenic bacteria? From their proteins.

In the case of pasteurized commercial milk, our immune systems will readily identify heat-killed microorganism cell parts and proteins and launch an immune response against these proteins as if it were being attacked by the microorganisms directly. This was shown in research from the University of Minnesota two decades ago (Takahashi *et al.* 1992).

It is thus not surprising that weak immune systems readily reject pasteurized cow's milk. In comparison, healthy cow raw milk has fewer pathogenic microorganisms and more probiotic organisms. This has been confirmed by tests done by a California organic milk farm, which compared test results of their raw organic milk against standardized state test results from conventional milk farms.

In addition, pasteurization breaks apart or denatures many of the proteins and sugar molecules. This was illustrated by researchers from Japan's Nagasaki International University (Nodake *et al.* 2010), who found that when beta-lactoglobulin is naturally conjugated with dextran-glycylglycine, its allergenicity is decreased. A dextran is a very long chain of glucose molecules—a polysaccharide. The dextran polysaccharide is naturally joined with the amino acid glycine in raw state. When pasteurized, beta-lactoglobulin is separated.

This is not surprising. Natural whole cow's milk also contains special polysaccharides called oligosaccharides. They are largely indigestible polysaccharides that feed our intestinal bacteria. Because of this trait, these indigestible sugars are called prebiotics.

Whole milk contains a number of these oligosaccharides, including oligogalactose, oligolactose, galactooligosaccharides (GOS) and transgalactooligosaccharides (TOS). Galactooligosaccharides are produced by conversion from enzymes in healthy cows and healthy mothers.

These polysaccharides provide a number of benefits. Not only are they some of the more preferred foods for probiotics: Research has also shown that they reduce the ability of pathogenic bacteria like *E. coli* to adhere to our intestinal cells.

These oligosaccharides also provide environments that reduce the availability of separated beta-lactoglobulin. This is accomplished through a combination of probiotic colonization and the availability of the long-chain polysaccharides that keep these complexes stabilized.

This reduced availability of beta-lactoglobulin has been directly observed in humans and animals following consistent supplementation with probiotics (Taylor *et al.* 2006; Adel-Patient *et al.* 2005; Prioult *et al.* 2003).

It is not surprising, given this information, that people with many digestive conditions—including GERD—have benefited from withdrawing from pasteurized milk and cheese. Raw milk, yogurt, kefir, goat's milk and cheese, along with soy and almond milk, are great alternatives.

Supplementing with Probiotics

As discussed earlier, clinical studies have shown that GERD, gastritis and other digestive issues are greatly benefited by probiotic supplementation.

The main consideration in probiotic supplementation is consuming *live* organisms. These are typically described as "CFU" which stands for *colony forming units*. In other words, live probiotics will produce new colonies once inside the intestines. Heat-killed ones are not as beneficial, although they can also stimulate the immune system. So the key is keeping the probiotics alive while in the capsule and supplement bottle, until we are ready to consume them. Here are a few considerations about probiotic supplements:

Capsules: Vegetable capsules contain less moisture than gelatin or enteric-coated capsules. Even a little moisture in the capsule can increase the possibility of waking up the probiotics while in the bottle. Once woken up, they can starve and die. Enteric coating can minimally protect the probiotics within the stomach, assuming they have survived in the bottle. Some manufactures use oils to help protect the probiotics in the stomach. In all cases, encapsulated freeze-dried probiotics should be refrigerated (no matter what the label says) at all times during shipping, at the store, and at home. Dark containers also better protect the probiotics from light exposure, which can kill them.

Powders of freeze-dried probiotics are subject to deterioration due to increased exposure to oxygen and light. Powders should be refrigerated in dark containers and sealed tightly to be kept viable. They should also be consumed with liquids or food, preferably dairy or fermented dairy. Powders can also be used as starters for homemade yogurt and kefir.

Caplets/Tablets: Some tablet/caplets have special coatings that provide viability through to the intestines without refrigeration. If not, those tablets would likely be in the same category as encapsulated products, requiring refrigeration.

Shells or Beads: These can provide longer shelf viability without refrigeration and better survive the stomach. However, because of the size of the shell, these typically come with less CFU quantity, increasing the cost per therapeutic dose. Another drawback may be that the intestines must dissolve this thick shell. An easy test is to examine the stool to be sure that the beads or shells aren't coming out the other end whole.

Lozenges: These are one of the best ways to get probiotics directly into the mucosal membranes of our mouth, sinuses, throat and airways. A correctly formulated chewable or lozenge can inoculate the mouth, nose and throat with beneficial bacteria to compete with and fight off pathogenic bacteria as they enter or reside in our mouth, nose, throat and airways of the lungs.

Probiotic supplements that survive well among the mucous membranes of the airways, sinuses and oral cavity include *L. reuteri, L. rhamnosus, L. plantarum, L. paracasei, and Streptococcus salivarius.* As we discussed in the research, several of these, notably *L. reuteri,* have been shown to increase airway health and decrease lung infections.

However, most of the probiotics in a lozenge will not likely survive the stomach acids and penetrate the intestines. (Therefore, intestinal probiotics in one of the forms above are recommended in addition to probiotic lozenges.)

As the research showed in the last chapter (see topic on oral probiotics), lozenges are an excellent way to help prevent new infections and sore throats during increased exposures. The bacteria in a good lozenge or chewable will allow the probiotics to colonize around our gums and throat, fending off microorganisms that threaten their welfare.

This type of supplement should still be kept sealed, airtight and cool. Refer to the author's book *Oral Probiotics* for detailed information regarding species, strategies and additional research on these probiotics.

Liquid Supplements: There are several probiotic supplements in small liquid form. One brand has a long tradition and a hardy, well-researched strain. A liquid probiotic should be in a light-sealed, refrigerated container. It should also contain some dairy or other probiotic-friendly substrate, giving the probiotics some food while awaiting delivery to the intestines.

Probiotic Dosage: A good dosage for intestinal probiotics for prevention and maintenance can be ten to fifteen billion CFU (*colony forming units*) per day. Total intake during an illness or therapeutic period, however, will often double or triple that dosage. Much of the research shown in this text utilized 20 billion to 40 billion CFU per day, about a third of that dose for children and a quarter of that dose for infants. (*B. infantis* is often the supplement of choice for babies.)

Supplemental oral probiotic dosages can be far less (100 million to two billion), especially when the formula contains the hardy *L. reuteri*.

People who must take antibiotics for life-threatening reasons can alternate doses of probiotics between their antibiotic dosing. The probiotic dose can be at least two hours before or after the antibiotic dose. (Always consult with the prescribing doctor.)

Remember that these dosages depend upon delivery to the intestines. Therefore, a product that passes into the stomach with little protection would likely not deliver many colonies to the intestines. Such a supplement would likely require higher dosage to achieve the desired effects.

Prebiotic Foods

One of the most important factors in establishing a healthy environment for our probiotic colonies is making sure they have the right mix of nutrients available. The nutrients our probiotic families favor are called prebiotics. In other words, some foods are particularly beneficial for *bifidobacteria, lactobacilli* and other probiotic populations.

These are the oligosaccharides, fructooligosaccharides, galactooligosaccharides, and transgalactooligosaccharides—also referred to as inulin, FOS, GOS and TOS. Even two or three grams of one of these prebiotics will dramatically increase probiotic populations assuming healthy colonies. Inulin, FOS, GOS and TOS are also antagonistic to toxic microorganism genera such as *Salmonella, Listeria, Campylobacter, Shigella* and *Vibrio.* These and other pathogenic bacteria tend to thrive from refined sugars as opposed to the complex saccharides of inulin, FOS, GOS and TOS.

Oligosaccharides are short stacks of simple yet mostly indigestible sugars (from the Greek *oligos*, meaning "few"). If the sugar molecule is fructose, the stacked molecule is called a fructooligosaccharide. If the sugar molecule is galactose, the stacked molecule is called a galactooligosaccharide. These molecules are very useful for human cells and probiotics because they can be processed directly for energy as well as be combined with fatty acids to create cell wall structures and cellular communication molecules. These nutrients also provide energy and nourishment to our probiotic colonies.

The oligosaccharides inulin and oligofructose are probably the most recognized prebiotics. Inulin is a naturally occurring carbohydrate used by plants for storage. It has been estimated that more than 36,000 plant species contain inulin in varying degrees (Carpita *et al.* 1989). The roots often contain the greatest amounts of inulin.

Commercial sources of inulin include Jerusalem artichoke, agave cactus and chicory. Chicory, the root of the Belgian endive, is known to contain some of the highest levels of both inulin at 15-20%, and oligofructose at 5-10%. Inulin from agave has been described as highly branched. This gives it a higher solubility and digestibility than inulin derived from Jerusalem artichoke or chicory.

Notable prebiotic FOS-containing foods include beets, leeks, bananas, tree fruits, soybeans, burdock root, asparagus, maple sugar, whole rye and whole wheat among many others. Bananas contain one of the highest levels of FOS. Bananas are thus a favorite food for both humans and probiotics.

GOS and TOS are natural byproducts of milk. They are produced as lactose is enzymatically converted or hydrolyzed within the digestive tract. This process can also be done commercially. Before much of the recent research on prebiotics was performed, nutritionists simply thought of GOS and TOS as indigestible byproducts of milk.

Another element in plant foods providing prebiotic nutrition for probiotics is the polyphenol group. Polyphenols are groups of biochemicals produced in plants such as lignans, tannins, reservatrol, and flavonoids. There is some uncertainty as to which of these are most helpful to probiotic populations.

Some prebiotics have interesting side effects. For example, there seems to be a relationship between oligofructose inulin and calcium absorption. Inulin has been shown to improve calcium absorption by 20%, and yogurt supplemented with TOS has increased calcium absorption by 16% (van den Heuvel *et al.* 2000)

Galactooligosaccharides have another side effect that is important to note. Dr. Kari Shoaf and fellow researchers at the University of Nebraska (Shoaf *et al.* 2006) found in laboratory tests that galactooligosaccharides reduce the ability of *E. coli* to attach to human cells within tissue cultures. This effect was isolated from GOS' ability to nourish probiotics. This means that GOS provides more than nutrition to our probiotic colonies. This once considered useless indigestible nutrient also helps keep *E. coli* and other pathogenic bacteria from attaching to our cells. A nice package deal indeed.

FOS and GOS have been known to cause digestive disturbance in rare cases. Such a digestive disturbance is likely caused by dysbiosis, however.

Conclusively, a preponderance of scientific literature indicates that probiotics thrive from a diet of plant-based natural foods with plenty of phytonutrients, while overly processed, sugary and meat diets tend to promote pathogenic bacteria and their disease-causing endotoxins.

Enzyme Strategies

Enzymes are critical components in breaking down our foods. When our enzymes are not adequate, our gastric emptying will slow. This will cause a back up of food into the esophagus as our meals will await the stomach's emptying before they can proceed.

One of the most critical types of enzymes for gastric emptying are proteases, also called proteolytic enzymes, because they break down proteins.

Proteolytic enzymes are produced by plant-based foods, probiotics, and our own gastric, liver and bile system. For those with compromised digestive systems, these enzymes may not be as available as they should. In these cases, the supplementation of natural enzymes can be extremely productive.

Other enzymes are produced by probiotic microorganisms. For example, chemical engineering researchers from Stanford University (Ehren *et al.* 2009) found that aspergillopepsin (ASP) is produced from *Aspergillus niger* and dipeptidyl peptidase IV (DPP-IV) produced from the probiotic *Aspergillus oryzae*. These two enzymes break down glutens and gluten-type proteins.

Here is a list of the major digestive enzymes and their function within the body:

Major Enzyme	Foods it Breaks Down
Amylase	Starches
Bromelain	Proteins
Carboxypeptidase	Proteins (terminal)
Cellulase	Plant fiber (cellulose)
Chymotrypsin	Proteins
Elastase	Proteins and elastins
Glucoamylase	Starches
Isomaltase	Isomaltose and Maltose
Lactase	Lactose
Lipase	Fats
Maltase	Maltose
Nuclease	Protein nucleotides
Pepsin	Proteins
Peptidase	Proteins
Rennin	Milk
Steapsin	Triglycerides
Sucrase	Sucrose
Tributyrase	Butter Fat

Trypsin	Proteins
Xylanase	Hemicellulose (plant fiber)

As mentioned some plant-based foods supply enzymes that are considered proteolytic. These include bromelain, papain and natto-kinase. These have also been shown to have anti-inflammatory properties.

Papain is derived directly from papayas. It is a rich source of proteolytic enzymes.

The nattokinase enzyme is produced by *Bacillus natto,* the bacterium used to ferment soy. Bromelain is another botanical enzyme with proteolytic and anti-inflammatory properties.

Bromelain is derived from pineapple.

Our liver and pancreas produce many of these enzymes, but probiotics also produce a significant number of our body's digestive enzymes. This is one reason why probiotics are so helpful for digestive issues, as we've discussed.

Weight Loss and GERD

Because many studies have found an association between GERD and obesity, it is assumed that losing weight will also help GERD. Well, yes and no.

Swedish researchers (Kjellin *et al.* 1996) found, in a study of 20 obese GERD patients, that losing a little over 10 kilograms (about 22 pounds) did not result in a reduction of GERD symptoms or pH changes.

However, University of Amsterdam researchers (Mathus-Vliegen and Tytgat 1996) found that many extremely obese people with GERD did improve or resolve their GERD with extreme weight loss. Some of those with moderate weight loss also improved.

The researchers in both studies assumed that the weight loss would need to be considerable—enough to effectively bring their weight and BMI down to normal levels.

In other words, it is not as simple as just losing a few pounds. We have to look at the whole person, and the mix of foods and other lifestyle choices, as we've been discussing in this book. These dietary changes will naturally result in sustained weight loss.

That said, there are a few simple strategies that can stimulate weight loss and ease the pressure on our esophageal sphincters:

> We can eat smaller meals, more than three times a day. "Healthy snacking" throughout the day can allow us more activity as well as reduced pressure on our sphincters.

> We can eat more fibrous foods. Fibrous foods will increase our feeling of satiety without as many calories. Satiety is a complex topic, but to summarize, it is based upon a combination of nutrients, calories, fiber, digestive potency and issues related to stress and anxiety.

> On that topic, eating when we anxious or depressed will typically result in higher calorie intake.

> Eating under stress is also quite common. If we are stressed, we probably should not eat—or eat only a little—until we have more time to relax and eat slowly.

> We might consider watching our late night eating. Eating earlier in the evening allows us to stimulate our digestion with movement. Taking a walk after dinner instead of plopping right onto the couch is a good strategy, for example.

> Eating slower and chewing our food better can deliver foods that get through our sphincters easier and digest faster once in the stomach and intestines. This increases our stomach emptying and reduces esophageal backfilling.

> Breathing while we are eating—but not while swallowing—can help prevent air from getting trapped between the esophagus. It can also allow us to eat with less stress.

> "Wolfing" down our foods or talking while eating, on the other hand, lowers our gastric emptying rate and reduces satiety. We end up eating more than we need to before our body can realize it.

> Avoiding liquids while eating is beneficial for both weight loss and digestion, as we are able to better metabolically handle our fats, proteins and sugars. This also goes for cereals with milk.

> Avoiding sugary sodas is a key to not only keeping weight down, but helping our sphincters. The combination combined with the sugar seems to be at issue here with GERD, and the sugar alone seems to be the issue with weight gain.

> A healthy diet rich in plant-based foods and cultured foods is the best long-term strategy for losing weight. See the author's book, *The Living Foods Diet* for more diet strategies.

Mucosal Hydration

Many cases of GERD are simply issues of dehydration, as we've discussed. When the body does not have enough liquids, it begins to ration. Its first priority is the blood, lymph, intercellular fluids, intracellular fluids and others. The mucosal membranes fall down to the bottom of the list. One reason for this is that we can typically easily tell when we are dehydrated, as our mouths become dry. So it is also a biofeedback element.

When the mouth is dry, our throat is dry and so is our esophagus. These symptoms provide the most immediate feedback, telling us to rehydrate immediately. For many GERD sufferers, this is precisely what that burning discomfort is trying to tell us.

Dr. Jethro Kloss' research (1939) found that the average person loses about 550 cubic centimeters of water through the skin, 440 cc through the lungs, 1550 cc through the urine, and another 150 cc through the stool. This adds up to 2650 cc per day, equivalent to a little over 2-½ quarts (about 85 fluid ounces).

Many suggest drinking eight 8-oz glasses per day is adequate. However, this 64 ounces would result in a state of dehydration for most of us.

In 2004, the National Academy of Sciences released a study indicating that women typically meet their hydration needs with approximately 91 ounces of water per day, while men meet their needs with about 125 ounces per day. This study also indicated that approximately 80% of water intake comes from water/beverages and 20% comes from food. Therefore, we can assume a minimum of 73 ounces of fresh water for the average adult woman and 100 ounces of fresh water for the average adult man should cover our hydration needs. That is significantly more water than the standard eight glasses per day—especially for men.

The data suggests that 50-75% of Americans have chronic dehydration. Fereydoon Batmanghelidj, M.D., probably the world's foremost researcher on water, suggests a ½ ounce of water per pound of body weight. Drinking an additional 16-32 ounces for each 45 minutes to an hour of strenuous activity is also a good idea, with some before and some after exercising. More water should accompany temperature and elevation extremes, extra sweating or fevers or increased physical activity. Note also that alcohol is dehydrating as mentioned earlier.

The best time to drink water, especially for GERD sufferers, is on an empty stomach. This is because the mucosal membranes can more easily be hydrated when the esophagus and stomach are clear of food and digestive processes. The water is also more easily assimilated into the bloodstream, and does not pose an interference to digestion.

On the other hand, it is unwise to drink much water or other liquids during a significant meal. This is because liquids will dilute our enzymes and gastric acids, which slow the digestive process, and slow down the rate of stomach emptying. As we've discussed, this is critical to a GERD sufferer, because a slower rate of emptying increases the likelihood of reflux, as the food and acids back up into the esophagus.

This is not to say that taking a small glass of liquids to help clear the pallet and throat occasionally while eating will be a big problem. No more than 2-3 ounces of fluids during a meal are advisable.

This also goes for milk. Having a tall glass of milk during dinner may seem appetizing, but it will severely hamper our digestion. This is even more so if the milk is pasteurized and homogenized. A small amount of raw milk during dinner is acceptable. Even better would be a heaping tablespoon or two of fresh yogurt during dinner.

A glass of room-temperature water first thing in the morning on an empty stomach can significantly help saturate and hydrate our mucosal membranes. This is actually an ancient Ayurvedic remedy for digestive discomfort or slow emptying—slow digestion.

To further stimulate digestion, the remedy calls for infusing the water with black pepper. Simply pour a half-teaspoon of finely ground black pepper into an 8 ounce glass of water, and drink first thing in the morning before brushing.

Then we should be drinking water throughout the day, in between meals, or in small increments. Our evening should accompany reduced water consumption, so our sleep is not disrupted by urination.

There are easy ways to tell whether we are dehydrated. A sensation of being thirsty indicates that we are already dehydrated. This is when mucosal membrane damage has already been accomplished. In other words, the GERD sufferer should never reach the stage of dehydration if at all possible.

Dark yellow urine also indicates dehydration. Our urine color should be either clear, or bright yellow if after taking multivitamins.

Drinking just any water is not advised. Municipal water and even bottled water can contain many contaminants that can burden the immune system, and damage our mucosal membranes. Care must be taken to drink water that has been filtered of most toxins yet is naturally mineralized. Research has confirmed that neither distilled water nor soft water are advisable. Filtered natural mineral water is best. Please refer to the author's book, *Pure Water* for more information on water content, filters and water treatment options.

Hot baths also have a great tradition of success among those with GERD and digestive ailments. There are two reasons for this. First, our bodies assimilate water through our skin pores, and through our lungs in the form of steam. Secondly, hot baths will relax the nerves, which will rebalance the vagus nerve, and help stimulate sphincter tone.

Hippocrates, known to western medicine as the father of medicine, stated that the hot bath "...*promotes expectoration, improves the respiration, and allays lassitude; for it soothes the joints and the outer skin, and is diuretic, removes heaviness of the heat and moistens the nose."*

Hot water calms the body and slows the heart rate, as the body's blood vessels relax and dilate in response to thermal radiation. A hot bath will open skin pores, allowing a hydration and exfoliation of skin cells. For sore or damaged muscle tissues, the dilation of capillaries and micro-capillaries speeds up the process of cleansing the tissues of lactic and carbonic acids—the byproducts of inadequate respiration.

Hot baths can also be medicated with a variety of mucosal herbs, as listed earlier. Simply make an infusion tea, strain it and pour it into the bath.

It should be noted that too much hot water for too long a period can lead to cardiovascular stress. Hot water can also lead to heat exhaustion. For best results, hot water applications should be limited to about 10-15 minutes at the hotter levels.

A fresh mineral water bath is best. Epson salts can be added to increase the bath's effects. If we are using a hot tub, it is best to limit the bath to about 10-20 minutes. For hot tubs, care should be taken to prevent chlorine and chlorine byproduct overload. The byproducts of chlorine breakdown are trihalomethanes (TTHM) and haloacetic acids (TAA5). Over-exposure to these can increase our toxin burden. Today there are healthier alternatives to chlorine, including bromine and salt water blends.

Hot Mineral Springs typically use geothermal heat from volcanic magma to charge aquifers with high temperatures and a variety of minerals. Many hot springs have a wholesome mixture of bicarbonates, iron, boron, silica, magnesium, copper, lithium, and many trace elements. Some contain exotic elements such as arsenic—believed to help heal skin issues and digestive issues. In other words, not all hot springs are alike.

Due to the earth's sulfur conveyor system, many of these hot spring waters are rich in sulfur in the form of hydrogen sulfide or sulfate. These can loosen phlegm and relax the airways, and soothe the mucous membranes within the esophagus.

Exercise Strategies

In recent review of clinical studies from around the world determined that exercise, and physical activity in general helped some people with GERD. The research also illustrated that exercise reduces the risk of colon cancer, gastrointestinal bleeding, and inflammatory bowel disease (Martin 2011).

However, the research has also found that many endurance athletes have GERD or at least GER. This result surprised the researchers, but other evidence has revealed that endurance athletes can also suffer higher risks of heart disease and inflammatory diseases.

The issue connects the stress put onto the body, but also against the diaphragm, which can put pressure on the lower esophageal sphincter.

Also, endurance running will produce a chronic inflammatory status within the body during the run. It can also severely dehydrate the tissues during the run. These can, over time, inflict harm upon the tissues, arteries, and in this case, upon the mucosal membranes of the esophagus and stomach. So there is a likely doubling effect on some athletes who do not address hydration and recuperation between runs.

Remember the research we discussed from Northwestern University's School of Medicine (Pandolfino *et al.* 2004). Among 20 people, 10 with GERD, vigorous exercise produced a 300% increase in stomach acid exposure in the esophagus.

This, they said, was reason for GERD sufferers to be aware of the "anatomical integrity" of the sphincters as they go about their exercises and lifestyles.

What did they mean by "anatomical integrity?"

This term refers to maintaining correct posture, and not putting pressure upon the upper abdomen. Putting pressure upon the upper abdomen can damage one or both of the esophageal sphincters, and in the case of the lower sphincter, result in a hiatal hernia—where part of the stomach wall pushes through the sphincter.

This of course relates to contact sports or other types of workouts where the upper abdomen may be impacted or put pressure upon. It also relates to extreme endurance or sprinting where the diaphragm is pushed to its limits. Here are a few activities that may put mechanical pressure upon the sphincters and/or esophagus and stomach:

- Wrestling
- Boxing
- Basketball
- Football
- Soccer (European Football)
- Rugby
- Palates ball exercises
- Certain hatha yoga positions
- Diving from cliffs or high boards
- Belly flops
- Surfing
- Certain weight lifting routines

This is just a short list, but hopefully the reader gets the idea. Any activity that results in an impact to the upper abdomen can be injurious to the tissues of the esophagus, sphincters and stomach.

That said, exercise is one of the best things that we can do to lower stress, detoxify and invigorate the body.

Regular exercise will boost our immunity and increase our mucosal health. Exercise helps us circulate those mucosal membrane contents, by heavy breathing, sweating, and in general, body fluid turnover.

This is based on the fact that exercise increases circulation and detoxification, stimulates the immune system, pumps the lymphatic system and increases lung capacity. Exercise is one of the most assured ways to strengthen the immune system and thus increase tolerance. When we exercise, we contract muscles.

Muscle contraction is what circulates (or pumps) lymph around the body through the lymph vessels. This is because the lymphatic system does not have a heart like the circulatory system has. The lymphatic system relies on muscle contraction for circulation.

Lymph circulation is critical for mucosal health because immune cells circulating through the blood and lymph break down and carry out of the body those broken-down toxins and cell parts.

And of course, exercise also circulates oxygen and nutrients throughout the body. Exercise also stimulates the thymus gland, and speeds up healing of the intestinal cell walls. In all, exercise is one of the best and cheapest therapies available to boost immunity and tolerance.

And for us vigorous athletes, this means we need to strengthen the resilience of our mucosal membranes through hydration, diet, lifestyle and eating habits as discussed above. Remember that having a leaking sphincter is not that big a deal unless we also have damaged and thinned mucosal membranes within the lower esophagus.

Infantile GERD Strategies

This section is by no means a thorough guide to GERD among infants, but it can offer a significant amount of information in the form of relevant research illustrating a few strategies that parents and their physicians can consider employing.

Researchers from Taiwan's Chang Gung University Medical College (Chao and Vandenplas 2007) gave 63 infants under six months old who had GERD symptoms—regurgitating and/or vomiting—either a formula thickened with cereal or placed the infants in an upright posture for 90 minutes after eating. This posture treatment has been advised to infants with GERD to allow for less leakage of stomach acids into the esophagus.

After 8 weeks, the group receiving the formula thickened with cereal had significantly fewer GERD symptoms, and had 25% more calorie consumption than the group receiving upright posture treatment. This also resulted in the cereal-eating infants growing faster than the other infants during the treatment period.

Scientists from The Children's Hospital of Philadelphia (Liacouras *et al.* 2005), followed 381 children diagnosed with eosinophilic esophagitis for ten years and multiple treatment regimens.

Of the group, 312 had active GERD symptoms, while 69 had dysphagia symptoms. They found corticosteroids effective at eliminating symptoms until the medication was withdrawn. After being withdrawn, the symptoms returned.

The only treatment they found with lasting effectiveness was a change in diet. Eliminating the foods each child was sensitive or allergic to improved symptoms and/or reversed the condition for a significant part of the group. They concluded that: "The removal of dietary antigens significantly improved clinical symptoms and esophageal histology in 98% of patients."

Research from the University of Southern Denmark (Nielsen *et al.* 2004) studied the association between GERD and cow's milk allergy/sensitivity. They tested 42 children with GERD using pH monitoring. Of the 18 children with severe cases of GERD, 10 had cow's milk "hypersensitivity." They concluded:

"An association between GERD and cow milk hypersensitivity was observed in both infants and children with severe GERD."

Siena University researchers (Garzi *et al.* 2002) found that a significant number of infants with GERD symptoms had cow's milk allergies, and improved with an "Extensively Hydrolyzed Cow's Milk Formula."

Researchers from the University of Arkansas Medical School and Children's Hospital (Paddock *et al.* 2012) found that milk allergies in children are related to various ear, nose and throat conditions, including GERD. The research studied 191 children with allergies to cow's milk. Among the group, 141 children suffered from ear, nose or throat infections.

Of that milk allergy group, 36% suffered from eosinophilic esophagitis, and 80% suffered from throat infections, and 27% also suffered from gastroesophageal reflux. The researchers then put 101 of the children on a milk elimination diet for two years, and 91% of the children had significant improvement.

Other research has confirmed the finding that fiber-thickened formulas decrease GERD symptoms among infants. Thickening agents have included pectin and cereal grains.

Researchers from Japan's Gunma University Medical School (Miyazawa *et al.* 2008) studied 18 children who had cerebral palsy and GERD. They took pH readings, and began to treat two groups of the children with either a high or low fruit pectin diet. After four weeks on the formula, those in the high-pectin group had fewer GERD episodes and less vomiting. Both pectin groups had less coughing, and the pH of the esophagus improved in the pectin groups.

Other types of pre-thickened infant formulas have been shown to resolve infantile GERD symptoms. University of Nebraska researchers found this out in a study of 104 infants (Vanderhoof *et al.* 2004). Five weeks on the formula significantly helped the thickened group.

Philadelphia researchers found that soy supplemented with fiber reduced GER-oriented regurgitation among infants (Ostrom *et al.* 2006).

An international study that included infant feeding in 17 countries (Alarcon *et al.* 2002) was conducted to compare the gastrointestinal responses of feeding infants formulas versus feeding them breast milk. In total, 6,999 healthy infants—who were, full-term and 28 to 98 days old—were given either a new infant formula (Similac Advance), an older infant formula (Enfalac or S-26), or breast milk.

Those receiving breast milk had softer, more frequent stools and less reflux and regurgitation than did either of the groups of infants being fed the formulas—although the newer formulas rendered stools that were closer to breast milk quality than the older formulas.

Acupuncture and Acupressure

Acupuncture is an ancient technique that has been shown to be useful in many cases of GERD.

Researchers from Germany's University Hospital in Regensburg (Pfab *et al.* 2011) tested acupuncture treatment for critically ill patients with GERD symptoms and delayed gastric empying. They gave the patients either acupoint stimulation or conventional medications for five days. After the five days, 80% of the acupuncture-treated GERD patients had increased appetites and the ability to tolerate foods, while some in the drug test group began to feel better after six days of drug therapy.

The doctors concluded: "Acupoint stimulation at Neiguan (PC-6) may be a convenient and inexpensive option (with few side effects) for the prevention and treatment of malnutrition in critically ill patients."

The point called Neiguan (PC-6) lies at the center of the inside right wrist, approximately two inches from where the hand meets the wrist (reword), between the two tendons: the flexor carpi radialis and the palmaris longus tendon. This point is frequently used to relieve nausea, and today there are a number of wristbands that can be worn that will apply pressure upon that point. This of course is not acupuncture, but rather, acupressure.

??drawing??

Sleeping Strategies

Getting a good night's sleep is critical for anyone. For a GERD sufferer it is even more critical. The author has written a book that provides extensive research and hundreds of recommendations on getting a good night's sleep *("Natural Sleep Solutions for Insomnia: The Science of Sleep, Dreaming, and Nature's Sleep Remedies")*. This book is recommended for those with sleep difficulties.

Specific to GERD sufferers, we might add a few suggestions:

Eating a meal late at night should be avoided. If a snack is eaten, it should be light an easy to digest. Nuts, pasteurized dairy (yogurt is okay), and other fatty, high protein foods are discouraged, as these are slower to digest, have a slower emptying rate, and have a higher risk of putting pressure on the lower esophageal sphincter. A banana and yogurt, or a little fibrous grain snack could be okay.

Stressful television or conversations should be avoided at night for a GERD sufferer. Better to ease into a comfortable, stress-free late night. This also means avoiding working on the computer or having a work-related phone call. Talking about money late at night should also be discouraged.

Turning down the lights within an hour of bedtime will ease our stress levels, increase our melatonin levels and aid our digestive process.

Putting blocks under the head-side of the bed to create a slightly slanted bed has helped many nighttime GERD sufferers. This slightly lifts up the head, discouraging reflux contents from flowing up towards to upper esophageal sphincter. Prone sleeping is discouraged for a GERD sufferer.

Prone sleeping (on the back) can also be dangerous for chronic GERD sufferers, because it can result in apnea as the upper sphincter is damaged by acids and toxins. Prone sleeping can also be dangerous for infants who regurgitate or drool with reflux. This is because they can choke on their reflux.

Sleeping recommendations for infants with GERD have been established by the American Academy of Pediatrics. Prone sleep positioning is discouraged, and only suggested when the risk of death and complications from GERD outweighs the increased risk of sudden infant death syndrome (SIDS).

A firm pillow is also advised for someone with GERD, to keep the head at a higher level than the stomach.

Sleeping on the stomach can put undue pressure on the upper and lower sphincters.

To help relieve some of the side crunching that occurs when sleeping on our side, we can put a firm pillow between our knees. This will keep the knees slightly separated, allowing us to more comfortably maintain the side-sleeping position.

Drinking water late at night should also be avoided, as this can wake us up during the night—reducing our all-important deep sleep time.

Stress Strategies

We've described the effects of stress and its relationship to GERD at length in this text. There are numerous techniques we can use to decrease stress. Let's summarize these:

Nature

Living around or at least visiting a natural setting such as a forest or beach has many advantages. For example, researchers from Japan's Chiba University (Park *et al.* 2010) conducted 24 field experiments using 280 subjects among 24 forests throughout Japan. In each of the tests, six subjects walked through a forest, while another six walked through a city. The next day the six that walked the city would walk the forest and vice versa.

The research concluded that forest environments reduce stress-related cortisol levels, lower heart rate, reduce blood pressure, lower anxiety and increase reaction time. The researchers concluded that: "These results will contribute to the development of a research field dedicated to forest medicine, which may be used as a strategy for preventive medicine."

Other studies have confirmed these results. One study found that people living in natural environments had lower levels of stress than those living in urban environments (Ulrich *et al.* 1991). Another, from Emory University, found that natural environments improve health conditions (Frumkin 2001).

Research has also found that even looking at natural environments, even in photos or through windows, enhances positive moods (Blood *et al.* 1999; Kaplan 2001).

All of these improvements, including lower stress levels, positive moods, lower blood pressure and reduced heart rate are all linked to mucosal health. Thus, we can conclude that living in a natural setting or spending some significant time in natural settings would be an important strategy to consider.

Sounds of Nature and Music

Music is an excellent way to help relax, assuming it is the right kind of music.

Research has shown that the right kind of music not only helps relaxation. It also helps sleep and sleep quality—critical for GERD sufferers. In a controlled, randomized study (Tan 2004), 86 fifth-graders either received music for 45 minutes near naptime or didn't, for three weeks. Those receiving music at naptime had significantly greater sleep quality. They also had higher scores among all six parameters of the Pittsburgh Sleep Quality Index (PSQI).

Like the sounds of nature, certain music resonates with our body's natural rhythms, making our body's metabolism more consistent and harmonizing. This in turn creates better sleep quality, and reduced stress.

Most of us have experienced the calming and rejuvenating effect of listening to morning birds singing outside our window. Oxford University research has found that natural sounds are relaxing because they have mostly $1/f$ spectra: gradual and gentle fluctuations in pitch and loudness. The researchers also found that human subjects tend to prefer melodies with $1/f$ distributions than the $1/f0$ (slower) or $1/f2$ (faster) fluctuations in loudness and pitch. The researchers also found that the auditory cortex responded more positively to the $1/f$ distributions.

The connection between music, cognition, and relaxation was extensively studied during the 1960s by Dr. Georgi Lozanov. Dr. Lozanov's early research investigated different types of music and their effects upon learning. He discovered that the body responded

255

differently to different beats and melodies. In particular, music with about sixty beats per minute—close to the average human resting pulse—substantially relaxed the body. This also had the effect of calming and synchronizing breathing rates.

Furthermore, Dr. Lozanov's research found that baroque-style music as composed by sixteenth, seventeenth, and eighteenth century composers such as Handel, Bach and Vivaldi had the greatest positive effects upon relaxation and memory. They appear to relax the body and focus the mind more than other types of music.

Later research found that it is not simply the 60 beats-per-minute (or 3,600 hertz) frequency rate that enables better memorization and physical relaxation. It is the 4/4 or 4/3 tempo that creates part of this effect. While numerous beats and intonations were tested in this research, few had the effect upon relaxation as music at around 3,600 hertz with a 4/4 or 4/3 tempo (Ostrander 1979).

Of course, different people like different types of music. At the same time, these parameters can be accomplished in practically every genre. Even some hard-rock bands will play a few acoustic versions with slower beats and tempos that will approach these relaxation parameters. Creative musicians of jazz, folk, indie, country and various rock genres all can reach these parameters as they blend different beats and tones into some of their music.

Our own experiences and observations clearly indicate that natural melodies can induce a calming effect, together with a higher level of alertness and mental activity. Biofeedback research confirms that these moods are connected to a preponderance of alpha brainwaves.

Playing a musical or percussion instrument appears to provide a special benefit for relaxation and sleep inducement. Playing music with the parameters mentioned promotes not only the hearing, but allows an expression of our own creative rhythm. If we are musically inclined, a few minutes of soft music playing during the evening can readily relax the body and mind, given we choose the right songs and we don't stress too much about how well we play.

In general, music with slower rhythms—slower than one's heart rate—will provide the most relaxation. Music with faster beats—faster than one's heart rate—tends to increase our energy and stimulate heat. Also, familiar music from the past seems to soothe anxiety and depression, especially as we get older.

Music has been shown to relax and induce sleep in a number of studies. Even children respond to music with better quality sleep. Researchers from Belgium's Katholieke University (Eggermont and Van den Buick 2006) studied sleep inducement among 2,546 children in the seventh and 10th grades. About 60% of the children fell asleep to music.

Guided Imagery

Guided imagery is the process of imagining that we are at a particular place or doing a particular thing. As we place ourselves at the location or scene, we look around and begin to picture the details. For example, we could imagine a beach with waves lapping onto the beach; a waterfall; clouds floating across the sky; or a quiet desert. These scenes have been used to induce sleep with great success. We could, for example, use the imagery of a secluded waterfall, imagining ourselves at that location, and seeing all the details of the waterfall.

This process of picturing all the details takes us away from the stresses and concerns of our waking world. It jump-starts our thinking and imagination process, which is critical for obtaining slow-wave and REM-stage sleep. The guided imagery process can be self-guided, or it can be guided by another person. It can also be guided by watching a video or listening to a voice recording.

As for the later technique, we can look at a picture and record our own voice as we describe what is in the picture, with all the details, talking in first person as though we were at the location of the picture. When we go to bed, we can turn on the tape. As we listen to it, we can picture the location in our mind as we drift off.

Books of landscapes can also be used for this purpose. We can sit in bed with a soft lamp and flip to a beautiful landscape before switching off the lights—then using visualization to picture ourselves at that location.

Breathing

Deep breathing can help reduce stress and encourage relaxation. However, we might remember how singers suffered from more GERD because of their extended breathing practices. So deep breathing here should emphasize relaxed and slow breathing, rather than forced breathing. For more information about breathing techniques, consider the author's book, *"Breathing to Heal."*

This book may also provide significant help for those singers, wind musicians and athletes who are pushing their diaphragms harshly and damaging their sphincters. Learning to breathe correctly will not only relax our bodies and lower our stress. It will also take pressure off our sphincters.

Color

Colors can significantly calm us. The best colors for calming are green, blue, indigo, violet, purple and pink. The other colors tend to increase stress levels.

Green stimulates brainwaves in the higher theta region, about six to seven cycles per second with a wavelength of 490 to 560 nanometers. Green is calming and balancing. It stimulates growth, love and a sense of security. It is connected to devotion and giving. Green is also a soothing color, stimulating healing response, particularly among ailments related to the cardiovascular system—and considered beneficial to the heart, blood pressure, and congestion.

Blue stimulates lower theta waves in the five to six hertz area at wavelengths of 450 to 490 nanometers. Blue is cooling and calming. It slows metabolism. The rhythm of blue is gentle and holistic. Blue is associated with creativity and communication on both a spiritual and physical level.

Indigo stimulates low delta waves around one cycle per second and wavelengths of 400 to 450 nanometers. Indigo is associated with clarity, intuition and intelligence. It is a color associated with decision-making and meditative thinking. The sinuses, vision, and the immune system are therefore stimulated by and resonate with indigo.

Violet stimulates higher delta waves from two to four hertz. These waves vibrate at a faster frequency than indigo, primarily because they are more stimulating. Violet activities are associated with deep meditation, inspiration, prayer, and spiritual insight.

Purple, blends the effects of indigo and violet.

Pink has been associated with sedative and muscle-relaxing effects. Color behavioral therapist Alexander Schauss, Ph.D. has reported that pink colors create a tranquilizing effect, preventing or slowing anger and anxiety. Interestingly, Dr. Schauss also reported this same effect among colorblind patients.

The cooler colors of violet and indigo slow and reduce energy levels, providing a relaxing meditative environment. Greens and the blues are also calming, but do not promote sleep—as was evidenced in blue-blocking research. Blues and greens are appropriate during the daytime hours, and significant exposure to these colors during the daylight hours will promote sleep at night.

This was evidenced by a study (Gammack and Burke 2009) of nursing home residents, who slept better when given more exposure to natural light. Nature's blues and greens are available in most locations. All we have to do is look outside.

Progressive Relaxation

This stress-reducing technique has been increasingly recommended by physicians and alternative practitioners alike.

The method is to alternate contraction and relaxation of the major muscle groups one by one, starting from one end of the body to the other. We can start at the head by contracting the facial muscles for 1-2 seconds, followed by complete relaxation of those muscles. Then we can move down to the arms, the chest, the abdomen, legs, and feet—alternatively contracting and then relaxing each part. This (or the opposite progression, from the feet up) has been used to bring on a state of relaxation and help ease us into sleep.

Meditation and Prayer

Meditation and prayer prior to or after going to bed can help relax body and mind. Prayers and chants can be used to focus the inner self and mind upon the more important aspects of life. This can relieve our stresses and anxiety over the petty details of this temporary physical world.

In a study by researchers from Spain's University of Malaga (Vera *et al.* 2009), 26 subjects—including 16 long-term yoga practitioners—were tested for sleep quality and hormone cycles. The long-term yoga practitioners had significantly better sleep quality and better-regulated hormone cycles.

The strict *Sanskrit* translation of the word *yoga* means "connecting with God." Finding our spiritual connection with the Supreme Being through heartfelt prayer, meditation, mantras or praises has been used by billions of people for thousands of years to reduce stress and see a deeper meaning in life.

Other Anti-GERD Strategies

Clearing the Sinuses

Occasionally clearing the sinuses is important to the health of our esophagus and our mucous membranes in general. When the sinuses are clogged, our mucous membranes are not draining properly. Mucous needs to be swept out, and if the mucous is too thick or crustified with waste matter, it will narrow our available airways. As we breathe and swallow, the thickened mucous migrates to our esophagus.

So how do we accomplish keeping the sinuses clear? Well, besides breathing in through the nose and general hygiene to help keep the nostrils clean—we might consider periodic nasal irrigation.

Nasal lavage is the first consideration. This can utilize a special Ayurvedic lavage device called the neti pot. Neti has been in practice for thousands of years. The pot is simply filled with warm weakly-salty water, and poured through each nostril. A small teapot can also be used.

The technique is to first mix about a quarter-teaspoon of non-iodized salt to about a cup of lukewarm water. A pinch of baking soda may also be added, especially if the salt is iodized or otherwise burns in any way.

Lean forward, over the sink. With the chin level with the nose, turn the head sideways so the nose on a plane parallel with the ground as much as possible.

The water is lightly poured into one nostril, traveling around the septum and out the other nostril. There is no force or pressure involved. There is no snuffing in or pulling in. The solution is simply poured into one nostril, and out through the other. Just hold the head still while it pours out.

Nasal Irrigation: This can also be accomplished by gently pushing warm saline (water and salt) into each nostril using a soft

260

squeeze bottle. Soft squeeze bottles designed for cleaning the nostrils are often available at most drug stores. After using the saline in the bottle, the bottle can be refilled. Care must be taken not to forcefully squirt the water through, which can get water into the upper sinuses.

Another technique is to sniff the water up the nose and back down through to the pharynx and throat, where it is spit out into the sink. This can provide a more complete cleansing of the pharynx and sinuses, but should not be overdone, and only if the sinuses are at least partially clear.

Nasal irrigation has been proven in research to aid in allergic conditions and sinusitis. For example, researchers from Taiwan's Chung Shan Medical University Hospital (Wang *et al.* 2009) gave nasal irrigation or not to 69 children with acute sinusitis. The saline irrigation group improved significantly better than the other group with regard to symptoms and quality of life.

Nasal irrigation was also effective in reducing sinus congestion, rhinorrhea, sneezing and nasal itching in a study by medical researchers from Italy's University of Milano (Garavello *et al.* 2010). In this study, 23 pregnant women with seasonal allergic rhinitis underwent either nasal irrigation or not for six weeks.

In another study, presented at the 50th Scientific Assembly of the American Academy of Family Physicians, Dr. Richard Ravizza and Dr. John Fornadley of Pennsylvania State University divided 294 students into three groups, one of which did nasal irrigation with salt water and the other two groups either took a placebo pill or did nothing. The nasal irrigation group experienced fewer colds during the treatment period compared to the other two groups.

To be fair, some have questioned whether daily regular nasal irrigation for long periods is necessarily good. In a study presented at a the American College of Allergy, Asthma and Immunology (Nsouli 2009), researchers tested 68 patients with a history of sinusitis, who had been using nasal irrigation daily. Of the total, 44 patients discontinued the irrigation while 24 continued the daily treatment. After a year, those who had discontinued the irrigation had 62% less sinusitis infections than the group who continued to use nasal irrigation daily. Dr. Tamal Nsouli commented that daily irrigation may deplete healthy mucous from the sinuses. As we've discussed, healthy mucous membranes also cover the sinuses, helping protect us from infection. Dr. Nsouli also commented that he is not opposed to irrigation for three or four times a week, but suggested avoiding daily irrigation for long periods.

We should note that the study details and protocol have yet to be published, and was only presented in abstract form at the conference. Diane Heatley, M.D., a Professor at the University of Wisconsin School of Medicine, questioned the report, stating, "nasal irrigation has previously been proven safe and effective for treatment of sinus symptoms in both adults and children in a number of studies already published in peer-reviewed journals."

An appropriate conclusion here is that regular nasal irrigation should still include some moderation. Using it during periods of congestion and sensitivity is certainly appropriate. Use after or during environmental conditions where there is an increased level of pollution and/or infectious agents is also appropriate. But we can remember that our mucous membranes also house important immune cells and probiotics, which help protect us. We don't want to flush those away needlessly.

Oral Health

There are several oral health strategies we can implement to help with GERD.

Brushing without peppermint toothpaste is probably a good idea, since peppermint additives have been shown to reduce sphincter tone. This may or may not relate to raw peppermint or peppermint tea, as the research has not established this with definition.

But toothpaste with peppermint flavorings or peppermint extract is a different story, as the research connecting peppermint candies and peppermint additive foods have been more firm. If we do brush with a mint toothpaste, we should consider thoroughly rinsing afterward, as it will likely migrate to the esophagus otherwise.

Using a tongue cleaner is a good way to lower our bacteria counts within our esophagus. Those bacteria at the back of our tongues will ride down the throat into the esophagus and colonize there. Tongue cleaners are now found at most health food stores, but plastic versions are not as good as metal types, made of either stainless steel or silver. Ayurvedic medicine has recommended silver tongue cleaners for a variety of infective digestive issues.

Flossing and using a water flossing device are suggested to clear out some of the oral bacteria described in our chapter on probiotics. Cleaning the gums behind the back molars are critical, as these can harbor numerous pathogenic bacteria that will be washed down into our esophagus with our meals and drinks.

Besides these, a good *rinsing of our mouth* after our meals, by vigorously swishing clean water through our teeth and gums is also a great idea.

Clearing the Esophagus

We can also consider clearing the pharynx/throat and esophagus regions. This is quite simple. We can gargle with warm salt water periodically to clear out and remove the build up of toxins, food wastes and thickened mucous.

It is also best to follow each meal with a small sip of clean water to clear food debris from along our throat and esophagus linings. This can help prevent the breakdown of these foods at those sites—and the possibility that those breakdown molecules harm our epithelial cells and/or sphincter tissues.

Avoiding Toxins

This naturally brings us to strategies to combat toxin intake. We talked about the forms of various toxins in the last chapter.

Avoiding them is not difficult, but requires we look around us and gauge the extent that these toxins may be getting into our systems.

Then we simply need to take *practical* steps to reduce our exposure to them to the degree possible. The more toxin build up we have, the more our immune systems and mucosal membranes will be burdened.

Conclusion

As we've discovered, GERD is not simply a digestive ailment. There are a variety of issues that can help promote GERD issues, including our diet, our water consumption, pharmaceuticals, toxins, stress, sleep and many others. The combined effects of these factors pile up within our bodies, effectively reducing our mucosal secretions. This in turn exposes our epithelial cells of our esophagus and sphincters to damage from our stomach acids, the toxins in our foods, the microorganisms such as *H. pylori* and the acids within our undigested foods.

That said, the GERD solution is not a one-size fits all solution. We each have unique lifestyles, diets, habits, and many other variables in our lives that each can provoke the issues that produce GERD.

Each GERD or heartburn sufferer has relative degrees of the condition as well. This doesn't mean that those with minor sporatic heartburn should not take their condition seriously. As we've shown, as GERD advances it can cause major damage within our esophagus, throat, lungs and sinuses. So it behooves us to take corrective action regardless of our GERD's state of progression.

Therefore, we each need to do a little investigating. Using the tools this book has laid out, we can now ascertain those issues that produce our particular case of GERD. Because most GERD symptoms are sporadic, this allows us to do a little experimenting with some of the research that this book has laid out.

This said, we should always work closely with our primary health care professional as we make any changes. We might consider showing our health professional this book, and together looking at some things we might consider eliminating or adding to our diets or lifestyles.

This recipe, in the opinion of the author, has the most likelihood of success. In this respect, we might remember Einstein's famous quip that insanity is doing the same thing over and over again and expecting different results.

Let's consider doing something different.

References and Bibliography

Abdureyim S, Amat N, Umar A, Upur H, Berke B, Moore N. Anti-inflammatory, immunomodulatory, and heme oxygenase-1 inhibitory activities of ravan napas, a formulation of uighur traditional medicine, in a rat model of allergic asthma. *Evid Based Complement Alternat Med.* 2011;2011. pii: 725926.

Aberg N, Hesselmar B, Aberg B, Eriksson B. Increase of asthma, allergic rhinitis and eczema in Swedish schoolchildren between 1979 and 1991. *Clin Exp Allergy.* 1995;25:815-819.

Abonia JP, Rothenberg ME. Eosinophilic esophagitis: rapidly advancing insights. *Annu Rev Med.* 2012 Feb 18;63:421-34.

Adel-Patient K, Ah-Leung S, Creminon C, Nouaille S, Chatel JM, Langella P, Wal JM. Oral administration of recombinant Lactococcus lactis expressing bovine beta-lactoglobulin partially prevents mice from sensitization. *Clin Exp Allergy.* 2005 Apr;35(4):539-46.

Agache I, Ciobanu C. Risk factors and asthma phenotypes in children and adults with seasonal allergic rhinitis. *Phys Sportsmed.* 2010 Dec;38(4):81-6.

Agarwal PK, Singh A, Gaurav K, Goel S, Khanna HD, Goel RK. Evaluation of wound healing activity of extracts of plantain banana (Musa sapientum var. paradisiaca) in rats. *Indian J Exp Biol.* 2009 Jan;47(1):32-40.

Agarwal SK, Singh SS, Verma S. Antifungal principle of sesquiterpene lactones from Anamirta cocculus. *Indian Drugs.* 1999;36:754-5.

Aggarwal BB, Harikumar KB. Potential therapeutic effects of curcumin, the anti-inflammatory agent, against neurodegenerative, cardiovascular, pulmonary, metabolic, autoimmune and neoplastic diseases. *Int J Biochem Cell Biol.* 2009 Jan;41(1):40-59.

Aggarwal BB, Sung B. Pharmacological basis for the role of curcumin in chronic diseases: an age-old spice with modern targets. *Trends Pharmacol Sci.* 2009 Feb;30(2):85-94.

Agostoni C, Fiocchi A, Riva E, Terracciano L, Sarratud T, Martelli A, Lodi F, D'Auria E, Zuccotti G, Giovannini M. Growth of infants with IgE-mediated cow's milk allergy fed different formulas in the complementary feeding period. *Pediatr Allergy Immunol.* 2007 Nov;18(7):599-606.

Aguirre C, Ruiz-Irastorza G, Egurbide MV. Gastroesophageal reflux disease. *N Engl J Med.* 2009 Feb 12;360(7):729; author reply 729-30.

Aho K, Koskenvuo M, Tuominen J, Kaprio J. Occurrence of rheumatoid arthritis in a nationwide series of twins. *J Rheumatol.* 1986 Oct;13(5):899-902.

Aiyer HS, Li Y, Losso JN, Gao C, Schiffman SC, Slone SP, Martin RC. Effect of freeze-dried berries on the development of reflux-induced esophageal adenocarcinoma. *Nutr Cancer.* 2011 Nov;63(8):1256-62.

Akinbami LJ, Moorman JE, Garbe PL, Sondik EJ. Status of childhood asthma in the United States, 1980-2007. *Pediatrics.* 2009;123:S131-45.

Alarcon PA, Tressler RL, Mulvaney A, Lam W, Comer GM. Gastrointestinal tolerance of a new infant milk formula in healthy babies: an international study conducted in 17 countries. *Nutrition.* 2002 Jun;18(6):484-9.

Alemán A, Sastre J, Quirce S, de las Heras M, Carnés J, Fernández-Caldas E, Pastor C, Blázquez AB, Vivanco F, Cuesta-Herranz J. Allergy to kiwi: a double-blind, placebo-controlled food challenge study in patients from a birch-free area. *J Allergy Clin Immunol.* 2004 Mar;113(3):543-50.

Alexander DD, Cabana MD. Partially hydrolyzed 100% whey protein infant formula and reduced risk of atopic dermatitis: a meta-analysis. *J Pediatr Gastroenterol Nutr.* 2010 Apr;50(4):422-30.

Alexandrakis M, Letourneau R, Kempuraj D, Kandere-Grzybowska K, Huang M, Christodoulou S, Boucher W, Seretakis D, Theoharides TC. Flavones inhibit proliferation and increase mediator content in human leukemic mast cells (HMC-1). *Eur J Haematol.* 2003 Dec;71(6):448-54.

Al-Harrasi A, Al-Saidi S. Phytochemical analysis of the essential oil from botanically certified oleogum resin of Boswellia sacra (Omani Luban). *Molecules.* 2008 Sep 16;13(9):2181-9.

Almqvist C, Garden F, Xuan W, Mihrshahi S, Leeder SR, Oddy W, Webb K, Marks GB; CAPS team. Omega-3 and omega-6 fatty acid exposure from early life does not affect atopy and asthma at age 5 years. *J Allergy Clin Immunol.* 2007 Jun;119(6):1438-44.

Amato R, Pinelli M, Monticelli A, Miele G, Cocozza S. Schizophrenia and Vitamin D Related Genes Could Have Been Subject to Latitude-driven Adaptation. *BMC Evol Biol.* 2010 Nov 11;10(1):351.

American Conference of Governmental Industrial Hygienists. *Threshold limit values for chemical substances and physical agents in the work environment.* Cincinnati, OH: ACGIH, 1986.

American Dietetic Association; Dietitians of Canada. Position of the American Dietetic Association and Dietitians of Canada: vegetarian diets. *Can J Diet Pract Res.* 2003 Summer;64(2):62-81.

Ammon HP. Boswellic acids (components of frankincense) as the active principle in treatment of chronic inflammatory diseases. *Wien Med Wochenschr.* 2002;152(15-16):373-8.

Ammon HP. Boswellic acids in chronic inflammatory diseases. *Planta Med.* 2006 Oct;72(12):1100-16.

Anand P, Thomas SG, Kunnumakkara AB, Sundaram C, Harikumar KB, Sung B, Tharakan ST, Misra K, Priyadarsini IK, Rajasekharan KN, Aggarwal BB. Biological activities of curcumin and its analogues (Congeners) made by man and Mother Nature. *Biochem Pharmacol.* 2008 Dec 1;76(11):1590-611.

Anastasiou D, Poulogiannis G, Asara JM, Boxer MB, Jiang JK, Shen M, Bellinger G, Sasaki AT, Locasale JW, Auld DS, Thomas CJ, Vander Heiden MG, Cantley LC. Inhibition of pyruvate kinase M2 by reactive oxygen species contributes to cellular antioxidant responses. *Science.* 2011 Dec 2;334(6060):1278-83.

Anderson JL, May HT, Horne BD, Bair TL, Hall NL, Carlquist JF, Lappé DL, Muhlestein JB; Intermountain Heart Collaborative (IHC) Study Group. Relation of vitamin D deficiency to cardiovascular risk factors, disease status, and incident events in a general healthcare population. *Am J Cardiol.* 2010 Oct 1;106(7):963-8.

Anderson M., Grissom C. Increasing the Heavy Atom Effect of Xenon by Adsorption to Zeolites: Photolysis of 2,3-Diazabicyclo[2.2.2]oct-2-ene. *J. Am. Chem. Soc.* 1996;118:9552-9556.

Anderson RC, Anderson JH. Acute respiratory effects of diaper emissions. *Arch Environ Health.* 1999 Sep-Oct;54(5):353-8.

Anderson RC, Anderson JH. Acute toxic effects of fragrance products. *Arch Environ Health.* 1998 Mar-Apr;53(2):138-46.

Anderson RC, Anderson JH. Respiratory toxicity in mice exposed to mattress covers. *Arch Environ Health.* 1999 May-Jun;54(3):202-9.

Anderson RC, Anderson JH. Respiratory toxicity of fabric softener emissions. *J Toxicol Environ Health.* 2000 May 26;60(2):121-36.

Anderson RC, Anderson JH. Respiratory toxicity of mattress emissions in mice. *Arch Environ Health.* 2000 Jan-Feb;55(1):38-43.

Anderson RC, Anderson JH. Sensory irritation and multiple chemical sensitivity. *Toxicol Ind Health.* 1999 Apr-Jun;15(3-4):339-45.

Anderson RC, Anderson JH. Toxic effects of air freshener emissions. *Arch Environ Health.* 1997 Nov-Dec;52(6):433-41.

Anderson SD, Charlton B, Weiler JM, Nichols S, Spector SL, Pearlman DS; A305 Study Group. Comparison of mannitol and methacholine to predict exercise-induced bronchoconstriction and a clinical diagnosis of asthma. *Respir Res.* 2009 Jan 23;10:4.

Andoh T, Zhang Q, Yamamoto T, Tayama M, Hattori M, Tanaka K, Kuraishi Y. Inhibitory Effects of the Methanol Extract of Ganoderma lucidum on Mosquito Allergy-Induced Itch-Associated Responses in Mice. *J Pharmacol Sci.* 2010 Oct 8.

André C, André F, Colin L. Effect of allergen ingestion challenge with and without cromoglycate cover on intestinal permeability in atopic dermatitis, urticaria and other symptoms of food allergy. *Allergy.* 1989;44 Suppl 9:47-51.

André C. Food allergy. Objective diagnosis and test of therapeutic efficacy by measuring intestinal permeability. *Presse Med.* 1986 Jan 25;15(3):105-8.

Andre F, Andre C, Feknous M, Colin L, Cavagna S. Digestive permeability to different-sized molecules and to sodium cromoglycate in food allergy. *Allergy Proc.* 1991 Sep-Oct;12(5):293-8.

Anim-Nyame N, Sooranna SR, Johnson MR, Gamble J, Steer PJ. Garlic supplementation increases peripheral blood flow: a role for interleukin-6? *J Nutr Biochem.* 2004 Jan;15(1):30-6.

Annweiler C, Schott AM, Berrut G, Chauviré V, Le Gall D, Inzitari M, Beauchet O. Vitamin D and ageing: neurological issues. *Neuropsychobiology.* 2010 Aug;62(3):139-50.

Antczak A, Nowak D, Shariati B, Król M, Piasecka G, Kurmanowska Z. Increased hydrogen peroxide and thiobarbituric acid-reactive products in expired breath condensate of asthmatic patients. *Eur Respir J.* 1997 Jun;10(6):1235-41.

Aoki T, Usuda Y, Miyakoshi H, Tamura K, Herberman RB. Low natural killer syndrome: clinical and immunologic features. *Nat Immun Cell Growth Regul.* 1987;6(3):116-28.

Apáti P, Houghton PJ, Kite G, Steventon GB, Kéry A. In-vitro effect of flavonoids from Solidago canadensis extract on glutathione S-transferase. *J Pharm Pharmacol.* 2006 Feb;58(2):251-6.

APHA (American Public Health Association). Opposition to the Use of Hormone Growth Promoters in Beef and Dairy Cattle Production. Policy Date: 11/10/2009. Policy Number: 20098. http://www.apha.org/advocacy/policy/id=1379. Accessed Nov. 24, 2010.

Araki K, Shinozaki T, Irie Y, Miyazawa Y. Trial of oral administration of Bifidobacterium breve for the prevention of rotavirus infections. *Kansenshogaku Zasshi.* 1999 Apr;73(4):305-10.

Aramini B, Mattioli S, Lugaresi M, Brusori S, Di Simone MP, D'Ovidio F. Prevalence and clinical picture of gastroesophageal prolapse in gastroesophageal reflux disease. *Dis Esophagus.* 2011 Nov 21.

Araujo AC, Aprile LR, Dantas RO, Terra-Filho J, Vianna EO. Bronchial responsiveness during esophageal acid infusion. *Lung.* 2008 Mar-Apr;186(2):123-8. 2008 Feb 23.

Arbes SJ Jr, Gergen PJ, Vaughn B, Zeldin DC. Asthma cases attributable to atopy: results from the Third National Health and Nutrition Examination Survey. *J Allergy Clin Immunol.* 2007 Nov;120(5):1139-45. 2007 Sep 24.

Argento A, Tiraferri E, Marzaloni M. Oral anticoagulants and medicinal plants. An emerging interaction. *Ann Ital Med Int.* 2000 Apr-Jun;15(2):139-43.

Arif AA, Delclos GL, Colmer-Hamood J. Association between asthma, asthma symptoms and C-reactive protein in US adults: data from the National Health and Nutrition Examination Survey, 1999-2002. *Respirology.* 2007 Sep;12(5):675-82. .

Arif AA, Shah SM. Association between personal exposure to volatile organic compounds and asthma among US adult population. *Int Arch Occup Environ Health.* 2007 Aug;80(8):711-9.

Armstrong D, Sifrim D. New pharmacologic approaches in gastroesophageal reflux disease. *Thorac Surg Clin.* 2011 Nov;21(4):557-74.

Arshad SH, Bateman B, Sadeghnejad A, Gant C, Matthews SM. Prevention of allergic disease during childhood by allergen avoidance: the Isle of Wight prevention study. *J Allergy Clin Immunol.* 2007 Feb;119(2):307-13.

Arslanoglu S, Moro GE, Schmitt J, Tandoi L, Rizzardi S, Boehm G. Early dietary intervention with a mixture of prebiotic oligosaccharides reduces the incidence of allergic manifestations and infections during the first two years of life. *J Nutr.* 2008 Jun;138(6):1091-5.

REFERENCES

Arslanoglu S, Moro GE, Schmitt J, Tandoi L, Rizzardi S, Boehm G. Early dietary intervention with a mixture of prebiotic oligosaccharides reduces the incidence of allergic manifestations and infections during the first two years of life. *J Nutr.* 2008 Jun;138(6):1091-5.

Arterburn LM, Oken HA, Bailey Hall E, Hamersley J, Kuratko CN, Hoffman JP. Algal-oil capsules and cooked salmon: nutritionally equivalent sources of docosahexaenoic acid. *J Am Diet Assoc.* 2008 Jul;108(7):1204-9.

Arterburn LM, Oken HA, Hoffman JP, Bailey-Hall E, Chung G, Rom D, Hamersley J, McCarthy D. Bioequivalence of Docosahexaenoic acid from different algal oils in capsules and in a DHA-fortified food. *Lipids.* 2007 Nov;42(11):1011-24.

Arvaniti F, Priftis KN, Panagiotakos DB. Dietary habits and asthma: a review. *Allergy Asthma Proc.* 2010 Mar;31(2):e1-10.

Asero R, Antonicelli L, Arena A, Bommarito L, Caruso B, Colombo G, Crivellaro M, De Carli M, Della Torre E, Della Torre F, Heffler E, Lodi Rizzini F, Longo R, Manzotti G, Marcotulli M, Melchiorre A, Minale P, Morandi P, Moreni B, Moschella A, Murzilli F, Nebiolo F, Poppa M, Randazzo S, Rossi G, Senna GE. Causes of food-induced anaphylaxis in Italian adults: a multi-centre study. *Int Arch Allergy Immunol.* 2009;150(3):271-7.

Asero R, Mistrello G, Roncarolo D, Amato S, Caldironi G, Barocci F, van Ree R. Immunological cross-reactivity between lipid transfer proteins from botanically unrelated plant-derived foods: a clinical study. *Allergy.* 2002 Oct;57(10):900-6.

Ashrafi K, Chang FY, Watts JL, Fraser AG, Kamath RS, Ahringer J, Ruvkun G. Genome-wide RNAi analysis of Caenorhabditis elegans fat regulatory genes. *Nature.* 2003 Jan 16;421(6920):268-72.

Atkinson W, Harris J, Mills P, Moffat S, White C, Lynch O, Jones M, Cullinan P, Newman Taylor AJ. Domestic aeroallergen exposures among infants in an English town. *Eur Respir J.* 1999 Mar;13(3):583-9.

Atsumi T, Tonosaki K. Smelling lavender and rosemary increases free radical scavenging activity and decreases cortisol level in saliva. *Psychiatry Res.* 2007 Feb 28;150(1):89-96.

Attar A. Digestive manifestations in systemic sclerosis. *Ann Med Interne (Paris).* 2002 Jun;153(4):260-4.

Ayazi S, Leers JM, Oezcelik A, Abate E, Peyre CG, Hagen JA, DeMeester SR, Banki F, Lipham JC, DeMeester TR, Crookes PF. Measurement of gastric pH in ambulatory esophageal pH monitoring. *Surg Endosc.* 2009 Sep;23(9):1968-73.

Ayazi S, Pearson J, Hashemi M. Gastroesophageal reflux and voice changes: objective assessment of voice quality and impact of antireflux therapy. *J Clin Gastroenterol.* 2012 Feb;46(2):119-23.

Bacopoulou F, Veltsista A, Vassi I, Gika A, Lekea V, Priftis K, Bakoula C. Can we be optimistic about asthma in childhood? A Greek cohort study. *J Asthma.* 2009 Mar;46(2):171-4.

Badar VA, Thawani VR, Wakode PT, Shrivastava MP, Gharpure KJ, Hingorani LL, Khiyani RM. Efficacy of Tinospora cordifolia in allergic rhinitis. *J Ethnopharmacol.* 2005 Jan 15;96(3):445-9.

Bae GS, Kim MS, Jung WS, Seo SW, Yun SW, Kim SG, Park RK, Kim EC, Song HJ, Park SJ. Inhibition of lipopolysaccharide-induced inflammatory responses by piperine. *Eur J Pharmacol.* 2010 Sep 10;642(1-3):154-62.

Bafadhel M, Singapuri A, Terry S, Hargadon B, Monteiro W, Green RH, Bradding PH, Wardlaw AJ, Pavord ID, Brightling CE. Body mass and fat mass in refractory asthma: an observational 1 year follow-up study. *J Allergy.* 2010;2010:251758. 2010 Dec 1.

Baker SM. *Detoxification and Healing.* Chicago: Contemporary Books, 2004.

Bakkeheim E, Mowinckel P, Carlsen KH, Håland G, Carlsen KC. Paracetamol in early infancy: the risk of childhood allergy and asthma. Acta Paediatr. 2011 Jan;100(1):90-6.

Balch P, Balch J. *Prescription for Nutritional Healing.* New York: Avery, 2000.

Ballentine R. *Diet & Nutrition: A holistic approach.* Honesdale, PA: Himalayan Int., 1978.

Ballentine R. *Radical Healing.* New York: Harmony Books, 1999.

Ballmer-Weber BK, Holzhauser T, Scibilia J, Mittag D, Zisa G, Ortolani C, Oesterballe M, Poulsen LK, Vieths S, Bindslev-Jensen C. Clinical characteristics of soybean allergy in Europe: a double-blind, placebo-controlled food challenge study. *J Allergy Clin Immunol.* 2007 Jun;119(6):1489-96.

Ballmer-Weber BK, Vieths S, Lüttkopf D, Heuschmann P, Wüthrich B. Celery allergy confirmed by double-blind, placebo-controlled food challenge: a clinical study in 32 subjects with a history of adverse reactions to celery root. *J Allergy Clin Immunol.* 2000 Aug;106(2):373-8.

Banno N, Akihisa T, Yasukawa K, Tokuda H, Tabata K, Nakamura Y, Nishimura R, Kimura Y, Suzuki T. Anti-inflammatory activities of the triterpene acids from the resin of Boswellia carteri. *J Ethnopharmacol.* 2006 Sep 19;107(2):249-53.

Bant A, Kruszewski J. Increased sensitization prevalence to common inhalant and food allergens in young adult Polish males. *Ann Agric Environ Med.* 2008 Jun;15(1):21-7.

Barak N, Ehrenpreis ED, Harrison JR, Sitrin MD. Gastro-oesophageal reflux disease in obesity: pathophysiological and therapeutic considerations. *Obes Rev.* 2002 Feb;3(1):9-15.

Barnes M, Cullinan P, Athanasaki P, MacNeill S, Hole AM, Harris J, Kalogeraki S, Chatzinikolaou M, Drakonakis N, Bibaki-Liakou V, Newman Taylor AJ, Bibakis I. Crete: does farming explain urban and rural differences in atopy? *Clin Exp Allergy.* 2001 Dec;31(12):1822-8.

Barnetson RS, Drummond H, Ferguson A. Precipitins to dietary proteins in atopic eczema. *Br J Dermatol.* 1983 Dec;109(6):653-5.

Barnett AG, Williams GM, Schwartz J, Neller AH, Best TL, Petroeschevsky AL, Simpson RW. Air pollution and child respiratory health: a case-crossover study in Australia and New Zealand. *Am J Respir Crit Care Med.* 2005 Jun 1;171(11):1272-8.

Barrager E, Veltmann JR Jr, Schauss AG, Schiller RN. A multicentered, open-label trial on the safety and efficacy of methylsulfonylmethane in the treatment of seasonal allergic rhinitis. *J Altern Complement Med.* 2002 Apr;8(2):167-73.

Barros R, Moreira A, Fonseca J, de Oliveira JF, Delgado L, Castel-Branco MG, Haahtela T, Lopes C, Moreira P. Adherence to the Mediterranean diet and fresh fruit intake are associated with improved asthma control. *Allergy.* 2008 Jul;63(7):917-23.

Basu A, Devaraj S, Jialal I. Dietary factors that promote or retard inflammation. *Arterioscler Thromb Vasc Biol.* 2006 May;26(5):995-1001.

Bateman B, Warner JO, Hutchinson E, Dean T, Rowlandson P, Gant C, Grundy J, Fitzgerald C, Stevenson J. The effects of a double blind, placebo controlled, artificial food colourings and benzoate preservative challenge on hyperactivity in a general population sample of preschool children. *Arch Dis Child.* 2004 Jun;89(6):506-11.

Bates DW, Cullen DJ, Laird N, Petersen LA, Small SD, Servi D, Laffel G, Sweitzer BJ, Shea BF, Hallisey R, *et al.* Incidence of adverse drug events and potential adverse drug events. Implications for prevention. ADE Prevention Study Group. *JAMA.* 1995 Jul 5;274(1):29-34.

Batista R, Martins I, Jeno P, Ricardo CP, Oliveira MM. A proteomic study to identify soya allergens—the human response to transgenic versus non-transgenic soya samples. *Int Arch Allergy Immunol.* 2007;144(1):29-38.

Batmanghelidj F. Neurotransmitter histamine: an alternative view point, *Science in Medicine Simplified.* Falls Church, VA: Foundation for the Simple in Medicine, 1990.

Batmanghelidj F. Pain: a need for paradigm change. *Anticancer Res.* 1987 Sep-Oct;7(5B):971-89.

Batmanghelidj F. *Your Body's Many Cries for Water.* 2nd Ed. Vienna, VA: Global Health, 1997.

Bax KC, Gupta SK. Allergic eosinophilic esophagitis. *Indian J Pediatr.* 2006 Oct;73(10):919-25.

Beasley R, Clayton T, Crane J, von Mutius E, Lai CK, Montefort S, Stewart A; ISAAC Phase Three Study Group. Association between paracetamol use in infancy and childhood, and risk of asthma, rhinoconjunctivitis, and eczema in children aged 6-7 years: analysis from Phase Three of the ISAAC programme. *Lancet.* 2008 Sep. 20;372(9643):1039-48.

Beaulieu A, Fessele K. Agent Orange: management of patients exposed in Vietnam. *Clin J Oncol Nurs.* 2003 May-Jun;7(3):320-3.

Becker KG, Simon RM, Bailey-Wilson JE, Freidlin B, Biddison WE, McFarland HF, Trent JM. Clustering of non-major histocompatibility complex susceptibility candidate loci in human autoimmune diseases. *Proc Natl Acad Sci U S A.* 1998 Aug 18;95(17):9979-84.

Beddoe AF. *Biologic Ionization as Applied to Human Nutrition.* Warsaw: Wendell Whitman, 2002.

Beecher GR. Phytonutrients' role in metabolism: effects on resistance to degenerative processes. *Nutr Rev.* 1999 Sep;57(9 Pt 2):S3-6.

Belcaro G, Cesarone MR, Errichi S, Zulli C, Errichi BM, Vinciguerra G, Ledda A, Di Renzo A, Stuard S, Dugall M, Pellegrini L, Gizzi G, Ippolito E, Ricci A, Cacchio M, Cipollone G, Ruffini I, Fano F, Hosoi M, Rohdewald P. Variations in C-reactive protein, plasma free radicals and fibrinogen values in patients with osteoarthritis treated with Pycnogenol. *Redox Rep.* 2008;13(6):271-6.

Bell IR, Baldwin CM, Schwartz GE, Illness from low levels of environmental chemicals: relevance to chronic fatigue syndrome and fibromyalgia. *Am J Med.* 1998;105 (suppl 3A).:74-82. S.

Bell SJ, Potter PC. Milk whey-specific immune complexes in allergic and non-allergic subjects. *Allergy.* 1988 Oct;43(7):497-503.

Ben, X.M., Zhou, X.Y., Zhao, W.H., Yu, W.L., Pan, W., Zhang, W.L., Wu, S.M., Van Beusekom, C.M., Schaafsma, A. (2004) Supplementation of milk formula with galactooligosaccharides improves intestinal micro-flora and fermentation in term infants. *Chin Med J.* 117(6):927-931, 2004.

Benard A, Desreumeaux P, Huglo D, Hoorelbeke A, Tonnel AB, Wallaert B. Increased intestinal permeability in bronchial asthma. *J Allergy Clin Immunol.* 1996 Jun;97(6):1173-8.

Bengmark S. Curcumin, an atoxic antioxidant and natural NFkappaB, cyclooxygenase-2, lipooxygenase, and inducible nitric oxide synthase inhibitor: a shield against acute and chronic diseases. *JPEN J Parenter Enteral Nutr.* 2006 Jan-Feb;30(1):45-51.

Bengmark S. Immunonutrition: role of biosurfactants, fiber, and probiotic bacteria. *Nutrition.* 1998 Jul-Aug;14(7-8):585-94.

Benlounes N, Dupont C, Candalh C, Blaton MA, Darmon N, Desjeux JF, Heyman M. The threshold for immune cell reactivity to milk antigens decreases in cow's milk allergy with intestinal symptoms. *J Allergy Clin Immunol.* 1996 Oct;98(4):781-9.

Bennett WD, Zeman KL, Jarabek AM. Nasal contribution to breathing and fine particle deposition in children versus adults. *J Toxicol Environ Health A.* 2008;71(3):227-37.

Ben-Shoshan M, Harrington DW, Soller L, Fragapane J, Joseph L, St Pierre Y, Godefroy SB, Elliot SJ, Clarke AE. A population-based study on peanut, tree nut, fish, shellfish, and sesame allergy prevalence in Canada. *J Allergy Clin Immunol.* 2010 Jun;125(6):1327-35.

Ben-Shoshan M, Kagan R, Primeau MN, Alizadehfar R, Turnbull E, Harada L, Dufresne C, Allen M, Joseph L, St Pierre Y, Clarke A. Establishing the diagnosis of peanut allergy in children never exposed to peanut or with an uncertain history: a cross-Canada study. *Pediatr Allergy Immunol.* 2010 Sep;21(6):920-6.

Bensky D, Gable A, Kaptchuk T (transl.). *Chinese Herbal Medicine Materia Medica.* Seattle: Eastland Press, 1986.

Bergner P. *The Healing Power of Garlic.* Prima Publishing, Rocklin CA 1996.

Berin MC, Yang PC, Ciok L, Waserman S, Perdue MH. Role for IL-4 in macromolecular transport across human intestinal epithelium. *Am J Physiol.* 1999 May;276(5 Pt 1):C1046-52.

Berkow R., (Ed.) *The Merck Manual of Diagnosis and Therapy.* 16th Edition. Rahway, N.J.: Merck Research Labs, 1992.

REFERENCES

Bernstein DI, Epstein T, Murphy-Berendts K, Liss GM. Surveillance of systemic reactions to subcutaneous immunotherapy injections: year 1 outcomes of the ACAAI and AAAAI collaborative study. *Ann Allergy Asthma Immunol.* 2010 Jun;104(6):530-5. .

Berseth CL, Mitmesser SH, Ziegler EE, Marunycz JD, Vanderhoof J. Tolerance of a standard intact protein formula versus a partially hydrolyzed formula in healthy, term infants. *Nutr J.* 2009 Jun 19;8:27.

Berteau O and Mulloy B. 2003. Sulfated fucans, fresh perspectives: structures, functions, and biological properties of sulfated fucans and an overview of enzymes active toward this class of polysaccharide. *Glycobiology.* Jun;13(6):29R-40R.

Best R, Lewis DA, Nasser N. The anti-ulcerogenic activity of the unripe plantain banana (Musa species). Br J Pharmacol. 1984 May;82(1):107-16.

Beyer K, Morrow E, Li XM, Bardina L, Bannon GA, Burks AW, Sampson HA. Effects of cooking methods on peanut allergenicity. *J Allergy Clin Immunol.* 2001;107:1077-81.

Beyer PL. Gastrointestinal disorders: roles of nutrition and the dietetics practitioner. *J Am Diet Assoc.* 1998 Mar;98(3):272-7.

Bhatia SJ, Reddy DN, Ghoshal UC, Jayanthi V, Abraham P, Choudhuri G, Broor SL, Ahuja V, Augustine P, Balakrishnan V, Bhasin DK, Bhat N, Chacko A, Dadhich S, Dhali GK, Dhawan PS, Dwivedi M, Goenka MK, Koshy A, Kumar A, Misra SP, Mukewar S, Raju EP, Shenoy KT, Singh SP, Sood A, Srinivasan R. Epidemiology and symptom profile of gastroesophageal reflux in the Indian population: report of the Indian Society of Gastroenterology Task Force. *Indian J Gastroenterol.* 2011 May;30(3):118-27.

Bhatia V, Tandon RK. Stress and the gastrointestinal tract. *J Gastroenterol Hepatol.* 2005 Mar;20(3):332-9.

Bielory BP, Perez VL, Bielory L. Treatment of seasonal allergic conjunctivitis with ophthalmic corticosteroids: in search of the perfect ocular corticosteroids in the treatment of allergic conjunctivitis. *Curr Opin Allergy Clin Immunol.* 2010 Oct;10(5):469-77.

Bielory L, Lupoli K. Herbal interventions in asthma and allergy. *J Asthma.* 1999;36:1-65.

Bielory L, Russin J, Zuckerman GB. Clinical efficacy, mechanisms of action, and adverse effects of complementary and alternative medicine therapies for asthma. *Allergy Asthma Proc.* 2004;25:283-91.

Bielory L. Complementary and alternative interventions in asthma, allergy, and immunology. *Ann Allergy Asthma Immunol.* 2004 Aug;93(2 Suppl 1):S45-54.

Bindslev-Jensen C, Skov PS, Roggen EL, Hvass P, Brinch DS. Investigation on possible allergenicity of 19 different commercial enzymes used in the food industry. *Food Chem Toxicol.* 2006 Nov;44(11):1909-15.

Birch EE, Khoury JC, Berseth CL, Castañeda YS, Couch JM, Bean J, Tamer R, Harris CL, Mitmesser SH, Scalabrin DM. The impact of early nutrition on incidence of allergic manifestations and common respiratory illnesses in children. *J Pediatr.* 2010 Jun;156(6):902-6, 906.e1. 2010 Mar 15.

Bisgaard H, Loland L, Holst KK, Pipper CB. Prenatal determinants of neonatal lung function in high-risk newborns. *J Allergy Clin Immunol.* 2009 Mar;123(3):651-7, 657.e1-4. 2009 Jan 18.

Bisset N.. *Herbal Drugs and Phytopharmaceuticals.* Stuttgart: CRC, 1994.

Bjarnason I, MacPherson A, Hollander D. Intestinal permeability: an overview. *Gastroenterology.* 1995 May;108(5):1566-81.

Blackhall K, Appleton S, Cates FJ. Ionisers for chronic asthma. *Cochrane Database Syst Rev* 2003;(3):CD002986.

Blood AJ, Zatorre RJ, Bermudez P, Evans AC. Emotional responses to pleasant and unpleasant music correlate with activity in paralimbic brain regions. *Nat Neurosci.* 1999;2:382-7.

Blumenthal M (ed.) *The Complete German Commission E Monographs.* Boston: Amer Botan Council, 1998.

Blumenthal M, Brinckmann J, Goldberg A (eds). *Herbal Medicine: Expanded Commission E Monographs.* Newton, MA: Integrative Med., 2000.

Boccafogli A, Vicentini L, Camerani A, Cogliati P, D'Ambrosi A, Scolozzi R. Adverse food reactions in patients with grass pollen allergic respiratory disease. *Ann Allergy.* 1994 Oct;73(4):301-8.

Bode C, Bode JC. Effect of alcohol consumption on the gut. *Best Pract Res Clin Gastroenterol.* 2003 Aug;17(4):575-92.

Bodinier M, Legoux MA, Pineau F, Triballeau S, Segain JP, Brossard C, Denery-Papini S. Intestinal translocation capabilities of wheat allergens using the Caco-2 cell line. *J Agric Food Chem.* 2007 May 30;55(11):4576-83.

Boehm, G., Lidestri, M., Casetta, P., Jelinek, J., Negretti, F., Stahl, B., Martini, A. (2002) Supplementation of a bovine milk formula with an oligosaccharide mixture increases counts of faecal bifidobacteria in preterm infants. *Arch Dis Child Fetal Neonatal Ed.* 86: F178-F181

Bolhaar ST, Tiemessen MM, Zuidmeer L, van Leeuwen A, Hoffmann-Sommergruber K, Bruijnzeel-Koomen CA, Taams LS, Knol EF, van Hoffen E, van Ree R, Knulst AC. Efficacy of birch-pollen immunotherapy on cross-reactive food allergy confirmed by skin tests and double-blind food challenges. *Clin Exp Allergy.* 2004 May;34(5):761-9.

Bolleddula J, Goldfarb J, Wang R, Sampson H, Li XM. Synergistic Modulation Of Eotaxin And Il-4 Secretion By Constituents Of An Anti-asthma Herbal Formula (ASHMI) In Vitro. *J Allergy Clin Immunol.* 2007;119:S172.

Bonfils P, Halimi P, Malinvaud D. Adrenal suppression and osteoporosis after treatment of nasal polyposis. *Acta Otolaryngol.* 2006 Dec;126(11):1195-200.

Bongaerts GP, Severijnen RS. Preventive and curative effects of probiotics in atopic patients. *Med Hypotheses.* 2005;64(6):1089-92.

Bongartz D, Hesse A. Selective extraction of quercetrin in vegetable drugs and urine by off-line coupling of boronic acid affinity chromatography and high-performance liquid chromatography. *J Chromatogr B Biomed Appl.* 1995 Nov 17;673(2):223-30.

Bonsignore MR, La Grutta S, Cibella F, Scichilone N, Cuttitta G, Interrante A, Marchese M, Veca M, Virzi' M, Bonanno A, Profita M, Morici G. Effects of exercise training and montelukast in children with mild asthma. *Med Sci Sports Exerc.* 2008 Mar;40(3):405-12.

Borchers AT, Hackman RM, Keen CL, Stern JS, Gershwin ME. Complementary medicine: a review of immunomodulatory effects of Chinese herbal medicines. *Am J Clin Nutr.* 1997 Dec;66(6):1303-12.

Borchert VE, Czyborra P, Fetscher C, Goepel M, Michel MC. Extracts from Rhois aromatica and Solidaginis virgaurea inhibit rat and human bladder contraction. *Naunyn Schmiedebergs Arch Pharmacol.* 2004 Mar;369(3):281-6.

Böttcher MF, Jenmalm MC, Voor T, Julge K, Holt PG, Björkstén B. Cytokine responses to allergens during the first 2 years of life in Estonian and Swedish children. *Clin Exp Allergy.* 2006 May;36(5):619-28.

Bottema RW, Kerkhof M, Reijmerink NE, Thijs C, Smit HA, van Schayck CP, Brunekreef B, van Oosterhout AJ, Postma DS, Koppelman GH. Gene-gene interaction in regulatory T-cell function in atopy and asthma development in childhood. *J Allergy Clin Immunol.* 2010 Aug;126(2):338-46, 346.e1-10.

Bouchez-Mahiout I, Pecquet C, Kerre S, Snégaroff J, Raison-Peyron N, Laurière M. High molecular weight entities in industrial wheat protein hydrolysates are immunoreactive with IgE from allergic patients. *J Agric Food Chem.* 2010 Apr 14;58(7):4207-15.

Bougault V, Turmel J, Boulet LP. Bronchial challenges and respiratory symptoms in elite swimmers and winter sport athletes: Airway hyperresponsiveness in asthma: its measurement and clinical significance. *Chest.* 2010 Aug;138(2 Suppl):31S-37S. 2010 Apr 2.

Bouin M, Savoye G, Hervé S, Hellot MF, Denis P, Ducrotté P. Does the supplementation of the formula with fibre increase the risk of gastro-oesophageal reflux during enteral nutrition? A human study. *Clin Nutr.* 2001 Aug;20(4):307-12.

Bourke B, Ceponis P, Chiba N, Czinn S, Ferraro R, Fischbach L, Gold B, Hyunh H, Jacobson K, Jones NL, Koletzko S, Lebel S, Moayyedi P, Ridell R, Sherman P, van Zanten S, Beck I, Best L, Boland M, Bursey F, Chaun H, Cooper G, Craig B, Creuzenet C, Critch J, Govender K, Hassall E, Kaplan A, Keelan M, Noad G, Robertson M, Smith L, Stein M, Taylor D, Walters T, Persaud R, Whitaker S, Woodland R; Canadian Helicobacter Study Group. Canadian Helicobacter Study Group Consensus Conference: Update on the approach to Helicobacter pylori infection in children and adolescents—an evidence-based evaluation. *Can J Gastroenterol.* 2005 Jul;19(7):399-408.

Boyce JA, Assa'ad A, Burks AW, Jones SM, Sampson HA, Wood RA, Plaut M, Cooper SF, Fenton MJ, Arshad SH, Bahna SL, Beck LA, Byrd-Bredbenner C, Camargo CA Jr, Eichenfield L, Furuta GT, Hanifin JM, Jones C, Kraft M, Levy BD, Lieberman P, Luccioli S, McCall KM, Schneider LC, Simon RA, Simons FE, Teach SJ, Yawn BP, Schwaninger JM. Guidelines for the diagnosis and management of food allergy in the United States: report of the NIAID-sponsored expert panel. *J Allergy Clin Immunol.* 2010 Dec;126(6 Suppl):S1-58.

Bråbäck L, Kjellman NI, Sandin A, Björkstén B. Atopy among schoolchildren in northern and southern Sweden in relation to pet ownership and early life events. *Pediatr Allergy Immunol.* 2001 Feb;12(1):4-10.

Bradette-Hébert ME, Legault J, Lavoie S, Pichette A. A new labdane diterpene from the flowers of Solidago canadensis. *Chem Pharm Bull.* 2008 Jan;56(1):82-4.

Brandtzaeg P. The mucosal immune system and its integration with the mammary glands. *J Pediatr.* 2010 Feb;156(2 Suppl):S8-15.

Bratus' VD, Pishchalenko NT, Tikhonenko VM, Musa A. New trends in the diagnosis and treatment of acute gastric hemorrhages. *Klin Khir.* 1980 Apr;(4):7-11.

Bredenoord AJ, Baron A, Smout AJ. Symptomatic gastro-oesophageal reflux in a patient with achlorhydria. *Gut.* 2006 Jul;55(7):1054-5.

Brehm JM, Schuemann B, Fuhlbrigge AL, Hollis BW, Strunk RC, Zeiger RS, Weiss ST, Litonjua AA; Childhood Asthma Management Program Research Group. Serum vitamin D levels and severe asthma exacerbations in the Childhood Asthma Management Program study. *J Allergy Clin Immunol.* 2010 Jul;126(1):52-8.e5. 2010 Jun 9.

Bresalier R. Barrett's Metaplasia: defining the problem. *Semin Oncol.* 2005 Dec;32(6 Suppl 8):21-4.

Brighenti F, Valtueña S, Pellegrini N, Ardigò D, Del Rio D, Salvatore S, Piatti P, Serafini M, Zavaroni I. Total antioxidant capacity of the diet is inversely and independently related to plasma concentration of high-sensitivity C-reactive protein in adult Italian subjects. *Br J Nutr.* 2005 May;93(5):619-25.

Brodtkorb TH, Zetterström O, Tinghög G. Cost-effectiveness of clean air administered to the breathing zone in allergic asthma. *Clin Respir J.* 2010 Apr;4(2):104-10.

Brody J. *Jane Brody's Nutrition Book.* New York: WW Norton, 1981.

Broekhuizen BD, Sachs AP, Hoes AW, Moons KG, van den Berg JW, Dalinghaus WH, Lammers E, Verheij TJ. Undetected chronic obstructive pulmonary disease and asthma in people over 50 years with persistent cough. *Br J Gen Pract.* 2010 Jul;60(576):489-94.

Brostoff J, Gamlin L, Brostoff J. *Food Allergies and Food Intolerance: The Complete Guide to Their Identification and Treatment.* Rochester, VT: Healing Arts, 2000.

Brownstein D. *Salt: Your Way to Health.* West Bloomfield, MI: Medical Alternatives, 2006.

Brown-Whitehorn TF, Spergel JM. The link between allergies and eosinophilic esophagitis: implications for management strategies. *Expert Rev Clin Immunol.* 2010 Jan;6(1):101-9.

Bruce S, Nyberg F, Melén E, James A, Pulkkinen V, Orsmark-Pietras C, Bergström A, Dahlén B, Wickman M, von Mutius E, Doekes G, Lauener R, Riedler J, Eder W, van Hage M, Pershagen G, Scheynius A, Kere J. The protective effect of farm animal exposure on childhood allergy is modified by NPSR1 polymorphisms. *J Med Genet.* 2009 Mar;46(3):159-67. 2008 Feb 19.

Bruneton J. *Pharmacognosy, Phytochemistry, Medicinal Plants.* Paris: Lavoisier, 1995.

270

REFERENCES

Bruton A, Lewith GT. The Buteyko breathing technique for asthma: a review. *Complement Ther Med.* 2005 Mar;13(1):41-6. 2005 Apr 18.

Bruton A, Thomas M. The role of breathing training in asthma management. *Curr Opin Allergy Clin Immunol.* 2011 Feb;11(1):53-7.

Bublin M, Pfister M, Radauer C, Oberhuber C, Bulley S, Dewitt AM, Lidholm J, Reese G, Vieths S, Breiteneder H, Hoffmann-Sommergruber K, Ballmer-Weber BK. Component-resolved diagnosis of kiwifruit allergy with purified natural and recombinant kiwifruit allergens. *J Allergy Clin Immunol.* 2010 Mar;125(3):687-94, 694.e1.

Buchanan TW, Lutz K, Mirzazade S, Specht K, Shah NJ, Zilles K, *et al.* Recognition of emotional prosody and verbal components of spoken language: an fMRI study. *Cogn Brain Res.* 2000;9:227-38.

Bucher X, Pichler WJ, Dahinden CA, Helbling A. Effect of tree pollen specific, subcutaneous immunotherapy on the oral allergy syndrome to apple and hazelnut. *Allergy.* 2004 Dec;59(12):1272-6.

Budzianowski J. Coumarins, caffeoyltartaric acids and their artifactual methyl esters from *Taraxacum officinale* leaves. *Planta Med.* 1997 Jun;63(3):288.

Bueso AK, Berntsen S, Mowinckel P, Andersen LF, Lodrup Carlsen KC, Carlsen KH. Dietary intake in adolescents with asthma - potential for improvement. *Pediatr Allergy Immunol.* 2010 Oct 20. doi: 10.1111/j.1399-3038.2010.01013.x.

Bundy R, Walker AF, Middleton RW, Booth J. Turmeric extract may improve irritable bowel syndrome symptomology in otherwise healthy adults: a pilot study. *J Altern Complement Med.* 2004 Dec;10(6):1015-8.

Burdge GC, Jones AE, Wootton SA. Eicosapentaenoic and docosapentaenoic acids are the principal products of alpha-linolenic acid metabolism in young men. *B J Nutr.* 2002 Oct;88(4):355-63.

Buret AG. How stress induces intestinal hypersensitivity. *Am J Pathol.* 2006 Jan;168(1):3-5.

Burgess CD, Bremner P, Thomson CD, Crane J, Siebers RW, Beasley R. Nebulized beta 2-adrenoceptor agonists do not affect plasma selenium or glutathione peroxidase activity in patients with asthma. *Int J Clin Pharmacol Ther.* 1994 Jun;32(6):290-2.

Burks W, Jones SM, Berseth CL, Harris C, Sampson HA, Scalabrin DM. Hypoallergenicity and effects on growth and tolerance of a new amino acid-based formula with docosahexaenoic acid and arachidonic acid. *J Pediatr.* 2008 Aug;153(2):266-71.

Burney PG, Luczynska C, Chinn S, Jarvis D. The European Community Respiratory Health Survey. *Eur Respir J.* 1994;7: 954-960.

Burr ML, Butland BK, King S, Vaughan-Williams E. Changes in asthma prevalence: two surveys 15 years apart. *Arch Dis Child.* 1989;64:1452-1456.

Busse PJ, Wen MC, Huang CK, Srivastava K, Zhang TF, Schofield B, Sampson HA, Li XM. Therapeutic effects of the Chinese herbal formula, MSSM-03d, on persistent airway hyperreactivity and airway remodeling. *J Allergy Clin Immunol.* 2004;113:S220.

Buxbaum JL, Eloubeidi MA. Endoscopic evaluation and treatment of esophageal cance. *Minerva Gastroenterol Dietol.* 2009 Dec;55(4):455-69.

Byrne AM, Malka-Rais J, Burks AW, Fleischer DM. How do we know when peanut and tree nut allergy have resolved, and how do we keep it resolved? *Clin Exp Allergy.* 2010 Sep;40(9):1303-11.

Cabanillas B, Pedrosa MM, Rodríguez J, González A, Muzquiz M, Cuadrado C, Crespo JF, Burbano C. Effects of enzymatic hydrolysis on lentil allergenicity. *Mol Nutr Food Res.* 2010 Mar 19.

Cadiot G. Consequences of achlorhydria secondary to antisecretory treatments. *Gastroenterol Clin Biol.* 1999 Jan;23(1 Pt 2):S110-20.

Caglar E, Kavaloglu SC, Kuscu OO, Sandalli N, Holgerson PL, Twetman S. Effect of chewing gums containing xylitol or probiotic bacteria on salivary mutans streptococci and lactobacilli. *Clin Oral Investig.* 2007 Dec;11(4):425-9.

Caglar E, Kuscu OO, Cildir SK, Kuvvetli SS, Sandalli N. A probiotic lozenge administered medical device and its effect on salivary mutans streptococci and lactobacilli. *Int J Paediatr Dent.* 2008 Jan;18(1):35-9.

Caglar E, Kuscu OO, Selvi Kuvvetli S, Kavaloglu Cildir S, Sandalli N, Twetman S. Short-term effect of ice-cream containing *Bifidobacterium lactis* Bb-12 on the number of salivary mutans streptococci and lactobacilli. *Acta Odontol Scand.* 2008 Jun;66(3):154-8.

Calder PC. Dietary modification of inflammation with lipids. *Proc Nutr Soc.* 2002 Aug;61(3):345-58.

Camargo CA Jr, Ingham T, Wickens K, Thadhani R, Silvers KM, Epton MJ, Town GI, Pattemore PK, Espinola JA, Crane J; New Zealand Asthma and Allergy Cohort Study Group. Cord blood 25 hydroxyvitamin D levels and risk of respiratory infection, wheezing, and asthma. *Pediatrics.* 2011 Jan;127(1):e180-7.

Caminiti L, Passalacqua G, Barberi S, Vita D, Barberio G, De Luca R, Pajno GB. A new protocol for specific oral tolerance induction in children with IgE-mediated cow's milk allergy. *Allergy Asthma Proc.* 2009 Jul-Aug;30(4):443-8.

Cammarota G, Masala G, Cianci R, Palli D, Bendinelli B, Galli J, Pandolfi F, Gasbarrini A, Landolfi R. Reflux symptoms in wind instrument players. *Aliment Pharmacol Ther.* 2010 Mar;31(5):593-600.

Cammarota G, Masala G, Cianci R, Palli D, Capaccio P, Schindler A, Cuoco L, Galli J, Ierardi E, Cannizzaro O, Caselli M, Dore MP, Bendinelli B, Gasbarrini G. Reflux symptoms in professional opera choristers. *Gastroenterology.* 2007 Mar;132(3):890-8.

Campbell TC, Campbell TM. *The China Study.* Dallas, TX: Benbella Books, 2006.

Canali R, Comitato R, Schonlau F, Virgili F. The anti-inflammatory pharmacology of Pycnogenol in humans involves COX-2 and 5-LOX mRNA expression in leukocytes. *Int Immunopharmacol.* 2009 Sep;9(10):1145-9.

Canani RB, Cirillo P, Roggero P, Romano C, Malamisura B, Terrin G, Passariello A, Manguso F, Morelli L, Guarino A; Working Group on Intestinal Infections of the Italian Society of Pediatric Gastroenterology, Hepatology and Nu-

271

trition (SIGENP). Therapy with gastric acidity inhibitors increases the risk of acute gastroenteritis and community-acquired pneumonia in children. *Pediatrics.* 2006 May;117(5):e817-20.

Canonica GW, Passalacqua G. Noninjection routes for immunotherapy. *J Allergy Clin Immunol.* 2003 Mar;111(3):437-48; quiz 449.

Cantani A, Micera M. Natural history of cow's milk allergy. An eight-year follow-up study in 115 atopic children. *Eur Rev Med Pharmacol Sci.* 2004 Jul-Aug;8(4):153-64.

Cantani A, Micera M. The prick by prick test is safe and reliable in 58 children with atopic dermatitis and food allergy. *Eur Rev Med Pharmacol Sci.* 2006 May-Jun;10(3):115-20.

Cao G, Alessio HM, Cutler RG. Oxygen-radical absorbance capacity assay for antioxidants. *Free Radic Biol Med.* 1993 Mar;14(3):303-11.

Cao G, Shukitt-Hale B, Bickford PC, Joseph JA, McEwen J, Prior RL. Hyperoxia-induced changes in antioxidant capacity and the effect of dietary antioxidants. *J Appl Physiol.* 1999 Jun;86(6):1817-22.

Caramia G. The essential fatty acids omega-6 and omega-3: from their discovery to their use in therapy. *Minerva Pediatr.* 2008 Apr;60(2):219-33.

Carey DG, Aase KA, Pliego GJ. The acute effect of cold air exercise in determination of exercise-induced bronchospasm in apparently healthy athletes. J Strength Cond Res. 2010 Aug;24(8):2172-8.

Carmona-Sánchez R, Solana-Sentíes S. Efficacy, diagnostic utility and tolerance of intraesophageal pH ambulatory determination with wireless pH-testing monitoring system. *Rev Gastroenterol Mex.* 2004 Apr-Jun;69(2):69-75.

Carroccio A, Cavataio F, Montalto G, D'Amico D, Alabrese L, Iacono G. Intolerance to hydrolysed cow's milk proteins in infants: clinical characteristics and dietary treatment. *Clin Exp Allergy.* 2000 Nov;30(11):1597-603.

Carroll D. *The Complete Book of Natural Medicines.* New York: Summit, 1980.

Carroll MW, Jacobson K. Gastroesophageal Reflux Disease in Children and Adolescents: When and How to Treat. *Paediatr Drugs.* 2011 Nov 22.

Caruso M, Frasca G, Di Giuseppe PL, Pennisi A, Tringali G, Bonina FP. Effects of a new nutraceutical ingredient on allergen-induced sulphidoleukotrienes production and CD63 expression in allergic subjects. *Int Immunopharmacol.* 2008 Dec 20;8(13-14):1781-6.

Casale TB, Amin BV. Allergic rhinitis/asthma interrelationship. *Clin Rev Allergy Immunol.* 2001;21:27-49.

Cats A, Kuipers EJ, Bosschaert MA, Pot RG, Vandenbroucke-Grauls CM, Kusters JG. Effect of frequent consumption of a Lactobacillus casei-containing milk drink in Helicobacter pylori-colonized subjects. *Aliment Pharmacol Ther.* 2003 Feb;17(3):429-35.

Catto-Smith AG. Gastroesophageal reflux in children. *Aust Fam Physician.* 1998 Jun;27(6):465-9, 472-3.

Caughey AB, Nicholson JM, Cheng YW, Lyell DJ, Washington AE. Induction of labor and Cesarean delivery by gestational age. *Am J Obstet Gynecol.* 2006 Sep;195(3):700-5.

Celakovská J, Ettlerová J, Ettlerová K, Ettler K, Bukac J. The role of atopy patch test in diagnosis of food allergy in atopic eczema/dermatitis syndrom in patients over 14 years of age. *Acta Medica (Hradec Kralove).* 2010;53(2):101-8.

Celikel S, Karakaya G, Yurtsever N, Sorkun K, Kalyoncu AF. Bee and bee products allergy in Turkish beekeepers: determination of risk factors for systemic reactions. *Allergol Immunopathol (Madr).* 2006 Sep-Oct;34(5):180-4.

Centers for Disease Control and Prevention (CDC). Obesity prevalence among low-income, preschool-aged children - United States, 1998-2008. *MMWR Morb Mortal Wkly Rep.* 2009 Jul 24;58(28):769-73.

Centers for Disease Control and Prevention (CDC). Vital signs: nonsmokers' exposure to secondhand smoke - United States, 1999-2008. *MMWR Morb Mortal Wkly Rep.* 2010 Sep 10;59(35):1141-6.

Centre for Molecular, Environmental, Genetic and Analytic Epidemiology, School of Population Health, The UniverGumowski P, Lech B, Chaves I, Girard JP. Chronic asthma and rhinitis due to Candida albicans, epidermophyton, and trichophyton. *Ann Allergy.* 1987 Jul;59(1):48-51.

Cereijido M, Contreras RG, Flores-Benítez D, Flores-Maldonado C, Larre I, Ruiz A, Shoshani L. New diseases derived or associated with the tight junction. *Arch Med Res.* 2007 Jul;38(5):465-78.

Cezard JP. Managing gastro-oesophageal reflux disease in children. *Digestion.* 2004;69 Suppl 1:3-8.

Chafen JJ, Newberry SJ, Riedl MA, Bravata DM, Maglione M, Suttorp MJ, Sundaram V, Paige NM, Towfigh A, Hulley BJ, Shekelle PG. Diagnosing and managing common food allergies: a systematic review. *JAMA.* 2010 May 12;303(18):1848-56.

Chahine BG, Bahna SL. The role of the gut mucosal immunity in the development of tolerance versus development of allergy to food. *Curr Opin Allergy Clin Immunol.* 2010 Aug;10(4):394-9.

Chaitow L, Trenev N. *Probiotics.* New York: Thorsons, 1990.

Chaitow L. *Conquer Pain the Natural Way.* San Francisco: Chronicle Books, 2002.

Chakŭrski I, Matev M, Koĭchev A, Angelova I, Stefanov G. Treatment of chronic colitis with an herbal combination of Taraxacum officinale, Hipericum perforatum, Melissa officinaliss, Calendula officinalis and Foeniculum vulgare. *Vutr Boles.* 1981;20(6):51-4.

Chan CK, Kuo ML, Shen JJ, See LC, Chang HH, Huang JL. Ding Chuan Tang, a Chinese herb decoction, could improve airway hyper-responsiveness in stabilized asthmatic children: a randomized, double-blind clinical trial. *Pediatr Allergy Immunol.* 2006;17:316-22.

Chandra RK. Prospective studies of the effect of breast feeding on incidence of infection and allergy. *Acta Paediatr Scand.* 1979 Sep;68(5):691-4.

Chaney M, Ross M. *Nutrition.* New York: Houghton Mifflin, 1971.

REFERENCES

Chang HT, Tseng LJ, Hung TJ, Kao BT, Lin WY, Fan TC, Chang MD, Pai TW. Inhibition of the interactions between eosinophil cationic protein and airway epithelial cells by traditional Chinese herbs. *BMC Syst Biol.* 2010 Sep 13;4 Suppl 2:S8.

Chang TT, Huang CC, Hsu CH. Clinical evaluation of the Chinese herbal medicine formula STA-1 in the treatment of allergic asthma. *Phytother Res.* 2006;20:342-7.

Chang TT, Huang CC, Hsu CH. Inhibition of mite-induced immunoglobulin E synthesis, airway inflammation, and hyperreactivity by herbal medicine STA-1. *Immunopharmacol Immunotoxicol.* 2006;28:683-95.

Chao A, Thun MJ, Connell CJ, McCullough ML, Jacobs EJ, Flanders WD, Rodriguez C, Sinha R, Calle EE. Meat consumption and risk of colorectal cancer. *JAMA.* 2005 Jan 12;293(2):172-82.

Chao HC, Vandenplas Y. Effect of cereal-thickened formula and upright positioning on regurgitation, gastric emptying, and weight gain in infants with regurgitation. *Nutrition.* 2007 Jan;23(1):23-8.

Characterization and quantitation of Antioxidant Constituents of Sweet Pepper (Capsicum annuum - Cayenne). *J Agric Food Chem.* 2004 Jun 16;52(12):3861-9.

Chattopadhyay S, Chaudhuri S, Ghosal S. Activation of peritoneal macrophages by sitoindoside-IV, an anti-ulcerogenic acylsterylglycoside from Musa paradisiaca. *Planta Med.* 1987 Feb;53(1):16-8.

Chatzi L, Apostolaki G, Bibakis I, Skypala I, Bibaki-Liakou V, Tzanakis N, Kogevinas M, Cullinan P. Protective effect of fruits, vegetables and the Mediterranean diet on asthma and allergies among children in Crete. *Thorax.* 2007 Aug;62(8):677-83.

Chatzi L, Torrent M, Romieu I, Garcia-Esteban R, Ferrer C, Vioque J, Kogevinas M, Sunyer J. Mediterranean diet in pregnancy is protective for wheeze and atopy in childhood. *Thorax.* 2008 Jun;63(6):507-13.

Chaves TC, de Andrade e Silva TS, Monteiro SA, Watanabe PC, Oliveira AS, Grossi DB. Craniocervical posture and hyoid bone position in children with mild and moderate asthma and mouth breathing. *Int J Pediatr Otorhinolaryngol.* 2010 Sep;74(9):1021-7.

Chehade M, Aceves SS. Food allergy and eosinophilic esophagitis. *Curr Opin Allergy Clin Immunol.* 2010 Jun;10(3):231-7.

Chellini E, Talassi F, Corbo G, Berti G, De Sario M, Rusconi F, Piffer S, Caranci N, Petronio MG, Sestini P, Dell'Orco V, Bonci E, Armenio L, La Grutta S; Gruppo Collaborativo SIDRIA-2. Environmental, social and demographic characteristics of children and adolescents, resident in different Italian areas. *Epidemiol Prev.* 2005 Mar-Apr;29(2 Suppl):14-23.

Chen HJ, Shih CK, Hsu HY, Chiang W. Mast cell-dependent allergic responses are inhibited by ethanolic extract of adlay (Coix lachryma-jobi L. var. ma-yuen Stapf) testa. *J Agric Food Chem.* 2010 Feb 24;58(4):2596-601.

Chen JX, Ji B, Lu ZL, Hu LS. Effects of chai hu (radix burpleuri) containing formulation on plasma beta-endorphin, epinephrine and dopamine on patients. *Am J Chin Med.* 2005;33(5):737-45.

Chen N, Huang L, Li H, Li DH, Li Y. Sputum analysis in patients with "disharmony of stomach". *Zhong Xi Yi Jie He Xue Bao.* 2004 Sep;2(5):343-5.

Chen WQ, He YT, Sun XB, Wen DG, Chen ZF, Zhao DL. Analysis of risk factors for upper gastrointestinal cancer in China: a multicentric population-based case-control study. *Zhonghua Yu Fang Yi Xue Za Zhi.* 2011 Mar;45(3):244-8.

Chen Y, Blaser MJ. Helicobacter pylori colonization is inversely associated with childhood asthma. *J Infect Dis.* 2008 Aug 15;198(4):553-60.

Chen Y, Blaser MJ. Inverse associations of Helicobacter pylori with asthma and allergy. *Arch Intern Med.* 2007 Apr 23;167(8):821-7.

Cheney G, Waxler SH, Miller IJ. Vitamin U therapy of peptic ulcer; experience at San Quentin Prison. *Calif Med.* 1956 Jan;84(1):39-42.

Chevallier A. *Encyclopedia of Medicinal Plants.* New York, NY: DK Publishing; 1996.

Chevrier MR, Ryan AE, Lee DY, Zhongze M, Wu-Yan Z, Via CS. Boswellia carterii extract inhibits TH1 cytokines and promotes TH2 cytokines in vitro. *Clin Diagn Lab Immunol.* 2005 May;12(5):575-80.

Chilton FH, Rudel LL, Parks JS, Arm JP, Seeds MC. Mechanisms by which botanical lipids affect inflammatory disorders. *Am J Clin Nutr.* 2008 Feb;87(2):498S-503S.

Chilton FH, Tucker L. *Win the War Within.* New York: Rodale, 2006.

Chin A Paw MJ, de Jong N, Pallast EG, Kloek GC, Schouten EG, Kok FJ. Immunity in frail elderly: a randomized controlled trial of exercise and enriched foods. *Med Sci Sports Exerc.* 2000 Dec;32(12):2005-11.

Choi BW, Yoo KH, Jeong JW, Yoon HJ, Kim SH, Park YM, Kim WK, Oh JW, Rha YH, Pyun BY, Chang SI, Moon HB, Kim YY, Cho SH. Easy diagnosis of asthma: computer-assisted, symptom-based diagnosis. *J Korean Med Sci.* 2007 Oct;22(5):832-8.

Choi SY, Sohn JH, Lee YW, Lee EK, Hong CS, Park JW. Characterization of buckwheat 19-kD allergen and its application for diagnosing clinical reactivity. *Int Arch Allergy Immunol.* 2007;144(4):267-74.

Choi SZ, Choi SU, Lee KR. Phytochemical constituents of the aerial parts from Solidago virga-aurea var. gigantea. *Arch Pharm Res.* 2004 Feb;27(2):164-8.

Chong Neto HJ, Rosário NA; Grupo EISL Curitiba (Estudio Internacional de Sibilancias en Lactantes). Risk factors for wheezing in the first year of life. *J Pediatr.* 2008 Nov-Dec;84(6):495-502.

Chopra RN, Nayar SL, Chopra IC, eds. *Glossary of Indian Medicinal plants.* New Delhi: CSIR, 1956.

Choudhry S, Seibold MA, Borrell LN, Tang H, Serebrisky D, Chapela R, Rodriguez-Santana JR, Avila PC, Ziv E, Rodriguez-Cintron W, Risch NJ, Burchard EG. Dissecting complex diseases in complex populations: asthma in latino americans. *Proc Am Thorac Soc.* 2007 Jul;4(3):226-33.

Christopher JR. *School of Natural Healing.* Springville UT: Christopher Publ, 1976.

Chu YF, Liu RH. Cranberries inhibit LDL oxidation and induce LDL receptor expression in hepatocytes. *Life Sci.* 2005;77(15):1892-1901. 27.

Chung SY, Butts CL, Maleki SJ, Champagne ET. Linking peanut allergenicity to the processes of maturation, curing, and roasting. *J Agric Food Chem.* 2003;51: 4273-4277.

Cibella F, Cuttitta G. Nocturnal asthma and gastroesophageal reflux. *Am J Med.* 2001 Dec 3;111 Suppl 8A:31S-36S.

Cingi C, Demirbas D, Songu M. Allergic rhinitis caused by food allergies. *Eur Arch Otorhinolaryngol.* 2010 Sep;267(9):1327-35.

Cisneros C, García-Río F, Romera D, Villasante C, Girón R, Ancochea J. Bronchial reactivity indices are determinants of health-related quality of life in patients with stable asthma. *Thorax.* 2010 Sep;65(9):795-800.

Clark S, Bock SA, Gaeta TJ, Brenner BE, Cydulka RK, Camargo CA; Multicenter Airway Research Collaboration-8 Investigators. Multicenter study of emergency department visits for food allergies. *J Allergy Clin Immunol.* 2004 Feb;113(2):347-52.

Clement YN, Williams AF, Aranda D, Chase R, Watson N, Mohammed R, Stubbs O, Williamson D. Medicinal herb use among asthmatic patients attending a specialty care facility in Trinidad. *BMC Complement Altern Med.* 2005 Feb 15;5:3.

Cobo Sanz JM, Mateos JA, Muñoz Conejo A. Effect of *Lactobacillus casei* on the incidence of infectious conditions in children. *Nutr Hosp.* 2006 Jul-Aug;21(4):547-51.

Codispoti CD, Levin L, LeMasters GK, Ryan P, Reponen T, Villareal M, Burkle J, Stanforth S, Lockey JE, Khurana Hershey GK, Bernstein DI. Breast-feeding, aeroallergen sensitization, and environmental exposures during infancy are determinants of childhood allergic rhinitis. *J Allergy Clin Immunol.* 2010 May;125(5):1054-1060.e1.

Cohen A, Goldberg M, Levy B, Leshno M, Katz Y. Sesame food allergy and sensitization in children: the natural history and long-term follow-up. *Pediatr Allergy Immunol.* 2007 May;18(3):217-23.

Cohen RT, Raby BA, Van Steen K, Fuhlbrigge AL, Celedón JC, Rosner BA, Strunk RC, Zeiger RS, Weiss ST; Childhood Asthma Management Program Research Group. In utero smoke exposure and impaired response to inhaled corticosteroids in children with asthma. *J Allergy Clin Immunol.* 2010 Sep;126(3):491-7. 2010 Jul 31. ; .

Colletti RB, Christie DL, Orenstein SR. Statement of the North American Society for Pediatric Gastroenterology and Nutrition (NASPGN). Indications for pediatric esophageal pH monitoring. *J Pediatr Gastroenterol Nutr.* 1995 Oct;21(3):253-62.

Collin P, Mustalahti K, Kyrönpalo S, Rasmussen M, Pehkonen E, Kaukinen K. Should we screen reflux oesophagitis patients for coeliac disease? *Eur J Gastroenterol Hepatol.* 2004 Sep;16(9):917-20.

Collipp PJ, Goldzier S 3rd, Weiss N, Soleymani Y, Snyder R. Pyridoxine treatment of childhood bronchial asthma. *Ann Allergy.* 1975 Aug;35(2):93-7.

Colombo P, Mangano M, Bianchi PA, Penagini R. Effect of calories and fat on postprandial gastro-oesophageal reflux. *Scand J Gastroenterol.* 2002 Jan;37(1):3-5.

Conio M, Filiberti R, Blanchi S, Ferraris R, Marchi S, Ravelli P, Lapertosa G, Iaquinto G, Sablich R, Gusmaroli R, Aste H, Giacosa A; Gruppo Operativo per lo Studio delle Precancerosi Esofagee (GOSPE). Risk factors for Barrett's esophagus: a case-control study. *Int J Cancer.* 2002 Jan 10;97(2):225-9.

Conquer JA, Holub BJ. Dietary docosahexaenoic acid as a source of eicosapentaenoic acid in vegetarians and omnivores. *Lipids.* 1997 Mar;32(3):341-5.

Contini S, Scarpignato C. Evaluation of clinical outcome after laparoscopic antireflux surgery in clinical practice: still a controversial issue. *Minim Invasive Surg.* 2011;2011:725472.

Cooper GS, Miller FW, Germolec DR: Occupational exposures and autoimmune diseases. *Int Immunopharm* 2002, 2:303-313.

Cooper K. *The Aerobics Program for Total Well-Being.* New York: Evans, 1980.

Corbe C, Boissin JP, Siou A. Light vision and chorioretinal circulation. Study of the effect of procyanidolic oligomers (Endotelon). *J Fr Ophtalmol.* 1988;11(5):453-60.

Corbo GM, Forastiere F, De Sario M, Brunetti L, Bonci E, Bugiani M, Chellini E, La Grutta S, Migliore E, Pistelli R, Rusconi F, Russo A, Simoni M, Talassi F, Galassi C; Sidria-2 Collaborative Group. Wheeze and asthma in children: associations with body mass index, sports, television viewing, and diet. *Epidemiology.* 2008 Sep;19(5):747-55.

Cortesini C, Marcuzzo G, Pucciani F. Relationship between mixed acid-alkaline gastroesophageal reflux and esophagitis. *Ital J Surg Sci.* 1985;15(1):9-15.

Cory S, Ussery-Hall A, Griffin-Blake S, Easton A, Vigeant J, Balluz L, Garvin W, Greenlund K; Centers for Disease Control and Prevention (CDC). Prevalence of selected risk behaviors and chronic diseases and conditions-steps communities, United States, 2006-2007. *MMWR Surveill Summ.* 2010 Sep 24;59(8):1-37.

Courtney R, Cohen M. Investigating the claims of Konstantin Buteyko, M.D., Ph.D.: the relationship of breath holding time to end tidal CO_2 and other proposed measures of dysfunctional breathing. *J Altern Complement Med.* 2008 Mar;14(2):115-23.

Couzy F, Kastenmayer P, Vigo M, Clough J, Munoz-Box R, Barclay DV. Calcium bioavailability from a calcium- and sulfate-rich mineral water, compared with milk, in young adult women. *Am J Clin Nutr.* 1995 Dec;62(6):1239-44.

Covar R, Gleason M, Macomber B, Stewart L, Szefler P, Engelhardt K, Murphy J, Liu A, Wood S, DeMichele S, Gelfand EW, Szefler SJ. Impact of a novel nutritional formula on asthma control and biomarkers of allergic airway inflammation in children. *Clin Exp Allergy.* 2010 Aug;40(8):1163-74. 2010 Jun 7.

Crane J, Ellis I, Siebers R, Grimmet D, Lewis S, Fitzharris P. A pilot study of the effect of mechanical ventilation and heat exchange on house-dust mites and Der p 1 in New Zealand homes. *Allergy.* 1998 Aug;53(8):755-62.

274

REFERENCES

Crescente M, Jessen G, Momi S, Höltje HD, Gresele P, Cerletti C, de Gaetano G. Interactions of gallic acid, resveratrol, quercetin and aspirin at the platelet cyclooxygenase-1 level. Functional and modelling studies. *Thromb Haemost.* 2009 Aug;102(2):336-46.

Crinnion WJ. Toxic effects of the easily avoidable phthalates and parabens. *Altern Med Rev.* 2010 Sep;15(3):190-6.

Cserhati E. Current view on the etiology of childhood bronchial asthma. *Orv Hetil.* 2000;141:759-760.

Cuesta-Herranz J, Barber D, Blanco C, Cistero-Bahíma A, Crespo JF, Fernández-Rivas M, Fernández-Sánchez J, Florido JF, Ibáñez MD, Rodríguez R, Salcedo G, Garcia BE, Lombardero M, Quiralte J, Rodriguez J, Sánchez-Monge R, Vereda A, Villalba M, Alonso Díaz de Durana MD, Basagaña M, Carrillo T, Fernández-Nieto M, Tabar AI. Differences among Pollen-Allergic Patients with and without Plant Food Allergy. *Int Arch Allergy Immunol.* 2010 Apr 23;153(2):182-192.

Cummings M. *Human Heredity: Principles and Issues.* St. Paul, MN: West, 1988.

Cuomo R, Sarnelli G, Savarese MF, Buyckx M. Carbonated beverages and gastrointestinal system: between myth and reality. *Nutr Metab Cardiovasc Dis.* 2009 Dec;19(10):683-9.

Custovic A, Simpson BM, Simpson A, Kissen P, Woodcock A; NAC Manchester Asthma and Allergy Study Group. Effect of environmental manipulation in pregnancy and early life on respiratory symptoms and atopy during first year of life: a randomised trial. *Lancet.* 2001 Jul 21;358(9277):188-93.

D'Anneo RW, Bruno ME, Falagiani P. Sublingual allergoid immunotherapy: a new 4-day induction phase in patients allergic to house dust mites. *Int J Immunopathol Pharmacol.* 2010 Apr-Jun;23(2):553-60.

D'Auria E, Sala M, Lodi F, Radaelli G, Riva E, Giovannini M. Nutritional value of a rice-hydrolysate formula in infants with cows' milk protein allergy: a randomized pilot study. *J Int Med Res.* 2003 May-Jun;31(3):215-22.

D'Orazio N, Ficoneri C, Riccioni G, Conti P, Theoharides TC, Bollea MR. Conjugated linoleic acid: a functional food? *Int J Immunopathol Pharmacol.* 2003 Sep-Dec;16(3):215-20.

D'Urbano LE, Pellegrino K, Artesani MC, Donnanno S, Luciano R, Riccardi C, Tozzi AE, Ravà L, De Benedetti F, Cavagni G. Performance of a component-based allergen-microarray in the diagnosis of cow's milk and hen's egg allergy. *Clin Exp Allergy.* 2010 Jul 13.

Dallinga JW, Robroeks CM, van Berkel JJ, Moonen EJ, Godschalk RW, Jöbsis Q, Dompeling E, Wouters EF, van Schooten FJ. Volatile organic compounds in exhaled breath as a diagnostic tool for asthma in children. *Clin Exp Allergy.* 2010 Jan;40(1):68-76.

Davidson T. *Rhinology: The Collected Writings of Maurice H. Cottle, M.D.* San Diego, CA: American Rhinologic Society, 1987.

Davies G. *Timetables of Medicine.* New York: Black Dog & Leventhal, 2000.

Davin JC, Forget P, Mahieu PR. Increased intestinal permeability to (51 Cr) EDTA is correlated with IgA immune complex-plasma levels in children with IgA-associated nephropathies. *Acta Paediatr Scand.* 1988 Jan;77(1):118-24.

de Boissieu D, Dupont C, Badoual J. Allergy to nondairy proteins in mother's milk as assessed by intestinal permeability tests. *Allergy.* 1994 Dec;49(10):882-4.

de Boissieu D, Matarazzo P, Rocchiccioli F, Dupont C. Multiple food allergy: a possible diagnosis in breastfed infants. *Acta Paediatr.* 1997 Oct;86(10):1042-6.

de la Loge C, Trudeau E, Marquis P, Kahrilas P, Stanghellini V, Talley NJ, Tack J, Revicki DA, Rentz AM, Dubois D. Cross-cultural development and validation of a patient self-administered questionnaire to assess quality of life in upper gastrointestinal disorders: the PAGI-QOL. *Qual Life Res.* 2004 Dec;13(10):1751-62.

De Lucca AJ, Bland JM, Vigo CB, Cushion M, Selitrennikoff CP, Peter J, Walsh TJ. CAY-I, a fungicidal saponin from Capsicum sp. fruit. *Med Mycol.* 2002 Apr;40(2):131-7.

de Martino M, Novembre E, Galli L, de Marco A, Botarelli P, Marano E, Vierucci A. Allergy to different fish species in cod-allergic children: in vivo and in vitro studies. *J Allergy Clin Immunol.* 1990;86:909-914.

De Smet PA. Herbal remedies. *N Engl J Med.* 2002;347:2046-2056.

Dean C. *Death by Modern Medicine.* Belleville, ON: Matrix Verite-Media, 2005.

Debley JS, Carter ER, Redding GJ. Prevalence and impact of gastroesophageal reflux in adolescents with asthma: a population-based study. *Pediatr Pulmonol.* 2006 May;41(5):475-81.

Dehlink E, Yen E, Leichtner AM, Hait EJ, Fiebiger E. First evidence of a possible association between gastric acid suppression during pregnancy and childhood asthma: a population-based register study. *Clin Exp Allergy.* 2009 Feb;39(2):246-53. 2008 Dec 9.

Dekker W, Sanders GT, Tytgat GN. Indications and methods for gastric acidity determination. *Ned Tijdschr Geneeskd.* 1973 May 12;117(19):744-7.

del Giudice MM, Leonardi S, Maiello N, Brunese FP. Food allergy and probiotics in childhood. *J Clin Gastroenterol.* 2010 Sep;44 Suppl 1:S22-5.

Delacourt C. Bronchial changes in untreated asthma. *Arch Pediatr.* 2004 Jun;11 Suppl 2:71s-73s.

Del-Rio-Navarro B, Berber A, Blandón-Vijil V, Ramírez-Aguilar M, Romieu I, Ramírez-Chanona N, Heras-Acevedo S, Serrano-Sierra A, Barraza-Villareal A, Baeza-Bacab M, Sienra-Monge JJ. Identification of asthma risk factors in Mexico City in an International Study of Asthma and Allergy in Childhood survey. *Allergy Asthma Proc.* 2006 Jul-Aug;27(4):325-33.

Dengate S, Ruben A. Controlled trial of cumulative behavioural effects of a common bread preservative. *J Paediatr Child Health.* 2002 Aug;38(4):373-6.

Dente FL, Bacci E, Bartoli ML, Cianchetti S, Costa F, Di Franco A, Malagrinò L, Vagaggini B, Paggiaro P. Effects of oral prednisone on sputum eosinophils and cytokines in patients with severe refractory asthma. *Ann Allergy Asthma Immunol.* 2010 Jun;104(6):464-70.

Derebery MJ, Berliner KI. Allergy and its relation to Meniere's disease. *Otolaryngol Clin North Am.* 2010 Oct;43(5):1047-58.

Desjeux JF, Heyman M. Milk proteins, cytokines and intestinal epithelial functions in children. *Acta Paediatr Jpn.* 1994 Oct;36(5):592-6.

DesRoches A, Infante-Rivard C, Paradis L, Paradis J, Haddad E. Peanut allergy: is maternal transmission of antigens during pregnancy and breastfeeding a risk factor? *J Investig Allergol Clin Immunol.* 2010;20(4):289-94.

Deutsche Gesellschaft für Ernährung. Drink distilled water? *Med. Mo. Pharm.* 1993;16:146.

Devaraj TL. *Speaking of Ayurvedic Remedies for Common Diseases.* New Delhi: Sterling, 1985.

Devirgiliis C, Zalewski PD, Perozzi G, Murgia C. Zinc fluxes and zinc transporter genes in chronic diseases. *Mutat Res.* 2007 Sep 1;622(1-2):84-93. 2007 Feb 17.

Dharmage SC, Erbas B, Jarvis D, Wjst M, Raherison C, Norbäck D, Heinrich J, Sunyer J, Svanes C. Do childhood respiratory infections continue to influence adult respiratory morbidity? *Eur Respir J.* 2009 Feb;33(2):237-44.

Di Gioacchino M, Cavallucci E, Di Stefano F, Paolini F, Ramondo S, Di Sciascio MB, Ciuffreda S, Riccioni G, Della Vecchia R, Romano A, Boscolo P. Effect of natural allergen exposure on non-specific bronchial reactivity in asthmatic farmers. *Sci Total Environ.* 2001 Apr 10;270(1-3):43-8.

Di Gioacchino M, Cavallucci E, Di Stefano F, Verna N, Ramondo S, Ciuffreda S, Riccioni G, Boscolo P. Influence of total IgE and seasonal increase of eosinophil cationic protein on bronchial hyperreactivity in asthmatic grass-sensitized farmers. *Allergy.* 2000 Nov;55(11):1030-4.

Di Lorenzo C, Benninga MA, Forbes D, Morais MB, Morera C, Rudolph C, Staiano A, Sullivan PB, Tobin J; North American Society for Pediatric Gastroenterology, Hepatology and Nutrition. Functional gastrointestinal disorders, gastroesophageal reflux and neurogastroenterology: Working Group report of the second World Congress of Pediatric Gastroenterology, Hepatology, and Nutrition. *J Pediatr Gastroenterol Nutr.* 2004 Jun;39 Suppl 2:S616-25.

Di Marco F, Santus P, Centanni S. Anxiety and depression in asthma. *Curr Opin Pulm Med.* 2011 Jan;17(1):39-44.

Diamond JA, Diamond WJ. Common functional bowel problems. What do homeopathy, Chinese medicine and nutrition have to offer? *Adv Nurse Pract.* 2005 May;13(5):31-4, 72.

Dierksen KP, Moore CJ, Inglis M, Wescombe PA, Tagg JR. The effect of ingestion of milk supplemented with salivaricin A-producing Streptococcus salivarius on the bacteriocin-like inhibitory activity of streptococcal populations on the tongue. *FEMS Microbiol Ecol.* 2007 Mar;59(3):584-91.

Diğrak M, Ilçim A, Hakki Alma M. Antimicrobial activities of several parts of Pinus brutia, Juniperus oxycedrus, Abies cilicia, Cedrus libani and Pinus nigra. *Phytother Res.* 1999 Nov;13(7):584-7.

DiMango E, Holbrook JT, Simpson E, Reibman J, Richter J, Narula S, Prusakowski N, Mastronarde JG, Wise RA; American Lung Association Asthma Clinical Research Centers. Effects of asymptomatic proximal and distal gastroesophageal reflux on asthma severity. *Am J Respir Crit Care Med.* 2009 Nov 1;180(9):809-16. 2009 Aug 6.

Din FV, Theodoratou E, Farrington SM, Tenesa A, Barnetson RA, Cetnarskyj R, Stark L, Porteous ME, Campbell H, Dunlop MG. Effect of aspirin and NSAIDs on risk and survival from colorectal cancer. *Gut.* 2010 Dec;59(12):1670-9.

Diop L, Guillou S, Durand H. Probiotic food supplement reduces stress-induced gastrointestinal symptoms in volunteers: a double-blind, placebo-controlled, randomized trial. *Nutr Res.* 2008 Jan;28(1):1-5.

Dixon AE, Kaminsky DA, Holbrook JT, Wise RA, Shade DM, Irvin CG. Allergic rhinitis and sinusitis in asthma: differential effects on symptoms and pulmonary function. *Chest.* 2006 Aug;130(2):429-35.

Dona A, Arvanitoyannis IS. Health risks of genetically modified foods. *Crit Rev Food Sci Nutr.* 2009 Feb;49(2):164-75.

Donato F, Monarca S, Premi S., and Gelatti, U. Drinking water hardness and chronic degenerative diseases. Part III. Tumors, urolithiasis, fetal malformations, deterioration of the cognitive function in the aged and atopic eczema. *Ann. Ig.* 2003;15:57-70.

Dooley, M.A. and Hogan S.L. Environmental epidemiology and risk factors for autoimmune disease. *Curr Opin Rheum.* 2003;15(2):99-103.

dos Santos LH, Ribeiro IO, Sánchez PG, Hetzel JL, Felicetti JC, Cardoso PF. Evaluation of pantoprazol treatment response of patients with asthma and gastroesophageal reflux: a randomized prospective double-blind placebo-controlled study. *J Bras Pneumol.* 2007 Apr;33(2):119-27.

Doshi A, Bernard-Stover L, Kuelbs C, Castillo E, Stucky E. Apparent life-threatening event admissions and gastroesophageal reflux disease: the value of hospitalization. *Pediatr Emerg Care.* 2012 Jan;28(1):17-21.

Dotolo Institute. *The Study of Colon Hydrotherapy.* Pinellas Park, FL: Dotolo, 2003.

Dove MS, Dockery DW, Connolly GN. Smoke-free air laws and asthma prevalence, symptoms, and severity among non-smoking youth. *Pediatrics.* 2011 Jan;127(1):102-9. 2010 Dec 13.

Dowd JB, Zajacova A, Aiello A. Early origins of health disparities: burden of infection, health, and socioeconomic status in U.S. children. *Soc Sci Med.* 2009 Feb;68(4):699-707. 2009 Jan 17.

Ducrotté P. Irritable bowel syndrome: from the gut to the brain-gut. *Gastroenterol Clin Biol.* 2009 Aug-Sep;33(8-9):703-12.

Duffey KJ, Gordon-Larsen P, Shikany JM, Guilkey D, Jacobs DR Jr, Popkin BM. Food price and diet and health outcomes: 20 years of the CARDIA Study. Arch Intern Med. 2010 Mar 8;170(5):420-6. Erratum in: *Arch Intern Med.* 2010 Jun 28;170(12):1089.

Duke J. *CRC Handbook of Medicinal Herbs.* Boca Raton: CRC; 1989.

Duke J. *The Green Pharmacy.* New York: St. Martins, 1997.

Dunjic BS, Svensson I, Axelson J, Adlercreutz P, Ar'Rajab A, Larsson K, Bengmark S. Green banana protection of gastric mucosa against experimentally induced injuries in rats. A multicomponent mechanism? *Scand J Gastroenterol.* 1993 Oct;28(10):894-8.

Dunne DP, Paterson WG. Acid-induced esophageal shortening in humans: a cause of hiatus hernia? *Can J Gastroenterol.* 2000 Nov;14(10):847-50.

Dunstan JA, Roper J, Mitoulas L, Hartmann PE, Simmer K, Prescott SL. The effect of supplementation with fish oil during pregnancy on breast milk immunoglobulin A, soluble CD14, cytokine levels and fatty acid composition. *Clin Exp Allergy.* 2004 Aug;34(8):1237-42.

Duong M, Subbarao P, Adelroth E, Obminski G, Strinich T, Inman M, Pedersen S, O'Byrne PM. Sputum eosinophils and the response of exercise-induced bronchoconstriction to corticosteroid in asthma. *Chest.* 2008 Feb;133(2):404-11. 2007 Dec 10.

Dupont C, Barau E, Molkhou P, Raynaud F, Barbet JP, Dehennin L. Food-induced alterations of intestinal permeability in children with cow's milk-sensitive enteropathy and atopic dermatitis. *J Pediatr Gastroenterol Nutr.* 1989 May;8(4):459-65.

Dupont C, Barau E, Molkhou P. Intestinal permeability disorders in children. *Allerg Immunol.* 1991 Mar;23(3):95-103.

Dupont C, Soulaines P, Lapillonne A, Donne N, Kalach N, Benhamou P. Atopy patch test for early diagnosis of cow's milk allergy in preterm infants. *J Pediatr Gastroenterol Nutr.* 2010 Apr;50(4):463-4.

Dupuy P, Cassé M, André F, Dhivert-Donnadieu H, Pinton J, Hernandez-Pion C. Low-salt water reduces intestinal permeability in atopic patients. *Dermatology.* 1999;198(2):153-5.

Duran-Tauleria E, Vignati G, Guedan MJ, Petersson CJ. The utility of specific immunoglobulin E measurements in primary care. *Allergy.* 2004 Aug;59 Suppl 78:35-41.

Duwiejua M, Zeitlin IJ, Waterman PG, Chapman J, Mhango GJ, Provan GJ. Anti-inflammatory activity of resins from some species of the plant family Burseraceae. *Planta Med.* 1993 Feb;59(1):12-6.

Dykewicz MS, Lemmon JK, Keaney DL. Comparison of the Multi-Test II and Skintestor Omni allergy skin test devices. *Ann Allergy Asthma Immunol.* 2007 Jun;98(6):559-62.

Eastham EJ, Walker WA. Effect of cow's milk on the gastrointestinal tract: a persistent dilemma for the pediatrician. *Pediatrics.* 1977 Oct;60(4):477-81.

Eaton KK, Howard M, Howard JM. Gut permeability measured by polyethylene glycol absorption in abnormal gut fermentation as compared with food intolerance. *J R Soc Med.* 1995 Feb;88(2):63-6.

Ebers GC, Kukay K, Bulman DE, Sadovnick AD, Rice G, Anderson C, Armstrong H, Cousin K, Bell RB, Hader W, Paty DW, Hashimoto S, Oger J, Duquette P, Warren S, Gray T, O'Connor P, Nath A, Auty A, Metz L, Francis G, Paulseth JE, Murray TJ, Pryse-Phillips W, Nelson R, Freedman H, Brunet D, Bouchard JP, Hinds D, Risch N. A full genome search in multiple sclerosis. *Nat Genet.* 1996 Aug;13(4):472-6.

Eccles R. Menthol and related cooling compounds. *J Pharm Pharmacol.* 1994 Aug;46(8):618-30.

ECRHS (2002) The European Community Respiratory Health Survey II. *Eur Respir J.* 20: 1071-1079.

Edgecombe K, Latter S, Peters S, Roberts G. Health experiences of adolescents with uncontrolled severe asthma. *Arch Dis Child.* 2010 Dec;95(12):985-91. 2010 Jul 30.

Edgell PG. The psychology of asthma. *Can Med Assoc J.* 1952 Aug;67(2):121-5.

Egan LJ, Myhre GM, Mays DC, Dierkhising RA, Kammer PP, Murray JA. CYP2C19 pharmacogenetics in the clinical use of proton-pump inhibitors for gastro-oesophageal reflux disease: variant alleles predict gastric acid suppression, but not oesophageal acid exposure or reflux symptoms. *Aliment Pharmacol Ther.* 2003 Jun 15;17(12):1521-8.

Egashira Y, Nagano H. A multicenter clinical trial of TJ-96 in patients with steroid-dependent bronchial asthma. A comparison of groups allocated by the envelope method. *Ann N Y Acad Sci.* 1993 Jun 23;685:580-3.

Ege MJ, Frei R, Bieli C, Schram-Bijkerk D, Waser M, Benz MR, Weiss G, Nyberg F, van Hage M, Pershagen G, Brunekreef B, Riedler J, Lauener R, Braun-Fahrländer C, von Mutius E; PARSIFAL Study team. Not all farming environments protect against the development of asthma and wheeze in children. *J Allergy Clin Immunol.* 2007 May;119(5):1140-7.

Ege MJ, Herzum I, Büchele G, Krauss-Etschmann S, Lauener RP, Roponen M, Hyvärinen A, Vuitton DA, Riedler J, Brunekreef B, Dalphin JC, Braun-Fahrländer C, Pekkanen J, Renz H, von Mutius E; Protection Against Allergy Study in Rural Environments (PASTURE) Study group. Prenatal exposure to a farm environment modifies atopic sensitization at birth. *J Allergy Clin Immunol.* 2008 Aug;122(2):407-12, 412.e1-4.

Eggermont E. Cow's milk protein allergy. *Tijdschr Kindergeneeskd.* 1981 Feb;49(1):16-20.

Eggermont S, Van den Bulck J. Nodding off or switching off? The use of popular media as a sleep aid in secondary-school children. *J Paediatr Child Health.* 2006 Jul-Aug;42(7-8):428-33.

Ehling S, Hengel M, Shibamoto T. Formation of acrylamide from lipids. *Adv Exp Med Biol* 2005, 561:223-233.

Ehnert B, Lau-Schadendorf S, Weber A, Buettner P, Schou C, Wahn U. Reducing domestic exposure to dust mite allergen reduces bronchial hyperreactivity in sensitive children with asthma. *J Allergy Clin Immunol.* 1992 Jul;90(1):135-8.

Ehren J, Morón B, Martin E, Bethune MT, Gray GM, Khosla C. A food-grade enzyme preparation with modest gluten detoxification properties. *PLoS One.* 2009 Jul 21;4(7):e6313.

Eijkemans M, Mommers M, de Vries SI, van Buuren S, Stafleu A, Bakker I, Thijs C. Asthmatic symptoms, physical activity, and overweight in young children: a cohort study. *Pediatrics.* 2008 Mar;121(3):e666-72.

Ekelund M, Oberg S, Peterli R, Frederiksen SG, Hedenbro JL. Gastroesophageal Reflux after Vertical Banded Gastroplasty is Alleviated by Conversion to Gastric Bypass. *Obes Surg.* 2011 Nov 4.

Eldridge MW, Peden DB. Allergen provocation augments endotoxin-induced nasal inflammation in subjects with atopic asthma. *J Allergy Clin Immunol.* 2000 Mar;105(3):475-81.

el-Ghazaly M, Khayyal MT, Okpanyi SN, Arens-Corell M. Study of the anti-inflammatory activity of Populus tremula, Solidago virgaurea and Fraxinus excelsior. *Arzneimittelforschung.* 1992 Mar;42(3):333-6.

Ellingwood F. *American Materia Medica, Therapeutics and Pharmacognosy.* Portland: Eclectic Medical Publ., 1983.

Elliott RB, Harris DP, Hill JP, Bibby NJ, Wasmuth HE. Type I (insulin-dependent) diabetes mellitus and cow milk: casein variant consumption. *Diabetologia.* 1999 Mar;42(3):292-6.

el-Serag HB, Sonnenberg A. Opposing time trends of peptic ulcer and reflux disease. *Gut.* 1998 Sep;43(3):327-33.

Elwood PC. Epidemiology and trace elements. *Clin Endocrinol Metab.* 1985 Aug;14(3):617-28.

Emmanouil E, Manios Y, Grammatikaki E, Kondaki K, Oikonomou E, Papadopoulos N, Vassilopoulou E. Association of nutrient intake and wheeze or asthma in a Greek pre-school population. *Pediatr Allergy Immunol.* 2010 Feb;21(1 Pt 1):90-5. 2009 Sep 9.

Engler RJ. Alternative and complementary medicine: a source of improved therapies for asthma? A challenge for redefining the specialty? *J Allergy Clin Immunol.* 2000;106:627-9.

Environmental Working Group. *Human Toxome Project.* 2007. http://www.ewg.org/sites/humantoxome/. Accessed: 2007 Sep.

EPA. *A Brief Guide to Mold, Moisture and Your Home.* Environmental Protection Agency, Office of Air and Radiation/Indoor Environments Division. EPA 2002;402-K-02-003.

Epstein GN, Halper JP, Barrett EA, Birdsall C, McGee M, Baron KP, Lowenstein S. A pilot study of mind-body changes in adults with asthma who practice mental imagery. *Altern Ther Health Med.* 2004 Jul-Aug;10(4):66-71.

Erkkola M, Kaila M, Nwaru BI, Kronberg-Kippilä C, Ahonen S, Nevalainen J, Veijola R, Pekkanen J, Ilonen J, Simell O, Knip M, Virtanen SM. Maternal vitamin D intake during pregnancy is inversely associated with asthma and allergic rhinitis in 5-year-old children. *Clin Exp Allergy.* 2009 Jun;39(6):875-82.

Ernst E. Frankincense: systematic review. *BMJ.* 2008 Dec 17;337:a2813.

Erwin EA, James HR, Gutekunst HM, Russo JM, Kelleher KJ, Platts-Mills TA. Serum IgE measurement and detection of food allergy in pediatric patients with eosinophilic esophagitis. *Ann Allergy Asthma Immunol.* 2010 Jun;104(6):496-502.

EuroPrevall. *WP 1.1 Birth Cohort Update.* 1st Quarter 2006. Berlin, Germany: Charité University Medical Centre.

Evans P, Forte D, Jacobs C, Fredhoi C, Aitchison E, Hucklebridge F, Clow A. Cortisol secretory activity in older people in relation to positive and negative well-being. *Psychoneuroendocrinology.* 2007 Aug 7

Everhart JE. *Digestive Diseases in the United States.* Darby, PA: Diane Pub, 1994.

FAAN. *Public Comment on 2005 Food Safety Survey: Docket No. 2004N-0516 (2005 FSS).* Fairfax, VA: Food Allergy & Anaphylaxis Network.

Fairchild SS, Shannon K, Kwan E, Mishell RI. T cell-derived glucosteroid response-modifying factor (GRMF): a unique lymphokine made by normal T lymphocytes and a T cell hybridoma. *J Immunol.* 1984 Feb;132(2):821-7.

Fajac I, Frossard N. Neuropeptides of the nasal innervation and allergic rhinitis. *Rev Mal Respir.* 1994;11(4):357-67.

Fallone CA, Mayrand S. Gastroesophageal reflux and hyperacidity in chronic renal failure. *Perit Dial Int.* 2001;21 Suppl 3:S295-9.

Fälth-Magnusson K, Kjellman NI, Magnusson KE, Sundqvist T. Intestinal permeability in healthy and allergic children before and after sodium-cromoglycate treatment assessed with different-sized polyethyleneglycols (PEG 400 and PEG 1000). *Clin Allergy.* 1984 May;14(3):277-86.

Fälth-Magnusson K, Kjellman NI, Odelram H, Sundqvist T, Magnusson KE. Gastrointestinal permeability in children with cow's milk allergy: effect of milk challenge and sodium cromoglycate as assessed with polyethyleneglycols (PEG 400 and PEG 1000). *Clin Allergy.* 1986 Nov;16(6):543-51.

Fan AY, Lao L, Zhang RX, Zhou AN, Wang LB, Moudgil KD, Lee DY, Ma ZZ, Zhang WY, Berman BM. Effects of an acetone extract of Boswellia carterii Birdw. (Burseraceae) gum resin on adjuvant-induced arthritis in lewis rats. *J Ethnopharmacol.* 2005 Oct 3;101(1-3):104-9.

Fanaro S, Marten B, Bagna R, Vigi V, Fabris C, Peña-Quintana, Argüelles F, Scholz-Ahrens KE, Sawatzki G, Zelenka R, Schrezenmeir J, de Vrese M and Bertino E. Galacto-oligosaccharides are bifidogenic and safe at weaning: A double-blind Randomized Multicenter study. *J Pediatr Gastroent Nutr.* 2009 48; 82-88

Fang SP, Tanaka T, Tago F, Okamoto T, Kojima S. Immunomodulatory effects of gyokuheifusan on INF-gamma/IL-4 (Th1/Th2) balance in ovalbumin (OVA)-induced asthma model mice. *Biol Pharm Bull.* 2005;28:829-33.

FAO/WHO Expert Committee. *Fats and Oils in Human Nutrition.* Food and Nutrition Paper. 1994;(57).

Fawell J, Nieuwenhuijsen MJ. Contaminants in drinking water. *Br Med Bull.* 2003;68:199-208.

Faxén-Irving G, Cederholm T. Energy dense oleic acid rich formula to newly admitted geriatric patients—feasibility and effects on energy intake. *Clin Nutr.* 2011 Apr;30(2):202-8.

Fecka I. Qualitative and quantitative determination of hydrolysable tannins and other polyphenols in herbal products from meadowsweet and dog rose. *Phytochem Anal.* 2009 May;20(3):177-90.

Federação Brasileira de Gastroenterologia; Sociedade Brasileira de Endoscopia Digestiva; Colégio Brasileiro de Cirurgia Digestiva; Sociedade Brasileira de Pneumologia e Tisiologia. Gastroesophageal reflux disease: diagnosis. *Rev Assoc Med Bras.* 2011 Oct;57(5):499-507.

Felley CP, Corthésy-Theulaz I, Rivero JL, Sipponen P, Kaufmann M, Bauerfeind P, Wiesel PH, Brassart D, Pfeifer A, Blum AL, Michetti P. Favourable effect of an acidified milk (LC-1) on Helicobacter pylori gastritis in man. *Eur J Gastroenterol Hepatol.* 2001 Jan;13(1):25-9.

Fernández-Rivas M, Garrido Fernández S, Nadal JA, Díaz de Durana MD, García BE, González-Mancebo E, Martín S, Barber D, Rico P, Tabar AI. Randomized double-blind, placebo-controlled trial of sublingual immunotherapy with a Pru p 3 quantified peach extract. *Allergy.* 2009 Jun;64(6):876-83.

Fernández-Rivas M, González-Mancebo E, Rodríguez-Pérez R, Benito C, Sánchez-Monge R, Salcedo G, Alonso MD, Rosado A, Tejedor MA, Vila C, Casas ML. Clinically relevant peach allergy is related to peach lipid transfer protein, Pru p 3, in the Spanish population. *J Allergy Clin Immunol.* 2003 Oct;112(4):789-95.

REFERENCES

Ferrari M, Benini L, Brotto E, Locatelli F, De Iorio F, Bonella F, Tacchella N, Corradini G, Lo Cascio V, Vantini I. Omeprazole reduces the response to capsaicin but not to methacholine in asthmatic patients with proximal reflux. *Scand J Gastroenterol.* 2007 Mar;42(3):299-307.

Ferrier L, Berard F, Debrauwer L, Chabo C, Langella P, Bueno L, Fioramonti J. Impairment of the intestinal barrier by ethanol involves enteric microflora and mast cell activation in rodents. *Am J Pathol.* 2006 Apr;168(4):1148-54.

Field RW, Krewski D, Lubin JH, Zielinski JM, Alavanja M, Catalan VS, Klotz JB, Létourneau EG, Lynch CF, Lyon JL, Sandler DP, Schoenberg JB, Steck DJ, Stolwijk JA, Weinberg C, Wilcox HB. An overview of the North American residential radon and lung cancer case-control studies. *J Toxicol Environ Health A.* 2006 Apr;69(7):599-631.

Field T, Henteleff T, Hernandez-Reif M, Martinez E, Mavunda K, Kuhn C, Schanberg S. Children with asthma have improved pulmonary functions after massage therapy. *J Pediatr.* 1998 May;132(5):854-8.

Finkelman FD, Boyce JA, Vercelli D, Rothenberg ME. Key advances in mechanisms of asthma, allergy, and immunology in 2009. *J Allergy Clin Immunol.* 2010 Feb;125(2):312-8.

Fiocchi A, Restani P, Bernardo L, Martelli A, Ballabio C, D'Auria E, Riva E. Tolerance of heat-treated kiwi by children with kiwifruit allergy. *Pediatr Allergy Immunol.* 2004 Oct;15(5):454-8.

Fiocchi A, Travaini M, D'Auria E, Banderali G, Bernardo L, Riva E. Tolerance to a rice hydrolysate formula in children allergic to cow's milk and soy. *Clin Exp Allergy.* 2003 Nov;33(11):1576-80.

Fiocchi, A; Restani, P; Riva, E; Qualizza, R; Bruni, P; Restelli, AR; Galli, CL. Meat allergy: I. Specific IgE to BSA and OSA in atopic, beef sensitive children. *J Am Coll Nutr.* 1995 14: 239-244.

Fjeld T, Veiersted B, Sandvik L, Riise G, Levy F. The Effect of Indoor Foliage Plants on Health and Discomfort Symptoms among Office Workers. *Ind Built Environ.* 1998 July;7(4): 204-209.

Flandrin, J, Montanari M. (eds.). *Food: A Culinary History from Antiquity to the Present.* New York: Penguin Books, 1999.

Fleischer DM, Conover-Walker MK, Christie L, Burks AW, Wood RA. Peanut allergy: recurrence and its management. *J Allergy Clin Immunol.* 2004 Nov;114(5):1195-201.

Flinterman AE, van Hoffen E, den Hartog Jager CF, Koppelman S, Pasmans SG, Hoekstra MO, Bruijnzeel-Koomen CA, Knulst AC, Knol EF. Children with peanut allergy recognize predominantly Ara h2 and Ara h6, which remains stable over time. *Clin Exp Allergy.* 2007 Aug;37(8):1221-8.

Florén CH, Johnsson F. Effect of fibre on acid gastro-oesophageal reflux. *J Intern Med.* 1989 Apr;225(4):287-8.

Foliaki S, Annesi-Maesano I, Tuuau-Potoi N, Waqatakirewa L, Cheng S, Douwes J, Pearce N. Risk factors for symptoms of childhood asthma, allergic rhinoconjunctivitis and eczema in the Pacific: an ISAAC Phase III study. *Int J Tuberc Lung Dis.* 2008 Jul;12(7):799-806.

Forbes EE, Groschwitz K, Abonia JP, Brandt EB, Cohen E, Blanchard C, Ahrens R, Seidu L, McKenzie A, Strait R, Finkelman FD, Foster PS, Matthaei KI, Rothenberg ME, Hogan SP. IL-9- and mast cell-mediated intestinal permeability predisposes to oral antigen hypersensitivity. *J Exp Med.* 2008 Apr 14;205(4):897-913.

Forestier C, Guelon D, Cluytens V, Gillart T, Sirot J, De Champs C. Oral probiotic and prevention of Pseudomonas aeruginosa infections: a randomized, double-blind, placebo-controlled pilot study in intensive care unit patients. *Crit Care.* 2008;12(3):R69.

Forget-Dubois N, Boivin M, Dionne G, Pierce T, Tremblay RE, Pérusse D. A longitudinal twin study of the genetic and environmental etiology of maternal hostile-reactive behavior during infancy and toddlerhood. *Infant Behav Dev.* 2007

Foster S, Hobbs C. *Medicinal Plants and Herbs.* Boston: Houghton Mifflin, 2002.

Fox RD, *Algoculture.* Doctorate Disseration, 1983 Jul.

Fox VL, Nurko S, Furuta GT. Eosinophilic esophagitis: it's not just kid's stuff. *Gastrointest Endosc.* 2002 Aug;56(2):260-70.

Francavilla R, Lionetti E, Castellaneta SP, Magistà AM, Maurogiovanni G, Bucci N, De Canio A, Indrio F, Cavallo L, Ierardi E, Miniello VL. Inhibition of Helicobacter pylori infection in humans by Lactobacillus reuteri ATCC 55730 and effect on eradication therapy: a pilot study. *Helicobacter.* 2008 Apr;13(2):127-34.

Francis H, Fletcher G, Anthony C, Pickering C, Oldham L, Hadley E, Custovic A, Niven R. Clinical effects of air filters in homes of asthmatic adults sensitised and exposed to pet allergens. *Clin Exp Allergy.* 2003 Jan;33(1):101-5.

Frank PI, Morris JA, Hazell ML, Linehan MF, Frank TL. Long term prognosis in preschool children with wheeze: longitudinal postal questionnaire study 1993-2004. *BMJ.* 2008 Jun 21;336(7658):1423-6. 2008 Jun 16.

Frawley D, Lad V. *The Yoga of Herbs.* Sante Fe: Lotus Press, 1986.

Freedman BJ. A dietary free from additives in the management of allergic disease. *Clin Allergy.* 1977 Sep;7(5):417-21.

Fremont S, Moneret-Vautrin DA, Franck P, Morisset M, Croizier A, Codreanu F, Kanny G. Prospective study of sensitization and food allergy to flaxseed in 1317 subjects. *Eur Ann Allergy Clin Immunol.* 2010 Jun;42(3):103-11.

Frias J, Song YS, Martínez-Villaluenga C, González de Mejia E, Vidal-Valverde C. Immunoreactivity and amino acid content of fermented soybean products. *J Agric Food Chem.* 2008 Jan 9;56(1):99-105.

Friedman G. Nutritional therapy of irritable bowel syndrome. *Gastroenterol Clin North Am.* 1989 Sep;18(3):513-24.

Friedman LS, Harvard Health Publ. Ed. *Controlling GERD and Chronic Heartburn.* Boston: Harvard Health, 2008.

Frumkin H. Beyond toxicity: human health and the natural environment. *Am J Prev Med.* 2001;20(3):234-40.

Fu G, Zhong Y, Li C, Li Y, Lin X, Liao B, Tsang EW, Wu K, Huang S. Epigenetic regulation of peanut allergen gene Ara h 3 in developing embryos. *Planta.* 2010 Apr;231(5):1049-60.

Fu JX. Measurement of MEFV in 66 cases of asthma in the convalescent stage and after treatment with Chinese herbs. *Zhong Xi Yi Jie He Za Zhi.* 1989 Nov;9(11):658-9, 644.

Fujii T, Ohtsuka Y, Lee T, Kudo T, Shoji H, Sato H, Nagata S, Shimizu T, Yamashiro Y. Bifidobacterium breve enhances transforming growth factor beta1 signaling by regulating Smad7 expression in preterm in-fants. *J Pediatr Gastroenterol Nutr.* 2006 Jul;43(1):83-8.

Fujiwara Y, Kubo M, Kohata Y, Machida H, Okazaki H, Yamagami H, Tanigawa T, Watanabe K, Watanabe T, Tominaga K, Arakawa T. Cigarette smoking and its association with overlapping gastroesophageal reflux disease, functional dyspepsia, or irritable bowel syndrome. *Intern Med.* 2011;50(21):2443-7.

Furuhjelm C, Warstedt K, Larsson J, Fredriksson M, Böttcher MF, Fälth-Magnusson K, Duchén K. Fish oil supplementation in pregnancy and lactation may decrease the risk of infant allergy. *Acta Paediatr.* 2009 Sep;98(9):1461-7.

Furuta T, Shirai N, Xiao F, Takashima M, Hanai H. Effect of Helicobacter pylori infection and its eradication on nutrition. *Aliment Pharmacol Ther.* 2002 Apr;16(4):799-806.

Gabory A, Attig L, Junien C. Sexual dimorphism in environmental epigenetic programming. *Mol Cell Endocrinol.* 2009 May 25;304(1-2):8-18. 2009 Mar 9.

Galli J, Frenguelli A, Calò L, Agostino S, Cianci R, Cammarota G. Role of gastroesophageal reflux in precancerous conditions and in squamous cell carcinoma of the larynx: our experience. *Acta Otorhinolaryngol Ital.* 2001 Dec;21(6):350-5.

Gamboa PM, Cáceres O, Antepara I, Sánchez-Monge R, Ahrazem O, Salcedo G, Barber D, Lombardero M, Sanz ML. Two different profiles of peach allergy in the north of Spain. *Allergy.* 2007 Apr;62(4):408-14.

Gammack JK, Burke JM. Natural light exposure improves subjective sleep quality in nursing home residents. *J Am Med Dir Assoc.* 2009 Jul;10(6):440-1.

Gao X, Wang W, Wei S, Li W. Review of pharmacological effects of Glycyrrhiza radix and its bioactive compounds. *Zhongguo Zhong Yao Za Zhi.* 2009 Nov;34(21):2695-700.

Garavello W, Somigliana E, Acaia B, Gaini L, Pignataro I, Gaini RM. Nasal lavage in pregnant women with seasonal allergic rhinitis: a randomized study. *Int Arch Allergy Immunol.* 2010;151(2):137-41. 2009 Sep 15. 19752567.

Garcia Gomez LJ, Sanchez-Muniz FJ. Review: cardiovascular effect of garlic (Allium sativum). *Arch Latinoam Nutr.* 2000 Sep;50(3):219-29.

García-Compeán D, González MV, Galindo G, Mar DA, Treviño JL, Martínez R, Bosques F, Maldonado H. Prevalence of gastroesophageal reflux disease in patients with extraesophageal symptoms referred from otolaryngology, allergy, and cardiology practices: a prospective study. *Dig Dis.* 2000;18(3):178-82.

Garcia-Marcos L, Canflanca IM, Garrido JB, Varela AL, Garcia-Hernandez G, Guillen Grima F, Gonzalez-Diaz C, Carvajal-Urueña I, Arnedo-Pena A, Busquets-Monge RM, Morales Suarez-Varela M, Blanco-Quiros A. Relationship of asthma and rhinoconjunctivitis with obesity, exercise and Mediterranean diet in Spanish schoolchildren. *Thorax.* 2007 Jun;62(6):503-8.

Gardner ML. Gastrointestinal absorption of intact proteins. Annu Rev Nutr. 1988;8:329-50.

Garnett WR. Considerations for long-term use of proton-pump inhibitors. *Am J Health Syst Pharm.* 1998 Nov 1;55(21):2268-79.

Gary WK, Fanny WS, David SC. Factors associated with difference in prevalence of asthma in children from three cities in China: multicentre epidemiological survey. *BMJ.* 2004;329:1-4.

Garzi A, Messina M, Frati F, Carfagna L, Zagordo L, Belcastro M, Parmiani S, Sensi L, Marcucci F. An extensively hydrolysed cow's milk formula improves clinical symptoms of gastroesophageal reflux and reduces the gastric emptying time in infants. *Allergol Immunopathol (Madr).* 2002 Jan-Feb;30(1):36-41.

Garzi A, Messina M, Frati F, Carfagna L, Zagordo L, Belcastro M, Parmiani S, Sensi L, Marcucci F. An extensively hydrolysed cow's milk formula improves clinical symptoms of gastroesophageal reflux and reduces the gastric emptying time in infants. *Allergol Immunopathol (Madr).* 2002 Jan-Feb;30(1):36-41.

Gazdik F, Horvathova M, Gazdikova K, Jahnova E. The influence of selenium supplementation on the immunity of corticoid-dependent asthmatics. *Bratisl Lek Listy.* 2002;103(1):17-21.

Gazdik F, Kadrabova J, Gazdikova K. Decreased consumption of corticosteroids after selenium supplementation in corticoid-dependent asthmatics. *Bratisl Lek Listy.* 2002;103(1):22-5.

Geha RS, Beiser A, Ren C, Patterson R, Greenberger PA, Grammer LC, Ditto AM, Harris KE, Shaughnessy MA, Yarnold PR, Corren J, Saxon A. Multicenter, double-blind, placebo-controlled, multiple-challenge evaluation of reported reactions to monosodium glutamate. *J Allergy Clin Immunol.* 2000 Nov;106(5):973-80.

Gerez IF, Shek LP, Chng HH, Lee BW. Diagnostic tests for food allergy. *Singapore Med J.* 2010 Jan;51(1):4-9.

Gergen PJ, Arbes SJ Jr, Calatroni A, Mitchell HE, Zeldin DC. Total IgE levels and asthma prevalence in the US population: results from the National Health and Nutrition Examination Survey 2005-2006. *J Allergy Clin Immunol.* 2009 Sep;124(3):447-53. 2009 Aug 3.

Ghadioungui P. (transl.) *The Ebers Papyrus.* Academy of Scientific Research. Cairo, 1987.

Ghoshal UC, Chourasia D. Gastroesophageal Reflux Disease and Helicobacter pylori: What May Be the Relationship? *J Neurogastroenterol Motil.* 2010 Jul;16(3):243-50.

Giampietro PG, Kjellman NI, Oldaeus G, Wouters-Wesseling W, Businco L. Hypoallergenicity of an extensively hydrolyzed whey formula. *Pediatr Allergy Immunol.* 2001 Apr;12(2):83-6.

Gibbons E. *Stalking the Healthful Herbs.* New York: David McKay, 1966.

Gibbons TE, Gold BD. The use of proton pump inhibitors in children: a comprehensive. *Paediatr Drugs.* 2003;5(1):25-40.

Gibson RA. Docosa-hexaenoic acid (DHA) accumulation is regulated by the polyunsaturated fat content of the diet: Is it synthesis or is it incorporation? *Asia Pac J Clin Nutr.* 2004;13(Suppl):S78.

Gilbert CR, Arum SM, Smith CM. Vitamin D deficiency and chronic lung disease. *Can Respir J.* 2009 May-Jun;16(3):75-80.

Gill HS, Rutherfurd KJ, Cross ML, Gopal PK. Enhancement of immunity in the elderly by dietary supplementation with the probiotic Bifidobacterium lactis HN019. *Am J Clin Nutr.* 2001 Dec;74(6):833-9.

Gillman A, Douglass JA. What do asthmatics have to fear from food and additive allergy? *Clin Exp Allergy.* 2010 Sep;40(9):1295-302.

Ginde AA, Mansbach JM, Camargo CA Jr. Association between serum 25-hydroxyvitamin D level and upper respiratory tract infection in the Third National Health and Nutrition Examination Survey. *Arch Intern Med.* 2009 Feb 23;169(4):384-90.

Glück U, Gebbers J. Ingested probiotics reduce nasal colonization with pathogenic bacteria (Staphylococcus aureus, Streptococcus pneumoniae, and b-hemolytic streptococci. *Am J. Clin. Nutr.* 2003;77:517-520.

Goedsche K, Förster M, Kroegel C, Uhlemann C. Repeated cold water stimulations (hydrotherapy according to Kneipp) in patients with COPD. *Forsch Komplementmed.* 2007 Jun;14(3):158-66.

Goel RK, Gupta S, Shankar R, Sanyal AK. Anti-ulcerogenic effect of banana powder (Musa sapientum var. paradisiaca) and its effect on mucosal resistance. *J Ethnopharmacol.* 1986 Oct;18(1):33-44.

Goel RK, Sairam K, Rao CV. Role of gastric antioxidant and anti-Helicobacter pylori activities in antiulcerogenic activity of plantain banana (Musa sapientum var. paradisiaca). *Indian J Exp Biol.* 2001 Jul;39(7):719-22.

Goel V, Dolan RJ. The functional anatomy of humor: segregating cognitive and affective components. *Nat Neurosci.* 2001;4:237-8.

Gohil K, Packer L. Bioflavonoid-Rich Botanical Extracts Show Antioxidant and Gene Regulatory Activity. *Ann N Y Acad Sci.* 2002:957:70-7.

Gold BD. Helicobacter pylori infection in children. *Curr Probl Pediatr Adolesc Health Care.* 2001 Sep;31(8):247-66.

Gold BD. New approaches to Helicobacter pylori infection in children. *Curr Gastroenterol Rep.* 2001 Jun;3(3):235-47.

Goldin BR, Adlercreutz H, Dwyer JT, Swenson L, Warram JH, Gorbach SL. Effect of diet on excretion of estrogens in pre- and postmenopausal women. *Cancer Res.* 1981 Sep;41(9 Pt 2):3771-3.

Goldin BR, Adlercreutz H, Gorbach SL, Warram JH, Dwyer JT, Swenson L, Woods MN. Estrogen excretion patterns and plasma levels in vegetarian and omnivorous women. *N Engl J Med.* 1982 Dec 16;307(25):1542-7.

Goldin BR, Swenson L, Dwyer J, Sexton M, Gorbach SL. Effect of diet and Lactobacillus acidophilus supplements on human fecal bacterial enzymes. *J Natl Cancer Inst.* 1980 Feb;64(2):255-61.

Goldman JA, Blanton WP, Hay DW, Wolfe MM. False-positive secretin stimulation test for gastrinoma associated with the use of proton pump inhibitor therapy. *Clin Gastroenterol Hepatol.* 2009 May;7(5):600-2.

Goldstein JL, Aisenberg J, Zakko SF, Berger MF, Dodge WE. Endoscopic ulcer rates in healthy subjects associated with use of aspirin (81 mg q.d.) alone or coadministered with celecoxib or naproxen: a randomized, 1-week trial. *Dig Dis Sci.* 2008 Mar;53(3):647-56.

Golub E. *The Limits of Medicine.* New York: Times Books, 1994.

Gonzales M, Malcoe LH, Myers OB, Espinoza J. Risk factors for asthma and cough among Hispanic children in the southwestern United States of America, 2003-2004. *Rev Panam Salud Publica.* 2007 May;21(5):274-81.

González Alvarez R, Arruzazabala ML. Current views of the mechanism of action of prophylactic antiallergic drugs. *Allergol Immunopathol (Madr).* 1981 Nov-Dec;9(6):501-8.

González J, Fernández M, García Fragoso L. Exclusive breastfeeding reduces asthma in a group of children from the Caguas municipality of Puerto Rico. *Bol Asoc Med P R.* 2010 Jan-Mar;102(1):10-2.

González Morales JE, Leal de Hernández L, González Spencer D. Asthma associated with gastroesophageal reflux. *Rev Alerg Mex.* 1998 Jan-Feb;45(1):16-21.

González-Pérez A, Aponte Z, Vidaurre CF, Rodríguez LA. Anaphylaxis epidemiology in patients with and patients without asthma: a United Kingdom database review. *J Allergy Clin Immunol.* 2010 May;125(5):1098-1104.e1.

González-Sánchez R, Trujillo X, Trujillo-Hernández B, Vásquez C, Huerta M, Elizalde A. Forskolin versus sodium cromoglycate for prevention of asthma attacks: a single-blinded clinical trial. *J Int Med Res.* 2006 Mar-Apr;34(2):200-7.

Gordon BR. Patch testing for allergies. *Curr Opin Otolaryngol Head Neck Surg.* 2010 Jun;18(3):191-4.

Gore KV, Rao AK, Guruswamy MN. Physiological studies with Tylophora asthmatica in bronchial asthma. *Indian J Med Res.* 1980 Jan;71:144-8.

Goren AI, Hellmann S. Changes prevalence of asthma among schoolchildren in Israel. *Eur Respir J.* 1997;10:2279-2284.

Gotteland M, Poliak L, Cruchet S, Brunser O. Effect of regular ingestion of Saccharomyces boulardii plus inulin or Lactobacillus acidophilus LB in children colonized by Helicobacter pylori. *Acta Paediatr.* 2005 Dec;94(12):1747-51.

Govindan S, Viswanathan S, Vijayasekaran V, Alagappan R. A pilot study on the clinical efficacy of Solanum xanthocarpum and Solanum trilobatum in bronchial asthma. *J Ethnopharmacol.* 1999 Aug;66(2):205-10.

Govindan S, Viswanathan S, Vijayasekaran V, Alagappan R. Further studies on the clinical efficacy of Solanum xanthocarpum and Solanum trilobatum in bronchial asthma. *Phytother Res.* 2004 Oct;18(10):805-9.

Grant WB, Holick MF. Benefits and requirements of vitamin D for optimal health: a review. *Altern Med Rev.* 2005 Jun;10(2):94-111.

Grant WB. Hypothesis—ultraviolet-B irradiance and vitamin D reduce the risk of viral infections and thus their sequelae, including autoimmune diseases and some cancers. *Photochem Photobiol.* 2008 Mar-Apr;84(2):356-65. 2008 Jan 7.

Gray H. *Anatomy, Descriptive and Surgical.* 15th Edition. New York: Random House, 1977.

Gray-Davison F. *Ayurvedic Healing.* New York: Keats, 2002.

Greskevitch M, Kullman G, Bang KM, Mazurek JM. Respiratory disease in agricultural workers: mortality and morbidity statistics. *J Agromedicine.* 2007;12(3):5-10.

Griffith HW. *Healing Herbs: The Essential Guide.* Tucson: Fisher Books, 2000.

Grimm T, Chovanová Z, Muchová J, Sumegová K, Liptáková A, Duracková Z, Högger P. Inhibition of NF-kappaB activation and MMP-9 secretion by plasma of human volunteers after ingestion of maritime pine bark extract (Pycnogenol). *J Inflamm (Lond).* 2006 Jan 27;3:1.

Grimm T, Schäfer A, Högger P. Antioxidant activity and inhibition of matrix metalloproteinases by metabolites of maritime pine bark extract (pycnogenol). *Free Radic Biol Med.* 2004 Mar 15;36(6):811-22.

Grimm T, Skrabala R, Chovanová Z, Muchová J, Sumegová K, Liptáková A, Duracková Z, Högger P. Single and multiple dose pharmacokinetics of maritime pine bark extract (pycnogenol) after oral administration to healthy volunteers. *BMC Clin Pharmacol.* 2006 Aug 3;6:4.

Gropper SS, Smith JL, Groff JL. *Advanced nutrition and human metabolism.* Belmonth, CA: Wadsworth Publ, 2008.

Groschwitz KR, Ahrens R, Osterfeld H, Gurish MF, Han X, Abrink M, Finkelman FD, Pejler G, Hogan SP. Mast cells regulate homeostatic intestinal epithelial migration and barrier function by a chymase/Mcpt4-dependent mechanism. *Proc Natl Acad Sci U S A.* 2009 Dec 29;106(52):22381-6.

Grosser BI, Monti-Bloch L, Jennings-White C, Berliner DL. Behavioral and electrophysiological effects of androstadienone, a human pheromone. *Psychoneuroendocrinology.* 2000 Apr;25(3):289-99.

Grzanna R, Lindmark L, Frondoza CG. Ginger—an herbal medicinal product with broad anti-inflammatory actions. *J Med Food.* 2005 Summer;8(2):125-32.

Guandalini S. The influence of gluten: weaning recommendations for healthy children and children at risk for celiac disease. *Nestle Nutr Workshop Ser Pediatr Program.* 2007;60:139-51; discussion 151-5.

Guaré RO, Ferreira MC, Leite MF, Rodrigues JA, Lussi A, Santos MT. Dental erosion and salivary flow rate in cerebral palsy individuals with gastroesophageal reflux. *J Oral Pathol Med.* 2011 Nov 14.

Guedon C. How to diagnose gastroesophageal reflux? Part 1. Diagnostic value of symptoms. Interpretation and role of endoscopy. *Gastroenterol Clin Biol.* 1999 Jan;23(1 Pt 2):S202-7.

Guerin M, Huntley ME, Olaizola M. Haematococcus astaxanthin: applications for human health and nutrition. *Trends Biotechnol.* 2003 May;21(5):210-6.

Guinot P, Brambilla C, Duchier J, Braquet P, Bonvoisin B, Cournot A. Effect of BN 52063, a specific PAF-acether antagonist, on bronchial provocation test to allergens in asthmatic patients. A preliminary study. *Prostaglandins.* 1987 Nov;34(5):723-31.

Gundermann KJ, Müller J. Phytodolor—effects and efficacy of a herbal medicine. *Wien Med Wochenschr.* 2007;157(13-14):343-7.

Guo J, Reside G, Cooper LF. Full-mouth rehabilitation of a patient with gastroesophageal reflux disease: a clinical report. *J Prosthodont.* 2011 Oct;20 Suppl 2:S9-13.

Gupta I, Gupta V, Parihar A, Gupta S, Lüdtke R, Safayhi H, Ammon HP. Effects of Boswellia serrata gum resin in patients with bronchial asthma: results of a double-blind, placebo-controlled, 6-week clinical study. *Eur J Med Res.* 1998 Nov 17;3(11):511-4.

Gupta R, Sheikh A, Strachan DP, Anderson HR (2006) Time trends in allergic disorders in the UK. *Thorax,* published online. doi: 10.1136/thx.2004.038844.

Gupta S, George P, Gupta V, Tandon VR, Sundaram KR. Tylophora indica in bronchial asthma—a double blind study. *Indian J Med Res.* 1979 Jun;69:981-9.

Gupte AR, Draganov PV. Eosinophilic esophagitis. *World J Gastroenterol.* 2009 Jan 7;15(1):17-24.

Gutmanis J. *Hawaiian Herbal Medicine.* Waipahu, HI: Island Heritage, 2001.

Haggag EG, Abou-Moustafa MA, Boucher W, Theoharides TC. The effect of a herbal water-extract on histamine release from mast cells and on allergic asthma. *J Herb Pharmacother.* 2003;3(4):41-54.

Haines JL, Ter-Minassian M, Bazyk A, Gusella JF, Kim DJ, Terwedow H, Pericak-Vance MA, Rimmler JB, Haynes CS, Roses AD, Lee A, Shaner B, Menold M, Seboun E, Fitoussi RP, Gartioux C, Reyes C, Ribierre F, Gyapay G, Weissenbach J, Hauser SL, Goodkin DE, Lincoln R, Usuku K, Oksenberg JR, *et al.* A complete genomic screen for multiple sclerosis underscores a role for the major histocompatability complex. The Multiple Sclerosis Genetics Group. *Nat Genet.* 1996 Aug;13(4):469-71..

Hajar N, Castell DO, Ghomrawi H, Rackett R, Hila A. Impedance pH Confirms the Relationship Between GERD and BMI. *Dig Dis Sci.* 2012 Mar 27.

Halász A, Cserháti E. The prognosis of bronchial asthma in childhood in Hungary: a long-term follow-up. *J Asthma.* 2002 Dec;39(8):693-9.

Halken S, Hansen KS, Jacobsen HP, Estmann A, Faelling AE, Hansen LG, Kier SR, Lassen K, Lintrup M, Mortensen S, Ibsen KK, Osterballe O, Høst A. Comparison of a partially hydrolyzed infant formula with two extensively hydrolyzed formulas for allergy prevention: a prospective, randomized study. *Pediatr Allergy Immunol.* 2000 Aug;11(3):149-61.

Halpern GM, Miller AH. *Medicinal Mushrooms: Ancient Remedies for Modern Ailments.* New York: M. Evans, 2002.

Hamasaki Y, Kobayashi I, Hayasaki R, Zaitu M, Muro E, Yamamoto S, Ichimaru T, Miyazaki S. The Chinese herbal medicine, shinpi-to, inhibits IgE-mediated leukotriene synthesis in rat basophilic leukemia-2H3 cells. *J Ethnopharmacol.* 1997 Apr;56(2):123-31.

Hamelmann E, Beyer K, Gruber C, Lau S, Matricardi PM, Nickel R, Niggemann B, Wahn U. Primary prevention of allergy: avoiding risk or providing protection? *Clin Exp Allergy.* 2008 Feb;38(2):233-45.

Hamilton RG. Clinical laboratory assessment of immediate-type hypersensitivity. *J Allergy Clin Immunol.* 2010 Feb;125(2 Suppl 2):S284-96.

Hammond BG, Mayhew DA, Kier LD, Mast RW, Sander WJ. Safety assessment of DHA-rich microalgae from Schizochytrium sp. *Regul Toxicol Pharmacol.* 2002 Apr;35(2 Pt 1):255-65.

Han ER, Choi IS, Kim HK, Kang YW, Park JG, Lim JR, Seo JH, Choi JH. Inhaled corticosteroid-related tooth problems in asthmatics. *J Asthma.* 2009 Mar;46(2):160-4.

Han SN, Leka LS, Lichtenstein AH, Ausman LM, Meydani SN. Effect of a therapeutic lifestyle change diet on immune functions of moderately hypercholesterolemic humans. *J Lipid Res.* 2003 Dec;44(12):2304-10.

REFERENCES

Hansen KS, Ballmer-Weber BK, Lüttkopf D, Skov PS, Wüthrich B, Bindslev-Jensen C, Vieths S, Poulsen LK. Roasted hazelnuts—allergenic activity evaluated by double-blind, placebo-controlled food challenge. *Allergy.* 2003 Feb;58(2):132-8.

Hansen KS, Ballmer-Weber BK, Sastre J, Lidholm J, Andersson K, Oberhofer H, Lluch-Bernal M, Ostling J, Mattsson L, Schocker F, Vieths S, Poulsen LK. Component-resolved in vitro diagnosis of hazelnut allergy in Europe. *J Allergy Clin Immunol.* 2009 May;123(5):1134-41, 1141.e1-3.

Hansen KS, Khinchi MS, Skov PS, Bindslev-Jensen C, Poulsen LK, Malling HJ. Food allergy to apple and specific immunotherapy with birch pollen. *Mol Nutr Food Res.* 2004 Nov;48(6):441-8.

Haranath PS, Shyamalakumari S. Experimental study on mode of action of Tylophora asthmatica in bronchial asthma. *Indian J Med Res.* 1975 May;63(5):661-70.

Harju EJ, Larmi TK. Effect of guar gum added to the diet of patients with duodenal ulcer. *JPEN J Parenter Enteral Nutr.* 1985 Jul-Aug;9(4):496-500.

Harrington JJ, Lee-Chiong T Jr. Sleep and older patients. *Clin Chest Med.* 2007 Dec;28(4):673-84, v.

Hartz C, Lauer I, Del Mar San Miguel Moncin M, Cistero-Bahima A, Foetisch K, Lidholm J, Vieths S, Scheurer S. Comparison of IgE-Binding Capacity, Cross-Reactivity and Biological Potency of Allergenic Non-Specific Lipid Transfer Proteins from Peach, Cherry and Hazelnut. *Int Arch Allergy Immunol.* 2010 Jun 17;153(4):335-346.

Haruma K, Manabe N, Kamada T, Shiotani A, Kusaka K. Helicobacter pylori infection and GERD. *Nihon Rinsho.* 2007 May;65(5):841-5.

Harvald B, Hauge M: Hereditary factors elucidated by twin studies. *In Genetics and the Epidemiology of Chronic Disease.* Edited by Neel JV, Shaw MV, Schull WJ. Washington, DC: Dept Health, Education and Welfare, 1965:64-76.

Hassan AM. Selenium status in patients with aspirin-induced asthma. *Ann Clin Biochem.* 2008 Sep;45(Pt 5):508-12.

Hasselmark L, Malmgren R, Zetterström O, Unge G. Selenium supplementation in intrinsic asthma. *Allergy.* 1993 Jan;48(1):30-6.

Hata K, Ishikawa K, Hori K, Konishi T. Differentiation-inducing activity of lupeol, a lupane-type triterpene from Chinese dandelion root (Hokouei-kon), on a mouse melanoma cell line. *Biol Pharm Bull.* 2000 Aug;23(8):962-7.

Hattori K, Sasai M, Yamamoto A, Taniuchi S, Kojima T, Kobayashi Y, Iwamoto H, Yaeshima T, Hayasawa H. Intestinal flora of infants with cow milk hypersensitivity fed on casein-hydrolyzed formula supplemented raffinose. *Arerugi.* 2000 Dec;49(12):1146-55.

Heaney LG, Brightling CE, Menzies-Gow A, Stevenson M, Niven RM; British Thoracic Society Difficult Asthma Network. Refractory asthma in the UK: cross-sectional findings from a UK multicentre registry. *Thorax.* 2010 Sep;65(9):787-94.

Heaney RP, Dowell MS. Absorbability of the calcium in a high-calcium mineral water. *Osteoporos Int.* 1994 Nov;4(6):323-4.

Heap GA, van Heel DA. Genetics and pathogenesis of coeliac disease. *Semin Immunol.* May 13 2009.

Hemmer W, Focke M, Marzban G, Swoboda I, Jarisch R, Laimer M. Identification of Bet v 1-related allergens in fig and other Moraceae fruits. *Clin Exp Allergy.* 2010 Apr;40(4):679-87.

Hendel B, Ferreira P. *Water & Salt: The Essence of Life.* Gaithersburg: Natural Resources, 2003.

Henry SM. Discerning differences: gastroesophageal reflux and gastroesophageal reflux disease in infants. *Adv Neonatal Care.* 2004 Aug;4(4):235-47.

Herbert V. Vitamin B12: Plant sources, requirements, and assay. *Am J Clin Nutr.* 1988;48:852-858.

Herman PM, Drost LM. Evaluating the clinical relevance of food sensitivity tests: a single subject experiment. *Altern Med Rev.* 2004 Jun;9(2):198-207.

Herrerías Gutiérrez JM. Gastroesophageal reflux and Helicobacter pylori. *An R Acad Nac Med (Madr).* 1999;116(4):793-811; discussion 811-3.

Herzog AM, Black KA, Fountaine DJ, Knotts TR. Reflection and attentional recovery as two distinctive benefits of restorative environments. *J Environ Psychol.* 1997;17:165-70.

Hess-Kosa K. *Indoor Air Quality: Sampling Methodologies.* Boca Rataon: CRC Press, 2002.

Heyman M, Grasset E, Ducroc R, Desjeux JF. Antigen absorption by the jejunal epithelium of children with cow's milk allergy. *Pediatr Res.* 1988 Aug;24(2):197-202.

Hide DW, Matthews S, Tariq S, Arshad SH. Allergen avoidance in infancy and allergy at 4 years of age. *Allergy.* 1996 Feb;51(2):89-93.

Hijazi Z, Molla AM, Al-Habashi H, Muawad WM, Molla AM, Sharma PN. Intestinal permeability is increased in bronchial asthma. *Arch Dis Child.* 2004 Mar;89(3):227-9.

Hill J, Micklewright A, Lewis S, Britton J. Investigation of the effect of short-term change in dietary magnesium intake in asthma. *Eur Respir J.* 1997 Oct;10(10):2225-9.

Hirose Y, Murosaki S, Yamamoto Y, Yoshikai Y, Tsuru T. Daily intake of heat-killed Lactobacillus plantarum L-137 augments acquired immunity in healthy adults. *J Nutr.* 2006 Dec;136(12):3069-73.

Hobbs C. *Medicinal Mushrooms.* Summertown, TN: Botanica Press, 2003.

Hobbs C. *Stress & Natural Healing.* Loveland, CO: Interweave Press, 1997.

Hoffmann D. *Holistic Herbal.* London: Thorsons, 2002.

Hofmann D, Hecker M, Völp A. Efficacy of dry extract of ivy leaves in children with bronchial asthma-a review of randomized controlled trials. *Phytomedicine.* 2003 Mar;10(2-3):213-20.

Höiby AS, Strand V, Robinson DS, Sager A, Rak S. Efficacy, safety, and immunological effects of a 2-year immunotherapy with Depigoid birch pollen extract: a randomized, double-blind, placebo-controlled study. *Clin Exp Allergy.* 2010 Jul;40(7):1062-70.

Holick MF. Sunlight and vitamin D for bone health and prevention of autoimmune diseases, cancers, and cardiovascular disease. *Am J Clin Nutr.* 2004 Dec;80(6 Suppl):1678S-88S.

Holick MF. The vitamin D deficiency pandemic and consequences for nonskeletal health: mechanisms of action. *Mol Aspects Med.* 2008 Dec;29(6):361-8

Holick MF. Vitamin D status: measurement, interpretation, and clinical application. *Ann Epidemiol.* 2009 Feb;19(2):73-8.

Holladay, S.D. Prenatal Immunotoxicant Exposure and Postnatal Autoimmune Disease. *Environ Health Perspect.* 1999; 107(suppl 5):687-691.

Holt GA. Food & Drug Interactions. Chicago: Precept Press, 1998, 83.

Homma M, Oka K, Niitsuma T, Itoh H. A novel 11 beta-hydroxysteroid dehydrogenase inhibitor contained in saiboku-to, a herbal remedy for steroid-dependent bronchial asthma. *J Pharm Pharmacol.* 1994 Apr;46(4):305-9.

Hönscheid A, Rink L, Haase H. T-lymphocytes: a target for stimulatory and inhibitory effects of zinc ions. *Endocr Metab Immune Disord Drug Targets.* 2009 Jun;9(2):132-44.

Hooper R, Calvert J, Thompson RL, Deetlefs ME, Burney P. Urban/rural differences in diet and atopy in South Africa. *Allergy.* 2008 Apr;63(4):425-31.

Hope BE, Massey DG, Fournier-Massey G. Hawaiian materia medica for asthma. *Hawaii Med J.* 1993 Jun;52(6):160-6.

Horak E, Morass B, Ulmer H. Association between environmental tobacco smoke exposure and wheezing disorders in Austrian preschool children. *Swiss Med Wkly.* 2007 Nov 3;137(43-44):608-13.

Horrobin DF. Effects of evening primrose oil in rheumatoid arthritis. *Ann Rheum Dis.* 1989 Nov;48(11):965-6.

Hospers IC, de Vries-Vrolijk K, Brand PL. Double-blind, placebo-controlled cow's milk challenge in children with alleged cow's milk allergies, performed in a general hospital: diagnosis rejected in two-thirds of the children. *Ned Tijdschr Geneeskd.* 2006 Jun 10;150(23):1292-7.

Hosseini S, Pishnamazi S, Sadrzadeh SM, Farid F, Farid R, Watson RR. Pycnogenol((R)) in the Management of Asthma. *J Med Food.* 2001 Winter;4(4):201-209.

Hougee S, Vriesema AJ, Wijering SC, Knippels LM, Folkerts G, Nijkamp FP, Knol J, Garssen J. Oral treatment with probiotics reduces allergic symptoms in ovalbumin-sensitized mice: a bacterial strain comparative study. *Int Arch Allergy Immunol.* 2010;151(2):107-17. 2009 Sep 15.

Houle CR, Leo HL, Clark NM. A developmental, community, and psychosocial approach to food allergies in children. *Curr Allergy Asthma Rep.* 2010 Sep;10(5):381-6.

Houssen ME, Ragab A, Mesbah A, El-Samanoudy AZ, Othman G, Moustafa AF, Badria FA. Natural anti-inflammatory products and leukotriene inhibitors as complementary therapy for bronchial asthma. *Clin Biochem.* 2010 Jul;43(10-11):887-90.

Hsieh KH. Evaluation of efficacy of traditional Chinese medicines in the treatment of childhood bronchial asthma: clinical trial, immunological tests and animal study. Taiwan Asthma Study Group. *Pediatr Allergy Immunol.* 1996 Aug;7(3):130-40.

Hsu CH, Lu CM, Chang TT. Efficacy and safety of modified Mai-Men-Dong-Tang for treatment of allergic asthma. *Pediatr Allergy Immunol.* 2005;16:76-81.

Hu C, Kitts DD. Antioxidant, prooxidant, and cytotoxic activities of solvent-fractionated dandelion (Taraxacum officinale) flower extracts in vitro. *J Agric Food Chem.* 2003 Jan 1;51(1):301-10.

Hu C, Kitts DD. Dandelion (Taraxacum officinale) flower extract suppresses both reactive oxygen species and nitric oxide and prevents lipid oxidation in vitro. *Phytomedicine.* 2005 Aug;12(8):588-97.

Hu C, Kitts DD. Luteolin and luteolin-7-O-glucoside from dandelion flower suppress iNOS and COX-2 in RAW264.7 cells. *Mol Cell Biochem.* 2004 Oct;265(1-2):107-13.

Huang D, Ou B, Prior RL. The chemistry behind antioxidant capacity assays. *J Agric Food Chem.* 2005 Mar 23;53(6):1841-56.

Huang M, Wang W, Wei S. Investigation on medicinal plant resources of Glycyrrhiza uralensis in China and chemical assessment of its underground part. *Zhongguo Zhong Yao Za Zhi.* 2010 Apr;35(8):947-52.

Huang RC, Forbes DA, Davies MW. Feed thickener for newborn infants with gastro-oesophageal reflux. *Cochrane Database Syst Rev.* 2002;(3):CD003211.

Huntley A, Ernst E: Herbal medicines for asthma: a systematic review. *Thorax.* 2000, 55:925-929.

Hur YM, Rushton JP. Genetic and environmental contributions to prosocial behaviour in 2- to 9-year-old South Korean twins. *Biol Lett.* 2007 Dec 22;3(6):664-6.

Husby S. Dietary antigens: uptake and humoral immunity in man. *APMIS Suppl.* 1988;1:1-40.

Hyndman SJ, Vickers LM, Htut T, Maunder JW, Peock A, Higenbottam TW. A randomized trial of dehumidification in the control of house dust mite. *Clin Exp Allergy.* 2000 Aug;30(8):1172-80.

Ibero M, Boné J, Martín B, Martínez J. Evaluation of an extensively hydrolysed casein formula (Damira 2000) in children with allergy to cow's milk proteins. *Allergol Immunopathol (Madr).* 2010 Mar-Apr;38(2):60-8.

Inbar O, Dotan R, Dlin RA, Neuman I, Bar-Or O. Breathing dry or humid air and exercise-induced asthma during swimming. *Eur J Appl Physiol Occup Physiol.* 1980;44(1):43-50.

Indrio F, Ladisa G, Mautone A, Montagna O. Effect of a fermented formula on thymus size and stool pH in healthy term infants. *Pediatr Res.* 2007 Jul;62(1):98-100.

Indrio F, Riezzo G, Raimondi F, Bisceglia M, Filannino A, Cavallo L, Francavilla R. Lactobacillus reuteri accelerates gastric emptying and improves regurgitation in infants. *Eur J Clin Invest.* 2011 Apr;41(4):417-22.

Innis SM, Hansen JW. Plasma fatty acid responses, metabolic effects, and safety of microalgal and fungal oils rich in arachidonic and docosahexaenoic acids in adults. *Am J Clin Nutr.* 1996 Aug;64(2):159-67.

Ionescu JG. New insights in the pathogenesis of atopic disease. *J Med Life.* 2009 Apr-Jun;2(2):146-54.

REFERENCES

Ip S, Chung M, Moorthy D, Yu WW, Lee J, Chan JA, Bonis PA, Lau J. Comparative Effectiveness of Management Strategies for Gastroesophageal Reflux Disease. Rockville (MD): *Agency for Healthcare Research and Quality*, 2011 Sep.

Iribarren C, Tolstykh IV, Miller MK, Eisner MD. Asthma and the prospective risk of anaphylactic shock and other allergy diagnoses in a large integrated health care delivery system. *Ann Allergy Asthma Immunol.* 2010 May;104(5):371-7.

ISAAC. The International Study of Asthma and Allergies in Childhood (ISAAC) Steering Committee. Worldwide variation in prevalence of symptoms of asthma, allergic rhinoconjunctivitis, and atopic eczema: ISAAC. *Lancet.* 1998;351:1225-1232.

Ishida Y, Nakamura F, Kanzato H, Sawada D, Hirata H, Nishimura A, Kajimoto O, Fujiwara S. Clinical effects of *Lactobacillus acidophilus* strain L-92 on perennial allergic rhinitis: a double-blind, placebo-controlled study. *J Dairy Sci.* 2005 Feb;88(2):527-33.

Ishtiaq M, Hanif W, Khan MA, Ashraf M, Butt AM. An ethnomedicinal survey and documentation of important medicinal folklore food phytonims of flora of Samahni valley, (Azad Kashmir) Pakistan. *Pak J Biol Sci.* 2007 Jul 1;10(13):2241-56.

Ivory K, Chambers SJ, Pin C, Prieto E, Arqués JL, Nicoletti C. Oral delivery of *Lactobacillus casei* Shirota modifies allergen-induced immune responses in allergic rhinitis. *Clin Exp Allergy.* 2008 Aug;38(8):1282-9.

Izbicki G, Chavko R, Banauch GI, Weiden MD, Berger KI, Aldrich TK, Hall C, Kelly KJ, Prezant DJ. World trade center "sarcoid-like" granulomatous pulmonary disease in New York City fire department rescue workers. *Chest.* 2007 May;131(5):1414-23.

Izquierdo JL, Martín A, de Lucas P, Rodríguez-González-Moro JM, Almonacid C, Paravisini A. Misdiagnosis of patients receiving inhaled therapies in primary care. *Int J Chron Obstruct Pulmon Dis.* 2010 Aug 9;5:241-9.

Izumi K, Aihara M, Ikezawa Z. Effects of non steroidal antiinflammatory drugs (NSAIDs) on immediate-type food allergy analysis of Japanese cases from 1998 to 2009. *Arerugi.* 2009 Dec;58(12):1629-39.

Jaber R. Respiratory and allergic diseases: from upper respiratory tract infections to asthma. *Prim Care.* 2002 Jun;29(2):231-61.

Jackson DJ, Lemanske RF Jr. The role of respiratory virus infections in childhood asthma inception. *Immunol Allergy Clin North Am.* 2010 Nov;30(4):513-22, vi.

Jacobs DE, Wilson J, Dixon SL, Smith J, Evens A. The relationship of housing and population health: a 30-year retrospective analysis. *Environ Health Perspect.* 2009 Apr;117(4):597-604. 2008 Dec 16.

Jadcherla SR, Chan CY, Moore R, Malkar M, Timan CJ, Valentine CJ. Impact of Feeding Strategies on the Frequency and Clearance of Acid and Nonacid Gastroesophageal Reflux Events in Dysphagic Neonates. JPEN J Parenter Enteral Nutr. 2011 Oct 30.

Jadcherla SR. Gastroesophageal reflux in the neonate. *Clin Perinatol.* 2002 Mar;29(1):135-58.

Jagetia GC, Aggarwal BB. "Spicing up" of the immune system by curcumin. *J Clin Immunol.* 2007 Jan;27(1):19-35.

Jagetia GC, Nayak V, Vidyasagar MS. Evaluation of the antineoplastic activity of guduchi (Tinospora cordifolia) in cultured HeLa cells. *Cancer Lett.* 1998 May 15;127(1-2):71-82.

Jagetia GC, Rao SK. Evaluation of Cytotoxic Effects of Dichloromethane Extract of Guduchi (Tinospora cordifolia Miers ex Hook F & THOMS) on Cultured HeLa Cells. *Evid Based Complement Alternat Med.* 2006 Jun;3(2):267-72.

Jahnova E, Horvathova M, Gazdik F, Weissova S. Effects of selenium supplementation on expression of adhesion molecules in corticoid-dependent asthmatics. *Bratisl Lek Listy.* 2002;103(1):12-6.

Jaiswal M, Prajapati PK, Patgiri BJ Ravishankar B. A Comparative Pharmaco - Clinical Study on Anti-Asthmatic Effect of Shirisharishta Prepared by Bark, Sapwood and Heartwood of Albizia Lebbeck. *J Res Ayurv.* 2006;27(3):67-74.

Jancin B. Gastroesophageal disease linked to long antacid use. *Fam Pract News.* 1996;26(13):1-2.

Jankowski J, Hopwood D, Pringle R, Wormsley KG. Increased expression of epidermal growth factor receptors in Barrett's esophagus associated with alkaline reflux: a putative model for carcinogenesis. *Am J Gastroenterol.* 1993 Mar;88(3):402-8.

Janson C, Anto J, Burney P, Chinn S, de Marco R, Heinrich J, Jarvis D, Kuenzli N, Leynaert B, Luczynska C, Neukirch F, Svanes C, Sunyer J, Wjst M; European Community Respiratory Health Survey II. The European Community Respiratory Health Survey: what are the main results so far? European Community Respiratory Health Survey II. *Eur Respir J.* 2001 Sep;18(3):598-611.

Jarocka-Cyrta E, Baniukiewicz A, Wasilewska J, Pawlak J, Kaczmarski M. Focal villous atrophy of the duodenum in children who have outgrown cow's milk allergy. Chromoendoscopy and magnification endoscopy evaluation. *Med Wieku Rozwoj.* 2007 Apr-Jun;11(2 Pt 1):123-7.

Jayaprakasam B, Doddaga S, Wang R, Holmes D, Goldfarb J, Li XM. Licorice flavonoids inhibit eotaxin-1 secretion by human fetal lung fibroblasts in vitro. *J Agric Food Chem.* 2009 Feb 11;57(3):820-5.

Jennings S, Prescott SL. Early dietary exposures and feeding practices: role in pathogenesis and prevention of allergic disease? *Postgrad Med J.* 2010 Feb;86(1012):94-9.

Jensen B. *Foods that Heal.* Garden City Park, NY: Avery Publ, 1988, 1993.

Jensen B. *Nature Has a Remedy.* Los Angeles: Keats, 2001.

Jensen RT. Consequences of long-term proton pump blockade: insights from studies of patients with gastrinomas. *Basic Clin Pharmacol Toxicol.* 2006 Jan;98(1):4-19.

Jeon HJ, Kang HJ, Jung HJ, Kang YS, Lim CJ, Kim YM, Park EH. Anti-inflammatory activity of Taraxacum officinale. J *Ethnopharmacol.* 2008 Jan 4;115(1):82-8.

Jianu CS, Lange OJ, Viset T, Qvigstad G, Martinsen TC, Fougner R, Kleveland PM, Fossmark R, Hauso O, Waldum HL. Gastric neuroendocrine carcinoma after long-term use of proton pump inhibitor. *Scand J Gastroenterol.* 2012 Jan;47(1):64-7.

285

Johansson G, Holmén A, Persson L, Högstedt B, Wassén C, Ottova L, Gustafsson JA. Long-term effects of a change from a mixed diet to a lacto-vegetarian diet on human urinary and faecal mutagenic activity. *Mutagenesis.* 1998 Mar;13(2):167-71.

Johansson G, Holmén A, Persson L, Högstedt B, Wassén C, Ottova L, Gustafsson JA. Dietary influence on some proposed risk factors for colon cancer: fecal and urinary mutagenic activity and the activity of some intestinal bacterial enzymes. *Cancer Detect Prev.* 1997;21(3):258-66.

Johansson G, Holmén A, Persson L, Högstedt R, Wassén C, Ottova L, Gustafsson JA. The effect of a shift from a mixed diet to a lacto-vegetarian diet on human urinary and fecal mutagenic activity. *Carcinogenesis.* 1992 Feb;13(2):153-7.

Johansson G, Ravald N. Comparison of some salivary variables between vegetarians and omnivores. *Eur J Oral Sci.* 1995 Apr;103(2 (Pt 1)):95-8.

Johari H. *Ayurvedic Massage: Traditional Indian Techniques for Balancing Body and Mind.* Rochester, VT: Healing Arts, 1996.

John M. Eisenberg Center for Clinical Decisions and Communications Science. Managing Chronic Gastroesophageal Reflux Disease. 2011 Sep 23. Comparative Effectiveness Review Summary Guides for Clinicians. Rockville (MD): *Agency for Healthcare Research and Quality,* 2007.

Johnson LM. Gitksan medicinal plants—cultural choice and efficacy. *J Ethnobiol Ethnomed.* 2006 Jun 21;2:29.

Johnson T, Gerson L, Hershcovici T, Stave C, Fass R. Systematic review: the effects of carbonated beverages on gastro-oesophageal reflux disease. *Aliment Pharmacol Ther.* 2010 Mar;31(6):607-14.

Jones MA, Silman AJ, Whiting S, *et al.* Occurrence of rheumatoid arthritis is not increased in the first degree relatives of a population based inception cohort of inflammatory polyarthritis. *Ann Rheum Dis.* 1996;55(2): 89-93.

Jones NL, Wine E. Pediatric gastrointestinal diseases: are drugs the answer? *Curr Opin Pharmacol.* 2005 Dec;5(6):604-9.

José RJ, Roberts J, Bakerly ND. The effectiveness of a social marketing model on case-finding for COPD in a deprived inner city population. *Prim Care Respir J.* 2010 Jun;19(2):104-8.

Joseph SP, Borrell LN, Shapiro A. Self-reported lifetime asthma and nativity status in U.S. children and adolescents: results from the National Health and Nutrition Examination Survey 1999-2004. *J Health Care Poor Underserved.* 2010 May;21(2 Suppl):125-39.

Jóźwiak S, Kossoff EH, Kotulska-Jóźwiak K. Dietary treatment of epilepsy: rebirth of an ancient treatment. *Neurol Neurochir Pol.* 2011 Jul-Aug;45(4):370-8.

Juergens UR, Dethlefsen U, Steinkamp G, Gillissen A, Repges R, Vetter H. Anti-inflammatory activity of 1.8-cineol (eucalyptol) in bronchial asthma: a double-blind placebo-controlled trial. *Respir Med.* 2003 Mar;97(3):250-6.

Julkunen-Tiitto R. A chemotaxonomic survey of phenolics in leaves of northern Salicaceae species. Phytochemistry. 1986;25(3):663-667.

Jung HA, Yokozawa T, Kim BW, Jung JH, Choi JS. Selective inhibition of prenylated flavonoids from Sophora flavescens against BACE1 and cholinesterases. *Am J Chin Med.* 2010;38(2):415-29.

Jurenka JS. Anti-inflammatory properties of curcumin, a major constituent of Curcuma longa: a review of preclinical and clinical research. *Altern Med Rev.* 2009 Feb;14(2):141-153.

Juvonen R, Bloigu A, Peitso A, Silvennoinen-Kassinen S, Saikku P, Leinonen M, Hassi J, Harju T. Training improves physical fitness and decreases CRP also in asthmatic conscripts. *J Asthma.* 2008 Apr;45(3):237-42.

Kähkönen MP, Hopia AI, Vuorela HJ, Rauha JP, Pihlaja K, Kujala TS, Heinonen M. Antioxidant activity of plant extracts containing phenolic compounds. *J Agric Food Chem.* 1999 Oct;47(10):3954-62.

Kaila M, Vanto T, Valovirta E, Koivikko A, Juntunen-Backman K. Diagnosis of food allergy in Finland: survey of pediatric practices. *Pediatr Allergy Immunol.* 2000 Nov;11(4):246-9.

Kalach N, Benhamou PH, Campeotto F, Dupont Ch. Anemia impairs small intestinal absorption measured by intestinal permeability in children. *Eur Ann Allergy Clin Immunol.* 2007 Jan;39(1):20-2.

Kaliner M, Shelhamer JH, Borson B, Nadel J, Patow C, Marom Z. Human respiratory mucus. *Am Rev Respir Dis.* 1986 Sep;134(3):612-21.

Kalliomäki M, Salminen S, Arvilommi H, Kero P, Koskinen P, Isolauri E. Probiotics in primary prevention of atopic disease: a randomised placebo-controlled trial. *Lancet.* 2001 Apr 7;357(9262):1076-9.

Kamdar T, Bryce PJ. Immunotherapy in food allergy. Immunotherapy. 2010 May;2(3):329-38.

Kandulski A, Malfertheiner P. Gastroesophageal reflux disease from reflux episodes to mucosal inflammation. *Nat Rev Gastroenterol Hepatol.* 2011 Nov 22;9(1):15-22. doi: 10.1038/nrgastro.2011.210.

Kang SK, Kim JK, Ahn SH, Oh JE, Kim JH, Lim DH, Son BK. Relationship between silent gastroesophageal reflux and food sensitization in infants and young children with recurrent wheeze. *J Korean Med Sci.* 2010 Mar;25(3):425-8.

Kanny G, Grignon G, Dauca M, Guedenet JC, Moneret-Vautrin DA. Ultrastructural changes in the duodenal mucosa induced by ingested histamine in patients with chronic urticaria. *Allergy.* 1996 Dec;51(12):935-9.

Kapil A, Sharma S. Immunopotentiating compounds from Tinospora cordifolia. *J Ethnopharmacol.* 1997 Oct;58(2):89-95.

Kaplan C. Indoor air pollution from unprocessed solid fuels in developing countries. *Rev Environ Health.* 2010 Jul-Sep;25(3):221-42.

Kaplan M, Mutlu EA, Benson M, Fields JZ, Banan A, Keshavarzian A. Use of herbal preparations in the treatment of oxidant-mediated inflammatory disorders. *Complement Ther Med.* 2007 Sep;15(3):207-16. 2006 Aug 21.

Kaplan R. The nature of the view from home: psychological benefits. *Environ Behav.* 2001;33(4):507-42.

Kaplan R. Wilderness perception and psychological benefits: an analysis of a continuing program. *Leisure Sci.* 1984;6(3):271-90.

Karkoulias K, Patouchas D, Alahiotis S, Tsiamita M, Vrodakis K, Spiropoulos K. Specific sensitization in wheat flour and contributing factors in traditional bakers. *Eur Rev Med Pharmacol Sci.* 2007 May-Jun;11(3):141-8.

REFERENCES

Karpińska J, Mikoluć B, Motkowski R, Piotrowska-Jastrzebska J. HPLC method for simultaneous determination of retinol, alpha-tocopherol and coenzyme Q10 in human plasma. *J Pharm Biomed Anal.* 2006 Sep 18;42(2):232-6.

Kashiwada Y, Takanaka K, Tsukada H, Miwa Y, Taga T, Tanaka S, Ikeshiro Y. Sesquiterpene glucosides from anti-leukotriene B4 release fraction of Taraxacum officinale. *J Asian Nat Prod Res.* 2001;3(3):191-7.

Kastelein F, Spaander MC, Biermann K, Vucelic B, Kuipers EJ, Bruno MJ. Role of acid suppression in the development and progression of dysplasia in patients with Barrett's esophagus. *Dig Dis.* 2011;29(5):499-506.

Katial RK, Strand M, Prasertsuntarasai T, Leung R, Zheng W, Alam R. The effect of aspirin desensitization on novel biomarkers in aspirin-exacerbated respiratory diseases. *J Allergy Clin Immunol.* 2010 Oct;126(4):738-44. 2010 Aug 21.

Kattan JD, Srivastava KD, Sampson HA, Li XM. Pharmacologic and Immunologic Effects of Individual Herbs of Food Allergy Herbal Formula 2 in a Murine Model of Peanut Allergy. *J Allergy Clin Immunol.* 2006;117(2):S34.

Kattan JD, Srivastava KD, Zou ZM, Goldfarb J, Sampson HA, Li XM. Pharmacological and immunological effects of individual herbs in the Food Allergy Herbal Formula-2 (FAHF-2) on peanut allergy. *Phytother Res.* 2008 May;22(5):651-9.

Katz DL, Cushman D, Reynolds J, Njike V, Treu JA, Walker J, Smith E, Katz C. Putting physical activity where it fits in the school day: preliminary results of the ABC (Activity Bursts in the Classroom) for fitness program. *Prev Chronic Dis.* 2010 Jul;7(4):A82. 2010 Jun 15.

Katz PO, Castell DO, Chen Y, Andersson T, Sostek MB. Intragastric acid suppression and pharmacokinetics of twice-daily esomeprazole: a randomized, three-way crossover study. *Aliment Pharmacol Ther.* 2004 Aug 15;20(4):399-406.

Katz Y, Rajuan N, Goldberg MR, Eisenberg E, Heyman E, Cohen A, Leshno M. Early exposure to cow's milk protein is protective against IgE-mediated cow's milk protein allergy. *J Allergy Clin Immunol.* 2010 Jul;126(1):77-82.e1.

Kawahara H, Kubota A, Hasegawa T, Okuyama H, Ueno T, Ida S, Fukuzawa M. Effects of rikkunshito on the clinical symptoms and esophageal acid exposure in children with symptomatic gastroesophageal reflux. *Pediatr Surg Int.* 2007 Oct;23(10):1001-5.

Kazaks AG, Uriu-Adams JY, Albertson TE, Shenoy SF, Stern JS. Effect of oral magnesium supplementation on measures of airway resistance and subjective assessment of asthma control and quality of life in men and women with mild to moderate asthma: a randomized placebo controlled trial. *J Asthma.* 2010 Feb;47(1):83-92.

Kazansky DB. MHC restriction and allogeneic immune responses. *J Immunotoxicol.* 2008 Oct;5(4):369-84.

Kazlowska K, Hsu T, Hou CC, Yang WC, Tsai GJ. Anti-inflammatory properties of phenolic compounds and crude extract from Porphyra dentata. *J Ethnopharmacol.* 2010 Mar 2;128(1):123-30.

Keita AV, Söderholm JD. The intestinal barrier and its regulation by neuroimmune factors. *Neurogastroenterol Motil.* 2010 Jul;22(7):718-33.

Kekkonen RA, Lummela N, Karjalainen H, Latvala S, Tynkkynen S, Jarvenpaa S, Kautiainen H, Julkunen I, Vapaatalo H, Korpela R. Probiotic intervention has strain-specific anti-inflammatory effects in healthy adults. *World J Gastroenterol.* 2008 Apr 7;14(13):2029-36.

Kekkonen RA, Sysi-Aho M, Seppanen-Laakso T, Julkunen I, Vapaatalo H, Oresic M, Korpela R. Effect of probiotic *Lactobacillus rhamnosus* GG intervention on global serum lipidomic profiles in healthy adults. *World J Gastroenterol.* 2008 May 28;14(20):3188-94.

Kekkonen RA, Vasankari TJ, Vuorimaa T, Haahtela T, Julkunen I, Korpela R. The effect of probiotics on respiratory infections and gastrointestinal symptoms during training in marathon runners. *Int J Sport Nutr Exerc Metab.* 2007 Aug;17(4):352-63.

Kelder P. *Ancient Secret of the Fountain of Youth.* New York: Doubleday, 1998.

Kelly HW, Van Natta ML, Covar RA, Tonascia J, Green RP, Strunk RC; CAMP Research Group. Effect of long-term corticosteroid use on bone mineral density in children: a prospective longitudinal assessment in the childhood Asthma Management Program (CAMP) study. *Pediatrics.* 2008 Jul;122(1):e53-61.

Kelly-Pieper K, Patil SP, Busse P, Yang N, Sampson H, Li XM, Wisnivesky JP, Kattan M. Safety and tolerability of an antiasthma herbal Formula (ASHMI) in adult subjects with asthma: a randomized, double-blinded, placebo-controlled, dose-escalation phase I study. *J Altern Complement Med.* 2009 Jul;15(7):735-43.

Kenia P, Houghton T, Beardsmore C. Does inhaling menthol affect nasal patency or cough? *Pediatr Pulmonol.* 2008 Jun;43(6):532-7.

Keogh JB, Grieger JA, Noakes M, Clifton PM. Flow-Mediated Dilatation Is Impaired by a High-Saturated Fat Diet but Not by a High-Carbohydrate Diet. *Arterioscler Thromb Vasc Biol.* 2005 Mar 17

Kerckhoffs DA, Brouns F, Hornstra G, Mensink RP. Effects on the human serum lipoprotein profile of beta-glucan, soy protein and isoflavones, plant sterols and stanols, garlic and tocotrienols. *J Nutr.* 2002 Sep;132(9):2494-505.

Kerkhof M, Postma DS, Brunekreef B, Reijmerink NE, Wijga AH, de Jongste JC, Gehring U, Koppelman GH. Toll-like receptor 2 and 4 genes influence susceptibility to adverse effects of traffic-related air pollution on childhood asthma. *Thorax.* 2010 Aug;65(8):690-7.

Key T, Appleby P, Davey G, Allen N, Spencer E, Travis R. Mortality in British vegetarians: review and preliminary results from EPIC-Oxford. *Amer. Jour. Clin. Nutr. Suppl.* 2003;78(3): 533S-538S.

Khan S. Management of pediatric eosinophilic esophagitis: an update. *Paediatr Drugs.* 2012 Feb 1;14(1):23-33.

Kharagezov AD, Glushchenkov VA. Treatment of alkaline reflux gastritis and esophagitis after proximal gastrectomy by the Smith-Payne method. *Klin Khir.* 1989;(8):77-8.

Khoshoo V, Zembo M, King A, Dhar M, Reifen R, Pencharz P. Incidence of gastroesophageal reflux with whey- and casein-based formulas in infants and in children with severe neurological impairment. *J Pediatr Gastroenterol Nutr.* 1996 Jan;22(1):48-55.

Khresheh R. Strategies used by Jordanian women to alleviate heartburn during pregnancy. *Midwifery.* 2011 Oct;27(5):603-6.

Kiefte-de Jong JC, Escher JC, Arends LR, Jaddoe VW, Hofman A, Raat H, Moll HA. Infant nutritional factors and functional constipation in childhood: the Generation R study. *Am J Gastroenterol.* 2010 Apr;105(4):940-5.

Kim HM, Shin HY, Lim KH, Ryu ST, Shin TY, Chae HJ, Kim HR, Lyu YS, An NH, Lim KS. Taraxacum officinale inhibits tumor necrosis factor-alpha production from rat astrocytes. *Immunopharmacol Immunotoxicol.* 2000 Aug;22(3):519-30.

Kim JH, An S, Kim JE, Choi GS, Ye YM, Park HS. Beef-induced anaphylaxis confirmed by the basophil activation test. *Allergy Asthma Immunol Res.* 2010 Jul;2(3):206-8.

Kim JH, Ellwood PE, Asher MI. Diet and asthma: looking back, moving forward. *Respir Res.* 2009 Jun 12;10:49.

Kim JH, Lee SY, Kim HB, Jin HS, Yu JH, Kim BJ, Kim BS, Kang MJ, Jang SO, Hong SJ. TBXA2R gene polymorphism and responsiveness to leukotriene receptor antagonist in children with asthma. *Clin Exp Allergy.* 2008 Jan;38(1):51-9.

Kim JY, Kim DY, Lee YS, Lee BK, Lee KH, Ro JY. DA-9601, Artemisia asiatica herbal extract, ameliorates airway inflammation of allergic asthma in mice. *Mol Cells.* 2006;22:104-12.

Kim NI, Jo Y, Ahn SB, Son BK, Kim SH, Park YS, Kim SH, Ju JE. A case of eosinophilic esophagitis with food hypersensitivity. *J Neurogastroenterol Motil.* 2010 Jul;16(3):315-8.

Kim SJ, Jung JY, Kim HW, Park T. Anti-obesity effects of Juniperus chinensis extract are associated with increased AMP-activated protein kinase expression and phosphorylation in the visceral adipose tissue of rats. *Biol Pharm Bull.* 2008 Jul;31(7):1415-21.

Kim TE, Park SW, Noh G, Lee S. Comparison of skin prick test results between crude allergen extracts from foods and commercial allergen extracts in atopic dermatitis by double-blind placebo-controlled food challenge for milk, egg, and soybean. *Yonsei Med J.* 2002 Oct;43(5):613-20.

Kim YH, Kim KS, Han CS, Yang HC, Park SH, Ko KI, Lee SH, Kim KH, Lee NH, Kim JM, Son K. Inhibitory effects of natural plants of Jeju Island on elastase and MMP-1 expression. *Int J Cosmet Sci.* 2007 Dec;29(6):487-8.

Kimata H. Effect of viewing a humorous vs. nonhumorous film on bronchial responsiveness in patients with bronchial asthma. *Physiol Behav.* 2004 Jun;81(4):681-4.

Kimata M, Inagaki N, Nagai H. Effects of luteolin and other flavonoids on IgE-mediated allergic reactions. *Planta Med.* 2000 Feb;66(1):25-9.

Kimata M, Shichijo M, Miura T, Serizawa I, Inagaki N, Nagai H. Effects of luteolin, quercetin and baicalein on immunoglobulin E-mediated mediator release from human cultured mast cells. *Clin Exp Allergy.* 2000 Apr;30(4):501-8.

Kimmatkar N, Thawani V, Hingorani L, Khiyani R. Efficacy and tolerability of Boswellia serrata extract in treatment of osteoarthritis of knee—a randomized double blind placebo controlled trial. *Phytomedicine.* 2003 Jan;10(1):3-7.

Kinaciyan T, Jahn-Schmid B, Radakovics A, Zwölfer B, Schreiber C, Francis JN, Ebner C, Bohle B. Successful sublingual immunotherapy with birch pollen has limited effects on concomitant food allergy to apple and the immune response to the Bet v 1 homolog Mal d 1. *J Allergy Clin Immunol.* 2007 Apr;119(4):937-43.

Kinross JM, von Roon AC, Holmes E, Darzi A, Nicholson JK. The human gut microbiome: implications for future health care. *Curr Gastroenterol Rep.* 2008 Aug;10(4):396-403.

Kippelen P, Larsson J, Anderson SD, Brannan JD, Dahlén B, Dahlén SE. Effect of sodium cromoglycate on mast cell mediators during hyperpnea in athletes. *Med Sci Sports Exerc.* 2010 Oct;42(10):1853-60.

Kirby M, Noel RJ. Nutrition and gastrointestinal tract assessment and management of children with dysphagia. *Semin Speech Lang.* 2007 Aug;28(3):180-9.

Kirjavainen PV, Salminen SJ, Isolauri E. Probiotic bacteria in the management of atopic disease: underscoring the importance of viability. *J Pediatr Gastroenterol Nutr.* 2003 Feb;36(2):223-7.

Kisiel W, Barszcz B. Further sesquiterpenoids and phenolics from Taraxacum officinale. *Fitoterapia.* 2000 Jun;71(3):269-73.

Kisiel W, Michalska K. Sesquiterpenoids and phenolics from Taraxacum hondoense. *Fitoterapia.* 2005 Sep;76(6):520-4.

Kjellin A, Ramel S, Rössner S, Thor K. Gastroesophageal reflux in obese patients is not reduced by weight reduction. *Scand J Gastroenterol.* 1996 Nov;31(11):1047-51.

Klein R, Landau MG. *Healing: The Body Betrayed.* Minneapolis: DCI:Chronimed, 1992.

Klein-Galczinsky C. Pharmacological and clinical effectiveness of a fixed phytogenic combination trembling poplar (Populus tremula), true goldenrod (Solidago virgaurea) and ash (Fraxinus excelsior) in mild to moderate rheumatic complaints. *Wien Med Wochenschr.* 1999;149(8-10):248-53.

Klemola T, Vanto T, Juntunen-Backman K, Kalimo K, Korpela R, Varjonen E. Allergy to soy formula and to extensively hydrolyzed whey formula in infants with cow's milk allergy: a prospective, randomized study with a follow-up to the age of 2 years. *J Pediatr.* 2002 Feb;140(2):219-24.

Kloss J. *Back to Eden.* Twin Oaks, WI: Lotus Press, 1939-1999.

Knutson TW, Bengtsson U, Dannaeus A, Ahlstedt S, Knutson L. Effects of luminal antigen on intestinal albumin and hyaluronan permeability and ion transport in atopic patients. *J Allergy Clin Immunol.* 1996 Jun;97(6):1225-32.

Ko J, Busse PJ, Shek L, Noone SA, Sampson HA, Li XM. Effect of Chinese Herbal Formulas on T Cell Responses in Patients with Peanut Allergy or Asthma. *J Allergy Clin Immunol.* 2005;115:S34.

Ko J, Lee JI, Munoz-Furlong A, Li XM, Sicherer SH. Use of complementary and alternative medicine by food-allergic patients. *Ann Allergy Asthma Immunol.* 2006;97:365-9.

Kobayashi I, Hamasaki Y, Sato R, Zaitu M, Muro E, Yamamoto S, Ichimaru T, Miyazaki S. Saiboku-To, a herbal extract mixture, selectively inhibits 5-lipoxygenase activity in leukotriene synthesis in rat basophilic leukemia-1 cells. *J Ethnopharmacol.* 1995 Aug 11;48(1):33-41.

Kokwaro JO. *Medicinal Plants of East Africa.* Nairobi: Univ of Neirobi Press, 2009.

REFERENCES

Kolarski V, Petrova-Shopova K, Vasileva E, Petrova D, Nikolov S. Erosive gastritis and gastroduodenitis—clinical, diagnostic and therapeutic studies. *Vutr Boles.* 1987;26(3):56-9.

Kong LF, Guo LH, Zheng XY. Effect of yiqi bushen huoxue herbs in treating children asthma and on levels of nitric oxide, endothelin-1 and serum endothelial cells. *Zhongguo Zhong Xi Yi Jie He Za Zhi.* 2001 Sep;21(9):667-9.

Koo HN, Hong SH, Song BK, Kim CH, Yoo YH, Kim HM. Taraxacum officinale induces cytotoxicity through TNF-alpha and IL-1alpha secretion in Hep G2 cells. *Life Sci.* 2004 Jan 16;74(9):1149-57.

Kootstra HS, Vlieg-Boerstra BJ, Dubois AE. Assessment of the reduced allergenic properties of the Santana apple. *Ann Allergy Asthma Immunol.* 2007 Dec;99(6):522-5.

Kotzampassi K, Giamarellos-Bourboulis EJ, Voudouris A, Kazamias P, Eleftheriadis E. Benefits of a synbiotic formula (Synbiotic 2000Forte) in critically Ill trauma patients: early results of a randomized controlled trial. *World J Surg.* 2006 Oct;30(10):1848-55.

Kovács T, Mette H, Per B, Kun L, Schmelczer M, Barta J, Jean-Claude D, Nagy J. Relationship between intestinal permeability and antibodies against food antigens in IgA nephropathy. *Orv Hetil.* 1996 Jan 14;137(2):65-9.

Kowalchik C, Hylton W (eds). *Rodale's Illustrated Encyclopedia of Herbs.* Emmaus, PA: 1987.

Kowalczyk E, Krzesiński P, Kura N, Niedworok J, Kowalski J, Blaszczyk J. Pharmacological effects of flavonoids from Scutellaria baicalensis. *Przegl Lek.* 2006;63(2):95-6.

Kozlowski LT, Mehta NY, Sweeney CT, Schwartz SS, Vogler GP, Jarvis MJ, West RJ. Filter ventilation and nicotine content of tobacco in cigarettes from Canada, the United Kingdom, and the United States. *Tob Control.* 1998 Winter;7(4):369-75.

Kreig M. *Black Market Medicine.* New York: Bantam, 1968.

Kremmyda LS, Vlachava M, Noakes PS, Diaper ND, Miles EA, Calder PC. Atopy Risk in Infants and Children in Relation to Early Exposure to Fish, Oily Fish, or Long-Chain Omega-3 Fatty Acids: A Systematic Review. *Clin Rev Allergy Immunol.* 2009 Dec 9.

Krogulska A, Dynowski J, Wasowska-Królikowska K. Bronchial reactivity in schoolchildren allergic to food. *Ann Allergy Asthma Immunol.* 2010 Jul;105(1):31-8.

Krogulska A, Wasowska-Królikowska K, Dynowski J. Evaluation of bronchial hyperreactivity in children with asthma undergoing food challenges. *Pol Merkur Lekarski.* 2007 Jul;23(133):30-5.

Krogulska A, Wasowska-Królikowska K, Polakowska E, Chrul S. Cytokine profile in children with asthma undergoing food challenges. *J Investig Allergol Clin Immunol.* 2009;19(1):43-8.

Krogulska A, Wasowska-Królikowska K, Polakowska E, Chrul S. Evaluation of receptor expression on immune system cells in the peripheral blood of asthmatic children undergoing food challenges. Int Arch Allergy Immunol. 2009;150(4):377-88. 2009 Jul 1.

Krogulska A, Wasowska-Królikowska K, Trzeźwińska B. Food challenges in children with asthma. *Pol Merkur Lekarski.* 2007 Jul;23(133):22-9.

Kroidl RF, Schwichtenberg U, Frank E. Bronchial asthma due to storage mite allergy. Pneumologie. 2007 Aug;61(8):525-30.

Krueger AP, Reed EJ. Biological impact of small air ions. *Science.* 1976 Sep 24;193(4259):1209-13.

Krüger P, Kanzer J, Hummel J, Fricker G, Schubert-Zsilavecz M, Abdel-Tawab M. Permeation of Boswellia extract in the Caco-2 model and possible interactions of its constituents KBA and AKBA with OATP1B3 and MRP2. *Eur J Pharm Sci.* 2009 Feb 15;36(2-3):275-84.

Kuitunen M, Kukkonen K, Juntunen-Backman K, Korpela R, Poussa T, Tuure T, Haahtela T, Savilahti E. Probiotics prevent IgE-associated allergy until age 5 years in Cesarean-delivered children but not in the total cohort. *J Allergy Clin Immunol.* 2009 Feb;123(2):335-41.

Kuitunen M, Savilahti E, Sarnesto A. Human alpha-lactalbumin and bovine beta-lactoglobulin absorption in infants. *Allergy.* 1994 May;49(5):354-60.

Kuitunen M, Savilahti E. Mucosal IgA, mucosal cow's milk antibodies, serum cow's milk antibodies and gastrointestinal permeability in infants. *Pediatr Allergy Immunol.* 1995 Feb;6(1):30-5.

Kukkonen K, Kuitunen M, Haahtela T, Korpela R, Poussa T, Savilahti E. High intestinal IgA associates with reduced risk of IgE-associated allergic diseases. *Pediatr Allergy Immunol.* 2010 Feb;21(1 Pt 1):67-73.

Kukkonen K, Savilahti E, Haahtela T, Juntunen-Backman K, Korpela R, Poussa T, Tuure T, Kuitunen M. Probiotics and prebiotic galacto-oligosaccharides in the prevention of allergic diseases: a randomized, double-blind, placebo-controlled trial. *J Allergy Clin Immunol.* 2007 Jan;119(1):192-8.

Kulka M. The potential of natural products as effective treatments for allergic inflammation: implications for allergic rhinitis. *Curr Top Med Chem.* 2009;9(17):1611-24.

Kull I, Bergström A, Lilja G, Pershagen G, Wickman M. Fish consumption during the first year of life and development of allergic diseases during childhood. *Allergy.* 2006 Aug;61(8):1009-15.

Kull I, Melen E, Alm J, Hallberg J, Svartengren M, van Hage M, Pershagen G, Wickman M, Bergström A. Breast-feeding in relation to asthma, lung function, and sensitization in young schoolchildren. *J Allergy Clin Immunol.* 2010 May;125(5):1013-9.

Kumar A, Panghal S, Mallapur SS, Kumar M, Ram V, Singh BK. Antiinflammatory Activity of Piper longum Fruit Oil. *Indian J Pharm Sci.* 2009 Jul;71(4):454-6.

Kumar A, Saluja AK, Shah UD, Mayavanshi AV. Pharmacological potential of Albizzia lebbeck: A Review. *Pharmacog.* 2007 Jan-May; 1(1) 171-174.

Kumar R, Singh BP, Srivastava P, Sridhara S, Arora N, Gaur SN. Relevance of serum IgE estimation in allergic bronchial asthma with special reference to food allergy. *Asian Pac J Allergy Immunol.* 2006 Dec;24(4):191-9.

Kummeling I, Mills EN, Clausen M, Dubakiene R, Pérez CF, Fernández-Rivas M, Knulst AC, Kowalski ML, Lidholm J, Le TM, Metzler C, Mustakov T, Popov T, Potts J, van Ree R, Sakellariou A, Töndury B, Tzannis K, Burney P. The EuroPrevall surveys on the prevalence of food allergies in children and adults: background and study methodology. *Allergy.* 2009 Oct;64(10):1493-7.

Kung HC, Hoyert DL, Xu J, Murphy SL. Deaths: Final Data for 2005. *National Vital Statistics Reports.* 2008;56(10). http://www.cdc.gov/nchs/data/ nvsr/nvsr56/nvsr56_10.pdf. Accessed: 2008 Jun.

Kunisawa J, Kiyono H. Aberrant interaction of the gut immune system with environmental factors in the development of food allergies. *Curr Allergy Asthma Rep.* 2010 May;10(3):215-21.

Kurth T, Barr RG, Gaziano JM, Buring JE. Randomised aspirin assignment and risk of adult-onset asthma in the Women's Health Study. *Thorax.* 2008 Jun;63(6):514-8. 2008 Mar 13.

Kusunoki T, Morimoto T, Nishikomori R, Yasumi T, Heike T, Mukaida K, Fujii T, Nakahata T. Breastfeeding and the prevalence of allergic diseases in schoolchildren: Does reverse causation matter? *Pediatr Allergy Immunol.* 2010 Feb;21(1 Pt 1):60-6.

Kuvaeva IB. Permeability of the gastrointestinal tract for macromolecules in health and disease. *Hum Physiol.* 1979 Mar-Apr;4(2):272-83.

Kuz'mina IaS, Vavilova NN. Kinesitherapy of patients with bronchial asthma and excessive body weight at the early stage of rehabilitation treatment. *Vopr Kurortol Fizioter Lech Fiz Kult.* 2009 Sep-Oct;(5):17-20.

Kuznetsova TA, Shevchenko NM, Besednova NN. Biological activity of fucoidans from brown algae and the prospects of their use in medicine]. *Antibiot Khimioter.* 2004;49(5):24-30.

Kvamme JM, Wilsgaard T, Florholmen J, Jacobsen BK. Body mass index and disease burden in elderly men and women: the Tromsø Study. *Eur J Epidemiol.* 2010 Mar;25(3):183-93. 2010 Jan 20.

Kwon YS, Oelschlager BK, Merati AL. Evaluation and treatment of laryngopharyngeal reflux symptoms. *Thorac Surg Clin.* 2011 Nov;21(4):477-87.

Lad V. *Ayurveda: The Science of Self-Healing.* Twin Lakes, WI: Lotus Press.

Lai LH, Sung JJ. Helicobacter pylori and benign upper digestive disease. *Best Pract Res Clin Gastroenterol.* 2007;21(2):261-79.

Lamaison JL, Carnat A, Petitjean-Freytet C. Tannin content and inhibiting activity of elastase in Rosaceae. *Ann Pharm Fr.* 1990;48(6):335-40.

Laney AS, Cragin LA, Blevins LZ, Sumner AD, Cox-Ganser JM, Kreiss K, Moffatt SG, Lohff CJ. Sarcoidosis, asthma, and asthma-like symptoms among occupants of a historically water-damaged office building. *Indoor Air.* 2009 Feb;19(1):83-90.

Lang CJ, Hansen M, Roscioli E, Jones J, Murgia C, Leigh Ackland M, Zalewski P, Anderson G, Ruffin R. Dietary zinc mediates inflammation and protects against wasting and metabolic derangement caused by sustained cigarette smoke exposure in mice. *Biometals.* 2011 Feb;24(1):23-39. 2010 Aug 29.

Lange NE, Rifas-Shiman SL, Camargo CA Jr, Gold DR, Gillman MW, Litonjua AA. Maternal dietary pattern during pregnancy is not associated with recurrent wheeze in children. *J Allergy Clin Immunol.* 2010 Aug;126(2):250-5, 255.e1-4.

Lappe FM. *Diet for a Small Planet.* New York: Ballantine, 1971.

Larenas-Linnemann D, Matta JJ, Shah-Hosseini K, Michels A, Mösges R. Skin prick test evaluation of Dermatophagoides pteronyssinus diagnostic extracts from Europe, Mexico, and the United States. *Ann Allergy Asthma Immunol.* 2010 May;104(5):420-5.

Lau BH, Riesen SK, Truong KP, Lau EW, Rohdewald P, Barreta RA. Pycnogenol as an adjunct in the management of childhood asthma. *J Asthma.* 2004;41(8):825-32.

Laubereau B, Filipiak-Pittroff B, von Berg A, Grübl A, Reinhardt D, Wichmann HE, Koletzko S; GINI Study Group. Caesarean section and gastrointestinal symptoms, atopic dermatitis, and sensitisation during the first year of life. *Arch Dis Child.* 2004 Nov;89(11):993-7.

Laurière M, Pecquet C, Bouchez-Mahiout I, Snégaroff J, Bayrou O, Raison-Peyron N, Vigan M. Hydrolysed wheat proteins present in cosmetics can induce immediate hypersensitivities. *Contact Dermatitis.* 2006 May;54(5):283-9.

LaValle JB. *The Cox-2 Connection.* Rochester, VT: Healing Arts, 2001.

Lazarou J, Pomeranz BH, Corey PN. Incidence of adverse drug reactions in hospitalized patients: a meta-analysis of prospective studies. *JAMA.* 1998 Apr.

Lean G. US study links more than 200 diseases to pollution. *London Independent.* 2004 Nov 14.

Leander M, Cronqvist A, Janson C, Uddenfeldt M, Rask-Andersen A. Health-related quality of life predicts onset of asthma in a longitudinal population study. *Respir Med.* 2009 Feb;103(2):194-200.

Lecheler J, Pfannebecker B, Nguyen DT, Petzold U, Munzel U, Kremer HJ, Maus J. Prevention of exercise-induced asthma by a fixed combination of disodium cromoglycate plus reproterol compared with montelukast in young patients. *Arzneimittelforschung.* 2008;58(6):303-9.

Lee E, Haa K, Yook JM, Jin MH, Seo CS, Son KH, Kim HP, Bae KH, Kang SS, Son JK, Chang HW. Anti-asthmatic activity of an ethanol extract from Saururus chinensis. *Biol Pharm Bull.* 2006 Feb;29(2):211-5.

Lee J, Yang DH, Suh JH, Kim U, Eom HY, Kim J, Lee MY, Kim J, Han SB. Species discrimination of Radix Bupleuri through the simultaneous determination of ten saikosaponins by high performance liquid chromatography with evaporative light scattering detection and electrospray ionization mass spectrometry. *J Chromatogr B Analyt Technol Biomed Life Sci.* 2011 Dec 15;879(32):3887-95.

Lee JH, Noh J, Noh G, Kim HS, Mun SH, Choi WS, Cho S, Lee S. Allergen-specific B cell subset responses in cow's milk allergy of late eczematous reactions in atopic dermatitis. *Cell Immunol.* 2010;262(1):44-51.

REFERENCES

Lee JY, Kim CJ. Determination of allergenic egg proteins in food by protein-, mass spectrometry-, and DNA-based methods. *J AOAC Int.* 2010 Mar-Apr;93(2):462-77.

Lee KH, Yeh MH, Kao ST, Hung CM, Chen BC, Liu CJ, Yeh CC. Xia-bai-san inhibits lipopolysaccharide-induced activation of intercellular adhesion molecule-1 and nuclear factor-kappa B in human lung cells. *J Ethnopharmacol.* 2009 Jul 30;124(3):530-8.

Lee YS, Kim SH, Jung SH, Kim JK, Pan CH, Lim SS. Aldose reductase inhibitory compounds from Glycyrrhiza uralensis. *Biol Pharm Bull.* 2010;33(5):917-21.

Lehmann B. The vitamin D3 pathway in human skin and its role for regulation of biological processes. *Photochem Photobiol.* 2005 Nov-Dec;81(6):1246-51.

Lehto M, Airaksinen L, Puustinen A, Tillander S, Hannula S, Nyman T, Toskala E, Alenius H, Lauerma A. Thaumatin-like protein and baker's respiratory allergy. *Ann Allergy Asthma Immunol.* 2010 Feb;104(2):139-46.

Leitzmann C. Vegetarian diets: what are the advantages? *Forum Nutr.* 2005;(57):147-56.

Leu YL, Shi LS, Damu AG. Chemical constituents of Taraxacum formosanum. *Chem Pharm Bull.* 2003 May;51(5):599-601.

Leu YL, Wang YL, Huang SC, Shi LS. Chemical constituents from roots of Taraxacum formosanum. *Chem Pharm Bull.* 2005 Jul;53(7):853-5.

Leung DY, Sampson HA, Yunginger JW, Burks AW Jr, Schneider LC, Wortel CH, Davis FM, Hyun JD, Shanahan WR Jr; Avon Longitudinal Study of Parents and Children Study Team. Effect of anti-IgE therapy in patients with peanut allergy. *N Engl J Med.* 2003 Mar 13;348(11):986-93.

Leung DY, Shanahan WR Jr, Li XM, Sampson HA. New approaches for the treatment of anaphylaxis. *Novartis Found Symp.* 2004;257:248-60; discussion 260-4, 276-85.

Lewerin C, Jacobsson S, Lindstedt G, Nilsson-Ehle H. Serum biomarkers for atrophic gastritis and antibodies against Helicobacter pylori in the elderly: Implications for vitamin B12, folic acid and iron status and response to oral vitamin therapy. *Scand J Gastroenterol.* 2008;43(9):1050-6.

Lewis DA, Fields WN, Shaw GP. A natural flavonoid present in unripe plantain banana pulp (Musa sapientum L. var. paradisiaca) protects the gastric mucosa from aspirin-induced erosions. *J Ethnopharmacol.* 1999 Jun;65(3):283-8.

Lewis SA, Grimshaw KE, Warner JO, Hourihane JO. The promiscuity of immunoglobulin E binding to peanut allergens, as determined by Western blotting, correlates with the severity of clinical symptoms. *Clin Exp Allergy.* 2005 Jun;35(6):767-73.

Lewis WH, Elvin-Lewis MPF. *Medical Botany: Plants Affecting Man's Health.* New York: Wiley, 1977.

Lewontin R. *The Genetic Basis of Evolutionary Change.* New York: Columbia Univ Press, 1974.

Leyel CF. *Culpeper's English Physician & Complete Herbal.* Hollywood, CA: Wilshire, 1971.

Leynadier F. Mast cells and basophils in asthma. Ann Biol Clin (Paris). 1989;47(6):351-6.

Li J, Sun B, Huang Y, Lin X, Zhao D, Tan G, Wu J, Zhao H, Cao L, Zhong N. A multicentre study assessing the prevalence of sensitizations in patients with asthma and/or rhinitis in China. *Allergy.* 2009;64:1083-1092.

Li MH, Zhang HL, Yang BY. Effects of ginkgo leaf concentrated oral liquor in treating asthma. *Zhongguo Zhong Xi Yi Jie He Za Zhi.* 1997 Apr;17(4):216-8. 5.

Li S, Li W, Wang Y, Asada Y, Koike K. Prenylflavonoids from Glycyrrhiza uralensis and their protein tyrosine phosphatase-1B inhibitory activities. *Bioorg Med Chem Lett.* 2010 Sep 15;20(18):5398-401.

Li XM, Huang CK, Zhang TF, Teper AA, Srivastava K, Schofield BH, Sampson HA. The chinese herbal medicine formula MSSM-002 suppresses allergic airway hyperreactivity and modulates TH1/TH2 responses in a murine model of allergic asthma. *J Allergy Clin Immunol.* 2000;106:660-8.

Li XM, Srivastava K. Traditional Chinese medicine for the therapy of allergic disorders. *Curr Opin Otolaryngol Head Neck Surg.* 2006 Jun;14(3):191-6.

Li XM, Zhang TF, Huang CK, Srivastava K, Teper AA, Zhang L, Schofield BH, Sampson HA. Food Allergy Herbal Formula-1 (FAHF-1) blocks peanut-induced anaphylaxis in a murine model. *J Allergy Clin Immunol.* 2001;108:639-46.

Li XM, Zhang TF, Sampson H, Zou ZM, Beyer K, Wen MC, Schofield B. The potential use of Chinese herbal medicines in treating allergic asthma. *Ann Allergy Asthma Immunol.* 2004;93:S35-S44.

Li XM. Beyond allergen avoidance: update on developing therapies for peanut allergy. *Curr Opin Allergy Clin Immunol.* 2005;5:287-92.

Li YQ, Yuan W, Zhang SL. Clinical and experimental study of xiao er ke cuan ling oral liquid in the treatment of infantile bronchopneumonia. *Zhongguo Zhong Xi Yi Jie He Za Zhi.* 1992 Dec;12(12):719-21, 737, 708.

Liacouras CA, Spergel JM, Ruchelli E, Verma R, Mascarenhas M, Semeao E, Flick J, Kelly J, Brown-Whitehorn T, Mamula P, Markowitz JE. Eosinophilic esophagitis: a 10-year experience in 381 children. *Clin Gastroenterol Hepatol.* 2005 Dec;3(12):1198-206.

Lied GA, Lillestol K, Valeur J, Berstad A. Intestinal B cell-activating factor: an indicator of non-IgE-mediated hypersensitivity reactions to food? *Aliment Pharmacol Ther.* 2010 Jul;32(1):66-73.

Lillestol K, Berstad A, Lind R, Florvaag E, Arslan Lied G, Tangen T. Anxiety and depression in patients with self-reported food hypersensitivity. *Gen Hosp Psychiatry.* 2010 Jan-Feb;32(1):42-8.

Lima JA, Fischer GB, Sarria EE, Mattiello R, Solé D. Prevalence of and risk factors for wheezing in the first year of life. *J Bras Pneumol.* 2010 Oct;36(5):525-31. English, Portuguese.

Limb SL, Brown KC, Wood RA, Wise RA, Eggleston PA, Tonascia J, Hamilton RG, Adkinson NF Jr. Adult asthma severity in individuals with a history of childhood asthma. *J Allergy Clin Immunol.* 2005 Jan;115(1):61-6.

Lin SR. Furthering the standardized clinical study on gastroesophageal reflux disease. *Zhonghua Nei Ke Za Zhi.* 2011 Aug;50(8):625.

Lindahl O, Lindwall L, Spångberg A, Stenram A, Ockerman PA. Vegan regimen with reduced medication in the treatment of bronchial asthma. *J Asthma.* 1985;22(1):45-55.

Ling WH, Hänninen O. Shifting from a conventional diet to an uncooked vegan diet reversibly alters fecal hydrolytic activities in humans. J Nutr. 1992 Apr;122(4):924-30.

Lininger S, Gaby A, Austin S, Brown D, Wright J, Duncan A. *The Natural Pharmacy.* New York: Three Rivers, 1999.

Linsalata M, Russo F, Berloco P, Caruso ML, Matteo GD, Cifone MG, Simone CD, Ierardi E, Di Leo A. The influence of Lactobacillus brevis on ornithine decarboxylase activity and polyamine profiles in Helicobacter pylori-infected gastric mucosa. Helicobacter. 2004 Apr;9(2):165-72.

Lipski E. *Digestive Wellness.* Los Angeles, CA: Keats, 2000.

Liu AH, Jaramillo R, Sicherer SH, Wood RA, Bock SA, Burks AW, Massing M, Cohn RD, Zeldin DC. National prevalence and risk factors for food allergy and relationship to asthma: results from the National Health and Nutrition Examination Survey 2005-2006. *J Allergy Clin Immunol.* 2010 Oct;126(4):798-806.e13.

Liu GM, Cao MJ, Huang YY, Cai QF, Weng WY, Su WJ. Comparative study of in vitro digestibility of major allergen tropomyosin and other food proteins of Chinese mitten crab (Eriocheir sinensis). *J Sci Food Agric.* 2010 Aug 15;90(10):1614-20.

Liu HY, Giday Z, Moore BF. Possible pathogenetic mechanisms producing bovine milk protein inducible malabsorption: a hypothesis. *Ann Allergy.* 1977 Jul;39(1):1-7.

Liu JY, Hu JH, Zhu QG, Li FQ, Wang J, Sun HJ. Effect of matrine on the expression of substance P receptor and inflammatory cytokines production in human skin keratinocytes and fibroblasts. *Int Immunopharmacol.* 2007 Jun;7(6):816-23.

Liu T, Valdez R, Yoon PW, Crocker D, Moonesinghe R, Khoury MJ. The association between family history of asthma and the prevalence of asthma among US adults: National Health and Nutrition Examination Survey, 1999-2004. *Genet Med.* 2009 May;11(5):323-8.

Liu X, Beaty TH, Deindl P, Huang SK, Lau S, Sommerfeld C, Fallin MD, Kao WH, Wahn U, Nickel R. Associations between specific serum IgE response and 6 variants within the genes IL4, IL13, and IL4RA in German children: the German Multicenter Atopy Study. *J Allergy Clin Immunol.* 2004 Mar;113(3):489-95.

Liu XJ, Cao MA, Li WH, Shen CS, Yan SQ, Yuan CS. Alkaloids from Sophora flavescens Aition. *Fitoterapia.* 2010 Sep;81(6):524-7.

Lloyd JU. *American Materia Medica, Therapeutics and Pharmacognosy.* Portland, OR: Eclectic Medical Publications, 1989-1983.

Lloyd-Still JD, Powers CA, Hoffman DR, Boyd-Trull K, Lester LA, Benisek DC, Arterburn LM. Bioavailability and safety of a high dose of docosahexaenoic acid triacylglycerol of algal origin in cystic fibrosis patients: a randomized, controlled study. *Nutrition.* 2006 Jan;22(1):36-46.

Locke GR 3rd, Talley NJ, Fett SL, Zinsmeister AR, Melton LJ 3rd. Prevalence and clinical spectrum of gastroesophageal reflux: a population-based study in Olmsted County, Minnesota. *Gastroenterology.* 1997 May;112(5):1448-56.

Lodato F, Azzaroli F, Di Girolamo M, Feletti V, Cecinato P, Lisotti A, Festi D, Roda E, Mazzella G. Proton pump inhibitors in cirrhosis: tradition or evidence based practice? *World J Gastroenterol.* 2008 May 21;14(19):2980-5.

Loehrl TA. Sinonasal problems and reflux. *Facial Plast Surg Clin North Am.* 2012 Feb;20(1):83-6.

Loizzo MR, Saab AM, Tundis R, Statti GA, Menichini F, Lampronti I, Gambari R, Cinatl J, Doerr HW. Phytochemical analysis and in vitro antiviral activities of the essential oils of seven Lebanon species. *Chem Biodivers.* 2008 Mar;5(3):461-70.

Lomax AR, Calder PC. Probiotics, immune function, infection and inflammation: a review of the evidence from studies conducted in humans. *Curr Pharm Des.* 2009;15(13):1428-518.

Longo G, Barbi E, Berti I, Meneghetti R, Pittalis A, Ronfani L, Ventura A. Specific oral tolerance induction in children with very severe cow's milk-induced reactions. *J Allergy Clin Immunol.* 2008 Feb;121(2):343-7.

Lopes EA, Fanelli-Galvani A, Prisco CC, Gonçalves RC, Jacob CM, Cabral AL, Martins MA, Carvalho CR. Assessment of muscle shortening and static posture in children with persistent asthma. *Eur J Pediatr.* 2007 Jul;166(7):715-21.

López N, de Barros-Mazón S, Vilela MM, Silva CM, Ribeiro JD. Genetic and environmental influences on atopic immune response in early life. *J Investig Allergol Clin Immunol.* 1999 Nov-Dec;9(6):392-8.

Lopez-Garcia E, Schulze MB, Meigs JB, Manson JE, Rifai N, Stampfer MJ, Willett WC, Hu FB. Consumption of trans fatty acids is related to plasma biomarkers of inflammation and endothelial dysfunction. *J Nutr.* 2005 Mar;135(3):562-6.

Lotan M, Zysman L. The digestive system and nutritional considerations for individuals with Rett syndrome. Scientific-WorldJournal. 2006 Dec 28;6:1737-49.

Lu MK, Shih YW, Chang Chien TT, Fang LH, Huang HC, Chen PS. α-Solanine inhibits human melanoma cell migration and invasion by reducing matrix metalloproteinase-2/9 activities. *Biol Pharm Bull.* 2010;33(10):1685-91.

Lucas A, Brooke OG, Cole TJ, Morley R, Bamford MF. Food and drug reactions, wheezing, and eczema in preterm infants. *Arch Dis Child.* 1990 Apr;65(4):411-5. 8; .

Lunardi AC, Marques da Silva CC, Rodrigues Mendes FA, Marques AP, Stelmach R, Fernandes Carvalho CR. Musculoskeletal dysfunction and pain in adults with asthma. *J Asthma.* 2011 Feb;48(1):105-10.

Lustig RH, Schmidt LA, Brindis CD. Public health: The toxic truth about sugar. *Nature.* 2012 Feb 1;482(7383):27-9.

Lykken DT, Tellegen A, DeRubeis R: Volunteer bias in twin research: the rule of two-thirds. Soc Biol 1978, 25(1): 1-9. Phillips DI: Twin studies in medical research: can they tell us whether diseases are genetically determined? *Lancet* 1993;341(8851): 1008-1009.

Ma J, Xiao L, Knowles SB. Obesity, insulin resistance and the prevalence of atopy and asthma in US adults. Allergy. 2010 Nov;65(11):1455-63.

Ma XP, Muzhapaer D. Efficacy of sublingual immunotherapy in children with dust mite allergic asthma. *Zhongguo Dang Dai Er Ke Za Zhi.* 2010 May;12(5):344-7.

Mabey R, ed. *The New Age Herbalist.* New York: Simon & Schuster, 1941.

Macdonald TT, Monteleone G. Immunity, inflammation, and allergy in the gut. *Science.* 2005 Mar 25;307(5717):1920-5.

Maciorkowska E, Kaczmarski M, Andrzej K. Endoscopic evaluation of upper gastrointestinal tract mucosa in children with food hypersensitivity. *Med Wieku Rozwoj.* 2000 Jan-Mar;4(1):37-48.

Mackerras D, Cunningham J, Hunt A, Brent P. Re: "effect of supplemental folic acid in pregnancy on childhood asthma: a prospective birth cohort study". *Am J Epidemiol.* 2010 Mar 15;171(6):746-7; author reply 747. 2010 Feb 9.

MacRedmond R, Singhera G, Attridge S, Bahzad M, Fava C, Lai Y, Hallstrand TS, Dorscheid DR. Conjugated linoleic acid improves airway hyper-reactivity in overweight mild asthmatics. *Clin Exp Allergy.* 2010 Jul;40(7):1071-8.

Macsali F, Real FG, Omenaas ER, Bjorge L, Janson C, Franklin K, Svanes C. Oral contraception, body mass index, and asthma: a cross-sectional Nordic-Baltic population survey. *J Allergy Clin Immunol.* 2009 Feb;123(2):391-7.

Madden JA, Plummer SF, Tang J, Garaiova I, Plummer NT, Herbison M, Hunter JO, Shimada T, Cheng L, Shirakawa T. Effect of probiotics on preventing disruption of the intestinal microflora following antibiotic therapy: a double-blind, placebo-controlled pilot study. *Int Immunopharmacol.* 2005 Jun;5(6):1091-7.

Maeda N, Inomata N, Morita A, Kirino M, Ikezawa Z. Correlation of oral allergy syndrome due to plant-derived foods with pollen sensitization in Japan. *Ann Allergy Asthma Immunol.* 2010 Mar;104(3):205-10.

Maes HH, Silberg JL, Neale MC, Eaves LJ. Genetic and cultural transmission of antisocial behavior: an extended twin parent model. *Twin Res Hum Genet.* 2007 Feb;10(1):136-50.

Mai XM, Kull I, Wickman M, Bergström A. Antibiotic use in early life and development of allergic diseases: respiratory infection as the explanation. *Clin Exp Allergy.* 2010 Aug;40(8):1230-7.

Mainardi T, Kapoor S, Bielory L. Complementary and alternative medicine: herbs, phytochemicals and vitamins and their immunologic effects. *J Allergy Clin Immunol.* 2009 Feb;123(2):283-94; quiz 295-6.

Majamaa H, Isolauri E. Probiotics: a novel approach in the management of food allergy. *J Allergy Clin Immunol.* 1997 Feb;99(2):179-85.

Makrides M, Neumann M, Gibson R. Effect of maternal docosahexaenoic acid (DHA) supplementation on breast milk composition. *Europ Jrnl of Clin Nutr.* 1996;50:352-357.

Maliakal PP, Wanwimolruk S. Effect of herbal teas on hepatic drug metabolizing enzymes in rats. *J Pharm Pharmacol.* 2001 Oct;53(10):1323-9.

Mälkönen T, Alanko K, Jolanki R, Luukkonen R, Aalto-Korte K, Lauerma A, Susitaival P. Long-term follow-up study of occupational hand eczema. Br J Dermatol. 2010 Aug 13.

Mallol J, Solé D, Baeza-Bacab M, Aguirre-Camposano V, Soto-Quiros M, Baena-Cagnani C; Latin American ISAAC Group. Regional variation in asthma symptom prevalence in Latin American children. *J Asthma.* 2010 Aug;47(6):644-50.

Manabe N, Haruma K, Ito M, Takahashi N, Takasugi H, Wada Y, Nakata H, Katoh T, Miyamoto M, Tanaka S. Efficacy of adding sodium alginate to omeprazole in patients with nonerosive reflux disease: a randomized clinical trial. *Dis Esophagus.* 2011 Nov 2.

Maneechotesuwan K, Supawita S, Kasetsinsombat K, Wongkajornsilp A, Barnes PJ. Sputum indoleamine-2, 3-dioxygenase activity is increased in asthmatic airways by using inhaled corticosteroids. *J Allergy Clin Immunol.* 2008 Jan;121(1):43-50.

Månsson HL. Fatty acids in bovine milk fat. *Food Nutr Res.* 2008;52. doi: 10.3402/fnr.v52i0.1821.

Manz F. Hydration and disease. *J Am Coll Nutr.* 2007 Oct;26(5 Suppl):535S-541S.

Marcucci F, Duse M, Frati F, Incorvaia C, Marseglia GL, La Rosa M. The future of sublingual immunotherapy. *Int J Immunopathol Pharmacol.* 2009 Oct-Dec;22(4 Suppl):31-3.

Margioris AN. Fatty acids and postprandial inflammation. *Curr Opin Clin Nutr Metab Care.* 2009 Mar;12(2):129-37.

Maria KW, Behrens T, Brasky TM. Are asthma and allergies in children and adolescents increasing? Results from ISAAC Phase I and Phase II surveys in Munster, Germany. Allergy. 2003;58:572-579.

Markowitz JE, Spergel JM, Ruchelli E, Liacouras CA. Elemental diet is an effective treatment for eosinophilic esophagitis in children and adolescents. *Am J Gastroenterol.* 2003 Apr;98(4):777-82.

Marteau P, Munck A, Moreau J, Navarro J. Digestive and nutritional management of adults with cystic fibrosis. *Rev Mal Respir.* 2000 Aug;17(3 Pt 2):785-97.

Martin D. Physical activity benefits and risks on the gastrointestinal system. *South Med J.* 2011 Dec;104(12):831-7.

Martin IR, Wickens K, Patchett K, Kent R, Fitzharris P, Siebers R, Lewis S, Crane J, Holbrook N, Town GI, Smith S. Cat allergen levels in public places in New Zealand. *N Z Med J.* 1998 Sep 25;111(1074):356-8.

Martinez M. Docosahexaenoic acid therapy in docosahexaenoic acid-deficient patients with disorders of peroxisomal biogenesis. *Versicherungsmedizin.* 1996;31 Suppl:145-152

Martínez-Augustin O, Boza JJ, Del Pino JI, Lucena J, Martínez-Valverde A, Gil A. Dietary nucleotides might influence the humoral immune response against cow's milk proteins in preterm neonates. *Biol Neonate.* 1997;71(4):215-23.

Martin-Venegas R, Roig-Perez S, Ferrer R, Moreno JJ. Arachidonic acid cascade and epithelial barrier function during Caco-2 cell differentiation. J Lipid Res. 2006 Apr;3.

Maslowski KM, Mackay CR. Diet, gut microbiota and immune responses. *Nat Immunol.* 2011 Jan;12(1):5-9.

Masoli M, Fabian D, Holt S, Beasley R. The global burden of asthma: executive summary of the GINA Dissemination Committee Report. *Allergy.* 2004;59:469-478.

Massey DG, Chien YK, Fournier-Massey G. Mamane: scientific therapy for asthma? *Hawaii Med J.* 1994;53:350-1. 363.

Massicot JG, Cohen SG. Epidemiologic and socioeconomic aspects of allergic diseases. *J Allergy Clin Immunol.* 1986 Nov;78(5 Pt 2):954-8.

Matasar MJ, Neugut AI. Epidemiology of anaphylaxis in the United States. *Curr Allergy Asthma Rep.* 2003;3:30-35.

Matheson MC, Haydn Walters E, Burgess JA, Jenkins MA, Giles GG, Hopper JL, Abramson MJ, Dharmage SC. Childhood immunization and atopic disease into middle-age—a prospective cohort study. *Pediatr Allergy Immunol.* 2010 Mar;21(2 Pt 1):301-6.

Mathieu N. Risk of long-term treatment with proton pump inhibitors. *Rev Prat.* 2008 Sep 15;58(13):1451-4.

Mathus-Vliegen LM, Tytgat GN. Twenty-four-hour pH measurements in morbid obesity: effects of massive overweight, weight loss and gastric distension. *Eur J Gastroenterol Hepatol.* 1996 Jul;8(7):635-40.

Matricardi PM, Bockelbrink A, Beyer K, Keil T, Niggemann B, Grüber C, Wahn U, Lau S. Primary versus secondary immunoglobulin E sensitization to soy and wheat in the Multi-Centre Allergy Study cohort. *Clin Exp Allergy.* 2008 Mar;38(3):493-500.

Matsui EC, Matsui W. Higher serum folate levels are associated with a lower risk of atopy and wheeze. *J Allergy Clin Immunol.* 2009 Jun;123(6):1253-9.e2. 2009 May 5.

Mayes MD. Epidemiologic studies of environmental agents and systemic autoimmune diseases. *Environ Health Perspect.* 1999 Oct;107 Suppl 5:743-8.

Mayne ST, Risch HA, Dubrow R, Chow WH, Gammon MD, Vaughan TL, Borchardt L, Schoenberg JB, Stanford JL, West AB, Rotterdam H, Blot WJ, Fraumeni JF Jr. Carbonated soft drink consumption and risk of esophageal adenocarcinoma. *J Natl Cancer Inst.* 2006 Jan 4;98(1):72-5.

McAlindon TE. Nutraceuticals: do they work and when should we use them? *Best Pract Res Clin Rheumatol.* 2006 Feb;20(1):99-115.

McCarney RW, Lasserson TJ, Linde K, Brinkhaus B. An overview of two Cochrane systematic reviews of complementary treatments for chronic asthma: acupuncture and homeopathy. *Respir Med.* 2004 Aug;98(8):687-96.

McCarney RW, Linde K, Lasserson TJ. Homeopathy for chronic asthma. *Cochrane Database Syst Rev.* 2004;(1):CD000353.

McCarthy DM. Adverse effects of proton pump inhibitor drugs: clues and conclusions. Curr Opin Gastroenterol. 2010 Nov;26(6):624-31. Clayton SB, Rife CC, Singh ER, Kalbfleisch JH, Castell DO. Twice-daily proton pump inhibitor therapy does not decrease the frequency of reflux episodes during nocturnal recumbency in patients with refractory GERD: analysis of 200 patients using multichannel intraluminal impedance-pH testing. *Dis Esophagus.* 2012 Jan 31.

McConnaughey E. *Sea Vegetables.* Happy Camp, CA: Naturegraph, 1985.

McDougall J, McDougall M. *The McDougal Plan.* Clinton, NJ: New Win, 1983.

McHugh MK, Symanski E, Pompeii LA, Delclos GL. Prevalence of asthma by industry and occupation in the U.S. working population. *Am J Ind Med.* 2010 May;53(5):463-75.

McHugh MK, Symanski E, Pompeii LA, Delclos GL. Prevalence of asthma among adult females and males in the United States: results from the National Health and Nutrition Examination Survey (NHANES), 2001-2004. *J Asthma.* 2009 Oct;46(8):759-66.

McKeever TM, Lewis SA, Cassano PA, Ocké M, Burney P, Britton J, Smit HA. Patterns of dietary intake and relation to respiratory disease, forced expiratory volume in 1 s, and decline in 5-y forced expiratory volume. *Am J Clin Nutr.* 2010 Aug;92(2):408-15. 2010 Jun 16.

McKenzie H, Main J, Pennington CR, Parratt D. Antibody to selected strains of Saccharomyces cerevisiae (baker's and brewer's yeast) and Candida albicans in Crohn's disease. *Gut.* 1990 May;31(5):536-8.

McLachlan CN. beta-casein A1, ischaemic heart disease mortality, and other illnesses. *Med Hypotheses.* 2001 Feb;56(2):262-72.

McNally ME, Atkinson SA, Cole DE. Contribution of sulfate and sulfoesters to total sulfur intake in infants fed human milk. *J Nutr.* 1991 Aug;121(8):1250-4.

McNamara D, O'Morain C. Gastro-oesophageal reflux disease and Helicobacter pylori: an intricate relation. *Gut.* 1999 Jul;45 Suppl 1:I13-7.

McNaught CE, Woodcock NP, Anderson AD, MacFie J. A prospective randomised trial of probiotics in critically ill patients. *Clin Nutr.* 2005 Apr;24(2):211-9.

Meglio P, Bartone E, Plantamura M, Arabito E, Giampietro PG. A protocol for oral desensitization in children with IgE-mediated cow's milk allergy. *Allergy.* 2004 Sep;59(9):980-7.

Mehra PN, Puri HS. Studies on Gaduchi satwa. *Indian J Pharm.* 1969;31:180-2.

Meier B, Shao Y, Julkunen-Tiitto R, Bettschart A, Sticher O. A chemotaxonomic survey of phenolic compounds in Swiss willow species. *Planta Med.* 1992;58:A698.

Meier B, Sticher O, Julkunen-Tiitto R. Pharmaceutical aspects of the use of willows in herbal remedies. *Planta Med.* 1988;54(6):559-560.

Melcion C, Verroust P, Baud L, Ardaillou N, Morel-Maroger L, Ardaillou R. Protective effect of procyanidolic oligomers on the heterologous phase of glomerulonephritis induced by anti-glomerular basement membrane antibodies. *C R Seances Acad Sci III.* 1982 Dec 6;295(12):721-6.

Mendes FA, Gonçalves RC, Nunes MP, Saraiva-Romanholo BM, Cukier A, Stelmach R, Jacob-Filho W, Martins MA, Carvalho CR. Effects of aerobic training on psychosocial morbidity and symptoms in patients with asthma: a randomized clinical trial. *Chest.* 2010 Aug;138(2):331-7. 2010 Apr 2.

Menezes MD, McCarter R, Greene EA, Bauman NM. Status of propranolol for treatment of infantile hemangioma and description of a randomized clinical trial. *Ann Otol Rhinol Laryngol.* 2011 Oct;120(10):686-95.

REFERENCES

Merchant RE and Andre CA. 2001. A review of recent clinical trials of the nutritional supplement Chlorella pyrenoidosa in the treatment of fibromyalgia, hypertension, and ulcerative colitis. *Altern Ther Health Med.* May-Jun;7(3):79-91.

Messina M. Insights gained from 20 years of soy research. *J Nutr.* 2010 Dec;140(12):2289S-2295S. 2010 Oct 27.

Metsälä J, Lundqvist A, Kaila M, Gissler M, Klaukka T, Virtanen SM. Maternal and perinatal characteristics and the risk of cow's milk allergy in infants up to 2 years of age: a case-control study nested in the Finnish population. *Am J Epidemiol.* 2010 Jun 15;171(12):1310-6

Meyer A, Kirsch H, Domergue F, Abbadi A, Sperling P, Bauer J, Cirpus P, Zank TK, Moreau H, Roscoe TJ, Zähringer U, Heinz E. Novel fatty acid elongases and their use for the reconstitution of docosahexaenoic acid biosynthesis. *J Lipid Res.* 2004 Oct;45(10):1899-909.

Meyer AL, Elmadfa I, Herbacek I, Micksche M. Probiotic, as well as conventional yogurt, can enhance the stimulated production of proinflammatory cytokines. *J Hum Nutr Diet.* 2007 Dec;20(6):590-8.

Michaelsen KF. Probiotics, breastfeeding and atopic eczema. *Acta Derm Venereol Suppl (Stockh).* 2005 Nov;(215):21-4.

Michail S. The role of probiotics in allergic diseases. Allergy Asthma Clin Immunol. 2009 Oct 22;5(1):5.

Michalska K, Kisiel W. Sesquiterpene lactones from Taraxacum obovatum. *Planta Med.* 2003 Feb;69(2):181-3.

Michelson PH, Williams LW, Benjamin DK, Barnato AE. Obesity, inflammation, and asthma severity in childhood: data from the National Health and Nutrition Examination Survey 2001-2004. *Ann Allergy Asthma Immunol.* 2009 Nov;103(5):381-5.

Mickleborough TD, Lindley MR, Ray S. Dietary salt, airway inflammation, and diffusion capacity in exercise-induced asthma. *Med Sci Sports Exerc.* 2005 Jun;37(6):904-14.

Mikoluc B, Motkowski R, Karpińska J, Piotrowska-Jastrzebska J. Plasma levels of vitamins A and E, coenzyme Q10, and anti-ox-LDL antibody titer in children treated with an elimination diet due to food hypersensitivity. *Int J Vitam Nutr Res.* 2009 Sep;79(5-6):328-36.

Miller AL. The etiologies, pathophysiology, and alternative/complementary treatment of asthma. *Altern Med Rev.* 2001 Feb;6(1):20-47.

Miller GT. *Living in the Environment.* Belmont, CA: Wadsworth, 1996.

Minami H, McCallum RW. The physiology and pathophysiology of gastric emptying in humans. *Gastroenterology.* 1984 Jun;86(6):1592-610.

Mindell E, Hopkins V. *Prescription Alternatives.* New Canaan, CT: Keats, 1998.

Miranda H, Outeiro TF. The sour side of neurodegenerative disorders: the effects of protein glycation. *J Pathol.* 2010 May;221(1):13-25.

Mitchell AE, Hong YJ, Koh E, Barrett DM, Bryant DE, Denison RF, Kaffka S. Ten-year comparison of the influence of organic and conventional crop management practices on the content of flavonoids in tomatoes. *J Agric Food Chem.* 2007 Jul 25;55(15):6154-9.

Mittag D, Akkerdaas J, Ballmer-Weber BK, Vogel L, Wensing M, Becker WM, Koppelman SJ, Knulst AC, Helbling A, Hefle SL, Van Ree R, Vieths S. Ara h 8, a Bet v 1-homologous allergen from peanut, is a major allergen in patients with combined birch pollen and peanut allergy. *J Allergy Clin Immunol.* 2004 Dec;114(6):1410-7.

Mittag D, Vieths S, Vogel L, Becker WM, Rihs HP, Helbling A, Wüthrich B, Ballmer-Weber BK. Soybean allergy in patients allergic to birch pollen: clinical investigation and molecular characterization of allergens. *J Allergy Clin Immunol.* 2004 Jan;113(1):148-54.

Miyake Y, Sasaki S, Tanaka K, Hirota Y. Dairy food, calcium and vitamin D intake in pregnancy, and wheeze and eczema in infants. *Eur Respir J.* 2010 Jun;35(6):1228-34. 2009 Oct 19.

Miyazawa R, Tomomasa T, Kaneko H, Arakawa H, Shimizu N, Morikawa A. Effects of pectin liquid on gastroesophageal reflux disease in children with cerebral palsy. *BMC Gastroenterol.* 2008 Apr 16;8:11.

Miyazawa T, Itahashi K, Imai T. Management of neonatal cow's milk allergy in high-risk neonates. *Pediatr Int.* 2009 Aug;51(4):544-7.

Moattari A, Aleyasin S, Arabpour M, Sadeghi S. Prevalence of Human Metapneumovirus (hMPV) in Children with Wheezing in Shiraz-Iran. *Iran J Allergy Asthma Immunol.* 2010 Dec;9(4):250-4.

Mochiki E, Yanai M, Ohno T, Kuwano H. The effect of traditional Japanese medicine (Kampo) on gastrointestinal function. *Surg Today.* 2010 Dec;40(12):1105-11.

Modlin IM, Goldenring JR, Lawton GP, Hunt R. Aspects of the theoretical basis and clinical relevance of low acid states. *Am J Gastroenterol.* 1994 Mar;89(3):308-18.

Mokhtar N, Chan SC. Use of complementary medicine amongst asthmatic patients in primary care. *Med J Malaysia.* 2006 Mar;61(1):125-7.

Monarca S. Zerbini I, Simonati C, Gelatti U. Drinking water hardness and chronic degenerative diseases. Part II. Cardiovascular diseases. *Ann. Ig.* 2003;15:41-56.

Moneret-Vautrin DA, Kanny G, Thévenin F. Asthma caused by food allergy. *Rev Med Interne.* 1996;17(7):551-7.

Moneret-Vautrin DA, Morisset M. Adult food allergy. *Curr Allergy Asthma Rep.* 2005 Jan;5(1):80-5.

Monks H, Gowland MH, Mackenzie H, Erlewyn-Lajeunesse M, King R, Lucas JS, Roberts G. How do teenagers manage their food allergies? *Clin Exp Allergy.* 2010 Aug 2.

Moorhead KJ, Morgan HC. *Spirulina: Nature's Superfood.* Kailua-Kona, HI: Nutrex, 1995.

Moreira A, Delgado L, Haahtela T, Fonseca J, Moreira P, Lopes C, Mota J, Santos P, Rytilä P, Castel-Branco MG. Physical training does not increase allergic inflammation in asthmatic children. Eur Respir J. 2008 Dec;32(6):1570-5.

Moreira P, Moreira A, Padrão P, Delgado L. The role of economic and educational factors in asthma: evidence from the Portuguese health survey. *Public Health.* 2008 Apr;122(4):434-9. 2007 Oct 17.

Morel AF, Dias GO, Porto C, Simionatto E, Stuker CZ, Dalcol II. Antimicrobial activity of extractives of Solidago mi-
croglossa. *Fitoterapia.* 2006 Sep;77(6):453-5.
Morisset M, Moneret-Vautrin DA, Guenard L, Cuny JM, Frentz P, Hatahet R, Hanss Ch, Beaudouin E, Petit N, Kanny G.
Oral desensitization in children with milk and egg allergies obtains recovery in a significant proportion of cases. A
randomized study in 60 children with cow's milk allergy and 90 children with egg allergy. *Eur Ann Allergy Clin Immunol.* 2007 Jan;39(1):12-9.
Morisset M, Moneret-Vautrin DA, Kanny G, Guénard L, Beaudouin E, Flabbée J, Hatahet R. Thresholds of clinical
reactivity to milk, egg, peanut and sesame in immunoglobulin E-dependent allergies: evaluation by double-blind or
single-blind placebo-controlled oral challenges. *Clin Exp Allergy.* 2003 Aug;33(8):1046-51.
Moussaieff A, Shein NA, Tsenter J, Grigoriadis S, Simeonidou C, Alexandrovich AG, Trembovler V, Ben-Neriah Y,
Schmitz ML, Fiebich BL, Munoz E, Mechoulam R, Shohami E. Incensole acetate: a novel neuroprotective agent
isolated from Boswellia carterii. *J Cereb Blood Flow Metab.* 2008 Jul;28(7):1341-52.
Moyle A. *Nature Cure for Asthma and Hay Fever.* Wellingborough, U.K.: Thorsons, 1978.
Mozaffarian D, Aro A, Willett WC. Health effects of trans-fatty acids: experimental and observational evidence. *Eur J Clin
Nutr.* 2009 May;63 Suppl 2:S5-21.
Murray M, Pizzorno J. *Encyclopedia of Natural Medicine.* 2nd Edition. Roseville, CA: Prima Publishing, 1998.
Nadkarni AK, Nadkarni KM. *Indian Materia Medica.* (Vols 1 and 2). Bombay, India: Popular Pradashan, 1908, 1976.
Nagai T, Arai Y, Emori M, Nunome SY, Yabe T, Takeda T, Yamada H. Anti-allergic activity of a Kampo (Japanese herbal)
medicine "Sho-seiryu-to (Xiao-Qing-Long-Tang)" on airway inflammation in a mouse model. *Int Immunopharmacol.*
2004 Oct;4(10-11):1353-65.
Nagel G, Linseisen J. Dietary intake of fatty acids, antioxidants and selected food groups and asthma in adults. *Eur J Clin
Nutr.* 2005 Jan;59(1):8-15.
Nagel G, Weinmayr G, Kleiner A, Garcia-Marcos L, Strachan DP; ISAAC Phase Two Study Group. Effect of diet on
asthma and allergic sensitisation in the International Study on Allergies and Asthma in Childhood (ISAAC) Phase
Two. Thorax. 2010 Jun;65(6):516-22.
Naghii MR, Samman S. The role of boron in nutrition and metabolism. *Prog Food Nutr Sci.* 1993 Oct-Dec;17(4):331-49.
Nair PK, Rodriguez S, Ramachandran R, Alamo A, Melnick SJ, Escalon E, Garcia PI Jr, Wnuk SF, Ramachandran C.
Immune stimulating properties of a novel polysaccharide from the medicinal plant Tinospora cordifolia. *Int Im-
munopharmacol.* 2004 Dec 15;4(13):1645-59.
Nakano T, Shimojo N, Morita Y, Arima T, Tomiita M, Kohno Y. Sensitization to casein and beta-lactoglobulin (BLG) in
children with cow's milk allergy (CMA). *Arerugi.* 2010 Feb;59(2):117-22.
Napoli, J.E., Brand-Miller, J.C., Conway, P. (2003) Bifidogenic effects of feeding infant formula containing galactooligo-
saccharides in healthy formula-fed infants. *Asia Pac J Clin Nutr.* 12(Suppl): S60
Nariya M, Shukla V, Jain S, Ravishankar B. Comparison of enteroprotective efficacy of triphala formulations (Indian
Herbal Drug) on methotrexate-induced small intestinal damage in rats. *Phytother Res.* 2009 Aug;23(8):1092-8.
Naruszewicz M, Johansson ML, Zapolska-Downar D, Bukowska H. Effect of Lactobacillus plantarum 299v on cardio-
vascular disease risk factors in smokers. *Am J Clin Nutr.* 2002 Dec;76(6):1249-55.
National Cooperation Group on Childhood Asthma. A nationwide survey in China on prevalence of asthma in urban
children. Chin J Pediatr. pp. 123-127.
Navarro Silvera SA, Mayne ST, Risch HA, Gammon MD, Vaughan T, Chow WH, Dubin JA, Dubrow R, Schoenberg J,
Stanford JL, West AB, Rotterdam H, Blot WJ. Principal component analysis of dietary and lifestyle patterns in rela-
tion to risk of subtypes of esophageal and gastric cancer. *Ann Epidemiol.* 2011 Jul;21(7):543-50.
NDL, BHNRC, ARS, USDA. *Oxygen Radical Absorbance Capacity (ORAC) of Selected Foods - 2007.* Beltsville, MD: USDA-
ARS. 2007.
Nemati S, Mojtahedi A, Naghavi SE, Banan R, Zia F. Investigating Helicobacter pylori in nasal polyposis using polymerase
chain reaction, urease test and culture. *Eur Arch Otorhinolaryngol.* 2011 Nov 25.
Nentwich I, Míchková E, Nevoral J, Urbanek R, Szépfalusi Z. Cow's milk-specific cellular and humoral immune responses
and atopy skin symptoms in infants from atopic families fed a partially (pHF) or extensively (eHF) hydrolyzed in-
fant formula. *Allergy.* 2001 Dec;56(12):1144-56.
Newall CA, Anderson LA, Phillipson JD (eds). *Herbal Medicines: A Guide for Health-Care Professionals.* London: Pharmaceut
Press; 1996.
Newmark T, Schulick P. *Beyond Aspirin.* Prescott, AZ: Holm, 2000.
Neyestani TR, Shariatzadeh N, Gharavi A, Kalayi A, Khalaji N. Physiological dose of lycopene suppressed oxidative stress
and enhanced serum levels of immunoglobulin M in patients with Type 2 diabetes mellitus: a possible role in the
prevention of long-term complications. *J Endocrinol Invest.* 2007 Nov;30(10):833-8.
Ngai SP, Jones AY, Hui-Chan CW, Ko FW, Hui DS. Effect of Acu-TENS on post-exercise expiratory lung volume in
subjects with asthma-A randomized controlled trial. *Respir Physiol Neurobiol.* 2009 Jul 31;167(3):348-53. 2009 Jun 18.
Nguyen TL, Uchida T, Tsukamoto Y, Trinh DT, Ta L, Mai BH, Le SH, Thai KD, Ho DD, Hoang HH, Matsuhisa T,
Okimoto T, Kodama M, Murakami K, Fujioka T, Yamaoka Y, Moriyama M. Helicobacter pylori infection and gas-
troduodenal diseases in Vietnam: a cross-sectional, hospital-based study. *BMC Gastroenterol.* 2010 Sep 30;10:114.
Nicholls SJ, Lundman P, Harmer JA, Cutri B, Griffiths KA, Rye KA, Barter PJ, Celermajer DS. Consumption of saturated
fat impairs the anti-inflammatory properties of high-density lipoproteins and endothelial function. *J Am Coll Cardiol.* 2006 Aug 15;48(4):715-20.

REFERENCES

Nicolaou N, Poorafshar M, Murray C, Simpson A, Winell H, Kerry G, Härlin A, Woodcock A, Ahlstedt S, Custovic A. Allergy or tolerance in children sensitized to peanut: prevalence and differentiation using component-resolved diagnostics. *J Allergy Clin Immunol.* 2010 Jan;125(1):191-7.e1-13.

Niederau C, Göpfert E. The effect of chelidonium- and turmeric root extract on upper abdominal pain due to functional disorders of the biliary system. Results from a placebo-controlled double-blind study. *Med Klin.* 1999 Aug 15;94(8):425-30.

Nielsen RG, Bindslev-Jensen C, Kruse-Andersen S, Husby S. Severe gastroesophageal reflux disease and cow milk hypersensitivity in infants and children: disease association and evaluation of a new challenge procedure. *J Pediatr Gastroenterol Nutr.* 2004 Oct;39(4):383-91.

Nielsen RG, Bindslev-Jensen C, Kruse-Andersen S, Husby S. Severe gastroesophageal reflux disease and cow milk hypersensitivity in infants and children: disease association and evaluation of a new challenge procedure. *J Pediatr Gastroenterol Nutr.* 2004 Oct;39(4):383-91.

Niggemann B, von Berg A, Bollrath C, Berdel D, Schauer U, Rieger C, Haschke-Becher E, Wahn U. Safety and efficacy of a new extensively hydrolyzed formula for infants with cow's milk protein allergy. *Pediatr Allergy Immunol.* 2008 Jun;19(4):348-54.

Nightingale JA, Rogers DF, Hart LA, Kharitonov SA, Chung KF, Barnes PJ. Effect of inhaled endotoxin on induced sputum in normal, atopic, and atopic asthmatic subjects. *Thorax.* 1998 Jul;53(7):563-71.

Niimi A, Nguyen LT, Usmani O, Mann B, Chung KF. Reduced pH and chloride levels in exhaled breath condensate of patients with chronic cough. *Thorax.* 2004 Jul;59(7):608-12.

Ninan TK, Russell G. Respiratory symptoms and atopy in Aberdeen schoolchildren: evidence from two surveys 25 years apart. BMJ. 1992;304:873-875.

Njoroge GN, Bussmann RW. Traditional management of ear, nose and throat (ENT) diseases in Central Kenya. *J Ethnobiol Ethnomed.* 2006 Dec 27;2:54.

Nobaek S, Johansson ML, Molin G, Ahrné S, Jeppsson B. Alteration of intestinal microflora is associated with reduction in abdominal bloating and pain in patients with irritable bowel syndrome. *Am J Gastroenterol.* 2000 May;95(5):1231-8.

Nodake Y, Fukumoto S, Fukasawa M, Sakakibara R, Yamasaki N. Reduction of the immunogenicity of beta-lactoglobulin from cow's milk by conjugation with a dextran derivative. *Biosci Biotechnol Biochem.* 2010;74(4):721-6.

Noel RJ, Tipnis NA. Eosinophilic esophagitis—a mimic of GERD. *Int J Pediatr Otorhinolaryngol.* 2006 Jul;70(7):1147-53.

Noh J, Lee JH, Noh G, Bang SY, Kim HS, Choi WS, Cho S, Lee SS. Characterisation of allergen-specific responses of IL-10-producing regulatory B cells (Br1) in Cow Milk Allergy. *Cell Immunol.* 2010;264(2):143-9.

Noorbakhsh R, Mortazavi SA, Sankian M, Shahidi F, Assarehzadegan MA, Varasteh A. Cloning, expression, characterization, and computational approach for cross-reactivity prediction of manganese superoxide dismutase allergen from pistachio nut. *Allergol Int.* 2010 Sep;59(3):295-304.

Nord HJ. Extraesophageal symptoms: what role for the proton pump inhibitors? *Am J Med.* 2004 Sep 6;117 Suppl 5A:56S-62S.

Norsett KG, Laegreid A, Kusnierczyk W, Langaas M, Ylving S, Fossmark R, Myhre S, Falkmer S, Waldum HL, Sandvik AK. Changes in gene expression of gastric mucosa during therapeutic acid inhibition. *Eur J Gastroenterol Hepatol.* 2008 Jul;20(7):613-23.

Novembre E, Dini L, Bernardini R, Resti M, Vierucci A. Unusual reactions to food additives. *Pediatr Med Chir.* 1992 Jan-Feb;14(1):39-42.

Nowak-Wegrzyn A, Fiocchi A. Is oral immunotherapy the cure for food allergies? *Curr Opin Allergy Clin Immunol.* 2010 Jun;10(3):214-9.

Nsouli TM. Long-term use of nasal saline irrigation: harmful or helpful? *Amer Acad of Allergy, Asthma and Immunol.* 2009; Abstract O32.

Nurmatov U, Devereux G, Sheikh A. Nutrients and foods for the primary prevention of asthma and allergy: Systematic review and meta-analysis. *J Allergy Clin Immunol.* 2010 Dec 23.

Nusem D, Panasoff J. Beer anaphylaxis. *Isr Med Assoc J.* 2009 Jun;11(6):380-1.

Nutrition in systemic sclerosis. Mochiki E, Yanai M, Ohno T, Kuwano H. The effect of traditional Japanese medicine (Kampo) on gastrointestinal function. *Surg Today.* 2010 Dec;40(12):1105-11.

Nwaru BI, Erkkola M, Ahonen S, Kaila M, Haapala AM, Kronberg-Kippilä C, Salmelin R, Veijola R, Ilonen J, Simell O, Knip M, Virtanen SM. Age at the introduction of solid foods during the first year and allergic sensitization at age 5 years. *Pediatrics.* 2010 Jan;125(1):50-9. 2009 Dec 7.

O'Connor J., Bensky D. (ed). *Shanghai College of Traditional Chinese Medicine: Acupuncture: A Comprehensive Text.* Seattle: Eastland Press, 1981.

O'Neil C, Helbling AA, Lehrer SB. Allergic reactions to fish. *Clin Rev Allergy.* 1993 Summer;11(2):183-200.

O'Neil C, Helbling AA, Lehrer SB. Allergic reactions to fish. *Clin Rev Allergy.* 1993;11(2):183-200.

Odamaki T, Xiao JZ, Iwabuchi N, Sakamoto M, Takahashi N, Kondo S, Miyaji K, Iwatsuki K, Togashi H, Enomoto T, Benno Y. Influence of Bifidobacterium longum BB536 intake on faecal microbiota in individuals with Japanese cedar pollinosis during the pollen season. *J Med Microbiol.* 2007 Oct;56(Pt 10):1301-8.

Oehme FW (ed.). *Toxicity of heavy metals in the environment. Part 1.* New York: M.Dekker, 1979.

Ogawa T, Hashikawa S, Asai Y, Sakamoto H, Yasuda K, Makimura Y. A new synbiotic, Lactobacillus casei subsp. casei together with dextran, reduces murine and human allergic reaction. *FEMS Immunol Med Microbiol.* 2006 Apr;46(3):400-9.

Oh CK, Lücker PW, Wetzelsberger N, Kuhlmann F. The determination of magnesium, calcium, sodium and potassium in assorted foods with special attention to the loss of electrolytes after various forms of food preparations. *Mag.-Bull.* 1986;8:297-302.

Oh SY, Chung J, Kim MK, Kwon SO, Cho BH. Antioxidant nutrient intakes and corresponding biomarkers associated with the risk of atopic dermatitis in young children. *Eur J Clin Nutr.* 2010 Mar;64(3):245-52. 2010 Jan 27.

Ok IS, Kim SH, Kim BK, Lee JC, Lee YC. Pinellia ternata, Citrus reticulata, and their combinational prescription inhibit eosinophil infiltration and airway hyperresponsiveness by suppressing CCR3+ and Th2 cytokines production in the ovalbumin-induced asthma model. *Mediators Inflamm.* 2009;2009:413270.

Oldak E, Kurzatkowska B, Stasiak-Barmuta A. Natural course of sensitization in children: follow-up study from birth to 6 years of age, I. Evaluation of total serum IgE and specific IgE antibodies with regard to atopic family history. *Rocz Akad Med Bialymst.* 2000;45:87-95.

Oreskovic NM, Sawicki GS, Kinane TB, Winickoff JP, Perrin JM. Travel patterns to school among children with asthma. *Clin Pediatr.* 2009 Jul;48(6):632-40. 2009 May 6.

Orsi M, Cohen-Sabban J, Grandi C, Donato MG, Lifschitz C, D'Agostino D. Non acid gastroesophageal reflux episodes decrease with age as determined by multichannel intraluminal impedance-ph monitoring in symptomatic children. Rev Fac Cien Med Univ Nac Cordoba. 2011 Mar;68(1):8-13. 1. *Reumatol Clin.* 2011 Dec 23.

Ortiz-Andrellucchi A, Sánchez-Villegas A, Rodríguez-Gallego C, Lemes A, Molero T, Soria A, Peña-Quintana L, Santana M, Ramírez O, García J, Cabrera F, Cobo J, Serra-Majem L. Immunomodulatory effects of the intake of fermented milk with Lactobacillus casei DN114001 in lactating mothers and their children. *Br J Nutr.* 2008 Oct;100(4):834-45.

Osguthorpe JD. Immunotherapy. *Curr Opin Otolaryngol Head Neck Surg.* 2010 Jun;18(3):206-12.

Ostrander S, Schroeder L, Ostrander N. *Super-Learning.* New York: Delta, 1979.

Ostrom KM, Jacobs JR, Merritt RJ, Murray RD. Decreased regurgitation with a soy formula containing added soy fiber. *Clin Pediatr (Phila).* 2006 Jan-Feb;45(1):29-36.

Otten MH. Intestinal infections due to inhibition of gastric acid secretion in reflux disease. *Ned Tijdschr Geneeskd.* 1999 Dec 11;143(50):2511-4.

Otto SJ, van Houwelingen AC, Hornstra G. The effect of supplementation with docosahexaenoic and arachidonic acid derived from single cell oils on plasma and erythrocyte fatty acids of pregnant women in the second trimester. *Prostaglandins Leukot Essent Fatty Acids.* 2000 Nov;63(5):323-8.

Ou CC, Tsao SM, Lin MC, Yin MC. Protective action on human LDL against oxidation and glycation by four organosulfur compounds derived from garlic. *Lipids.* 2003 Mar;38(3):219-24.

Ouwehand AC, Bergsma N, Parhiala R, Lahtinen S, Gueimonde M, Finne-Soveri H, Strandberg T, Pitkälä K, Salminen S. Bifidobacterium microbiota and parameters of immune function in elderly subjects. *FEMS Immunol Med Microbiol.* 2008 Jun;53(1):18-25.

Ouwehand AC, Nermes M, Collado MC, Rautonen N, Salminen S, Isolauri E. Specific probiotics alleviate allergic rhinitis during the birch pollen season. *World J Gastroenterol.* 2009 Jul 14;15(26):3261-8.

Ouwehand AC, Tiihonen K, Saarinen M, Putaala H, Rautonen N. Influence of a combination of Lactobacillus acidophilus NCFM and lactitol on healthy elderly: intestinal and immune parameters. *Br J Nutr.* 2009 Feb;101(3):367-75.

Ozdemir O. Any benefits of probiotics in allergic disorders? *Allergy Asthma Proc.* 2010 Mar;31(2):103-11.

Paddack A, Gibbons T, Smith C, Patil S, Richter GT. Food Hypersensitivity and Otolaryngologic Conditions in Young Children. *Otolaryngol Head Neck Surg.* 2012 Mar 23.

Paganelli R, Pallone F, Montano S, Le Moli S, Matricardi PM, Fais S, Paoluzi P, D'Amelio R, Aiuti F. Isotypic analysis of antibody response to a food antigen in inflammatory bowel disease. *Int Arch Allergy Appl Immunol.* 1985;78(1):81-5.

Pahud JJ, Schwarz K. Research and development of infant formulae with reduced allergenic properties. *Ann Allergy.* 1984 Dec;53(6 Pt 2):609-14.

Pakhale S, Doucette S, Vandemheen K, Boulet LP, McIvor RA, Fitzgerald JM, Hernandez P, Lemiere C, Sharma S, Field SK, Alvarez GG, Dales RE, Aaron SD. A comparison of obese and nonobese people with asthma: exploring an asthma-obesity interaction. *Chest.* 2010 Jun;137(6):1316-23. 2010 Feb 12.

Palacin A, Bartra J, Muñoz R, Diaz-Perales A, Valero A, Salcedo G. Anaphylaxis to wheat flour-derived foodstuffs and the lipid transfer protein syndrome: a potential role of wheat lipid transfer protein Tri a 14. *Int Arch Allergy Immunol.* 2010;152(2):178-83.

Palacios R, Sugawara I. Hydrocortisone abrogates proliferation of T cells in autologous mixed lymphocyte reaction by rendering the interleukin-2 Producer T cells unresponsive to interleukin-1 and unable to synthesize the T-cell growth factor. *Scand J Immunol.* 1982 Jan;15(1):25-31. 7.

Palacios R. HLA-DR antigens render interleukin-2-producer T lymphocytes sensitive to interleukin-1. *Scand J Immunol.* 1981 Sep;14(3):321-6.

Palmer DJ, Gold MS, Makrides M. Effect of cooked and raw egg consumption on ovalbumin content of human milk: a randomized, double-blind, cross-over trial. *Clin Exp Allergy.* 2005 Feb;35(2):173-8.

Paluska SA. Current concepts: recognition and management of common activity-related gastrointestinal disorders. *Phys Sportsmed.* 2009 Apr;37(1):54-63.

Pandolfino JE, Bianchi LK, Lee TJ, Hirano I, Kahrilas PJ. Esophagogastric junction morphology predicts susceptibility to exercise-induced reflux. *Am J Gastroenterol.* 2004 Aug;99(8):1430-6.

Panghal S, Mallapur SS, Kumar M, Ram V, Singh BK. Antiinflammatory Activity of Piper longum Fruit Oil. *Indian J Pharm Sci.* 2009 Jul;71(4):454-6.

Panzani R, Ariano R, Mistrello G. Cypress pollen does not cross-react to plant-derived foods. *Eur Ann Allergy Clin Immunol.* 2010 Jun;42(3):125-6.

REFERENCES

Parcell S. Sulfur in human nutrition and applications in medicine. *Altern Med Rev.* 2002 Feb;7(1):22-44.

Park BJ, Tsunetsugu Y, Kasetani T, Kagawa T, Miyazaki Y. The physiological effects of Shinrin-yoku (taking in the forest atmosphere or forest bathing): evidence from field experiments in 24 forests across Japan. *Environ Health Prev Med.* 2010 Jan;15(1):18-26.

Parra D, De Morentin BM, Cobo JM, Mateos A, Martinez JA. Monocyte function in healthy middle-aged people receiving fermented milk containing Lactobacillus casei. *J Nutr Health Aging.* 2004;8(4):208-11.

Parra MD, Martínez de Morentin BE, Cobo JM, Mateos A, Martínez JA. Daily ingestion of fermented milk containing Lactobacillus casei DN114001 improves innate-defense capacity in healthy middle-aged people. *J Physiol Biochem.* 2004 Jun;60(2):85-91.

Partridge MR, Dockrell M, Smith NM. The use of complementary medicines by those with asthma. Respir Med 2003; 97:436-438.

Pastorello EA, Farioli L, Conti A, Pravettoni V, Bonomi S, Iametti S, Fortunato D, Scibilia J, Bindslev-Jensen C, Ballmer-Weber B, Robino AM, Ortolani C. Wheat IgE-mediated food allergy in European patients: alpha-amylase inhibitors, lipid transfer proteins and low-molecular-weight glutenins. Allergenic molecules recognized by double-blind, placebo-controlled food challenge. *Int Arch Allergy Immunol.* 2007;144(1):10-22.

Pastorello EA, Pompei C, Pravettoni V, Farioli L, Calamari AM, Scibilia J, Robino AM, Conti A, Iametti S, Fortunato D, Bonomi S, Ortolani C. Lipid-transfer protein is the major maize allergen maintaining IgE-binding activity after cooking at 100 degrees C, as demonstrated in anaphylactic patients and patients with positive double-blind, placebo-controlled food challenge results. *J Allergy Clin Immunol.* 2003 Oct;112(4):775-83.

Patchett K, Lewis S, Crane J, Fitzharris P. Cat allergen (Fel d 1) levels on school children's clothing and in primary school classrooms in Wellington, New Zealand. *J Allergy Clin Immunol.* 1997 Dec;100(6 Pt 1):755-9.

Patel DS, Rafferty GF, Lee S, Hannam S, Greenough A. Work of breathing and volume targeted ventilation in respiratory distress. *Arch Dis Child Fetal Neonatal Ed.* 2010 Nov;95(6):F443-6.

Patriarca G, Nucera E, Pollastrini E, Roncallo C, De Pasquale T, Lombardo C, Pedone C, Gasbarrini G, Buonomo A, Schiavino D. Oral specific desensitization in food-allergic children. *Dig Dis Sci.* 2007 Jul;52(7):1662-72.

Patriarca G, Nucera E, Roncallo C, Pollastrini E, Bartolozzi F, De Pasquale T, Buonomo A, Gasbarrini G, Di Campli C, Schiavino D. Oral desensitizing treatment in food allergy: clinical and immunological results. *Aliment Pharmacol Ther.* 2003 Feb;17(3):459-65.

Patwardhan B, Gautam M. Botanical immunodrugs: scope and opportunities. *Drug Discov Today.* 2005 Apr 1;10(7):495-502.

Pauwels A, Decraene A, Blondeau K, Mertens V, Farre R, Proesmans M, Van Bleyenbergh P, Sifrim D, Dupont LJ. Bile acids in sputum and increased airway inflammation in patients with cystic fibrosis. *Chest.* 2011 Dec 1.

Payment P, Franco E, Richardson L, Siemiatyck, J. Gastrointestinal health effects associated with the consumption of drinking water produced by point-of-use domestic reverse-osmosis filtration units. *Appl. Environ. Microbiol.* 1991;57:945-948.

Peat JK, van den Berg RH, Green WF, Mellis CM, Leeder SR, Woolcock AJ. Changing prevalence of asthma in Australian children. *BMJ.* 1994;308:1591-1596.

Pehl C, Pfeiffer A, Waizenhoefer A, Wendl B, Schepp W. Effect of caloric density of a meal on lower oesophageal sphincter motility and gastro-oesophageal reflux in healthy subjects. *Aliment Pharmacol Ther.* 2001 Feb;15(2):233-9.

Pehl C, Waizenhoefer A, Wendl B, Schmidt T, Schepp W, Pfeiffer A. Effect of low and high fat meals on lower esophageal sphincter motility and gastroesophageal reflux in healthy subjects. *Am J Gastroenterol.* 1999 May;94(5):1192-6.

Pehowich DJ, Gomes AV, Barnes JA. Fatty acid composition and possible health effects of coconut constituents. *West Indian Med J.* 2000 Jun;49(2):128-33.

Pereira Rde S. Regression of gastroesophageal reflux disease symptoms using dietary supplementation with melatonin, vitamins and aminoacids: comparison with omeprazole. *J Pineal Res.* 2006 Oct;41(3):195-200.

Perez-Galvez A, Martin HD, Sies H, Stahl W. Incorporation of carotenoids from paprika oleoresin into human chylomicrons. *Br J Nutr.* 2003 Jun;89(6):787-93.

Perez-Pena R. Secrets of the Mummy's Medicine Chest. *NY Times.* 2005 Sept 10.

Pessi T, Sütas Y, Hurme M, Isolauri E. Interleukin-10 generation in atopic children following oral Lactobacillus rhamnosus GG. *Clin Exp Allergy.* 2000 Dec;30(12):1804-8.

Peters JI, McKinney JM, Smith B, Wood P, Forkner E, Galbreath AD. Impact of obesity in asthma: evidence from a large prospective disease management study. *Ann Allergy Asthma Immunol.* 2011 Jan;106(1):30-5.

Peterson CG, Hansson T, Skott A, Bengtsson U, Ahlstedt S, Magnussons J. Detection of local mast-cell activity in patients with food hypersensitivity. *J Investig Allergol Clin Immunol.* 2007;17(5):314-20.

Peterson KA, Samuelson WM, Ryujin DT, Young DC, Thomas KL, Hilden K, Fang JC. The role of gastroesophageal reflux in exercise-triggered asthma: a randomized controlled trial. *Dig Dis Sci.* 2009 Mar;54(3):564-71. 2008 Aug 8.

Petlevski R, Hadzija M, Slijepcević M, Juretić D, Petrik J. Glutathione S-transferases and malondialdehyde in the liver of NOD mice on short-term treatment with plant mixture extract P-9801091. *Phytother Res.* 2003 Apr;17(4):311-4.

Pfab F, Winhard M, Nowak-Machen M, Napadow V, Irnich D, Pawlik M, Bein T, Hansen E. Acupuncture in critically ill patients improves delayed gastric emptying: a randomized controlled trial. *Anesth Analg.* 2011 Jan;112(1):150-5.

Pfefferle PI, Sel S, Ege MJ, Büchele G, Blümer N, Krauss-Etschmann S, Herzum I, Albers CE, Lauener RP, Roponen M, Hirvonen MR, Vuitton DA, Riedler J, Brunekreef B, Dalphin JC, Braun-Fahrländer C, Pekkanen J, von Mutius E, Renz H; PASTURE Study Group. Cord blood allergen-specific IgE is associated with reduced IFN-gamma production by cord blood cells: the Protection against Allergy-Study in Rural Environments (PASTURE) Study. *J Allergy Clin Immunol.* 2008 Oct;122(4):711-6.

Pfundstein B, El Desouky SK, Hull WE, Haubner R, Erben G, Owen RW. Polyphenolic compounds in the fruits of Egyptian medicinal plants (Terminalia bellerica, Terminalia chebula and Terminalia horrida): characterization, quantitation and determination of antioxidant capacities. *Phytochemistry.* 2010 Jul;71(10):1132-48.

Physicians' Desk Reference. Montvale, NJ: Thomson, 2003-2008.

Piche T, des Varannes SB, Sacher-Huvelin S, Holst JJ, Cuber JC, Galmiche JP. Colonic fermentation influences lower esophageal sphincter function in gastroesophageal reflux disease. *Gastroenterology.* 2003 Apr;124(4):894-902.

Pierce SK, Klinman NR. Antibody-specific immunoregulation. *J Exp Med.* 1977 Aug 1;146(2):509-19.

Piesman M, Hwang I, Maydonovitch C, Wong RK. Nocturnal reflux episodes following the administration of a standardized meal. Does timing matter? *Am J Gastroenterol.* 2007 Oct;102(10):2128-34.

Piirainen L, Haahtela S, Helin T, Korpela R, Haahtela T, Vaarala O. Effect of Lactobacillus rhamnosus GG on rBet v1 and rMal d1 specific IgA in the saliva of patients with birch pollen allergy. *Ann Allergy Asthma Immunol.* 2008 Apr;100(4):338-42.

Pike MG, Heddle RJ, Boulton P, Turner MW, Atherton DJ. Increased intestinal permeability in atopic eczema. *J Invest Dermatol.* 1986 Feb;86(2):101-4.

Pines JM, Prabhu A, Hilton JA, Hollander JE, Datner EM. The effect of emergency department crowding on length of stay and medication treatment times in discharged patients with acute asthma. *Acad Emerg Med.* 2010 Aug;17(8):834-9.

Pitten FA, Scholler M, Krüger U, Effendy I, Kramer A. Filamentous fungi and yeasts on mattresses covered with different encasings. Eur J Dermatol. 2001 Nov-Dec;11(6):534-7.

Pitt-Rivers R, Trotter WR. *The Thyroid Gland.* London: Butterworth Publ, 1954.

Plaschke P, Janson C, Norrman E, Björnsson E, Ellbjär S, Järvholm B. Association between atopic sensitization and asthma and bronchial hyperresponsiveness in swedish adults: pets, and not mites, are the most important allergens. *J Allergy Clin Immunol.* 1999 Jul;104(1):58-65.

Plaut TE, Jones TB. *Dr. Tom Plaut's Asthma guide for people of all ages.* Amherst, MA: Pedipress, 1999.

Plaza V, Miguel E, Bellido-Casado J, Lozano MP, Ríos L, Bolíbar I. [Usefulness of the Guidelines of the Spanish Society of Pulmonology and Thoracic Surgery (SEPAR) in identifying the causes of chronic cough]. Arch Bronconeumol. 2006 Feb;42(2):68-73.

Plohmann B, Bader G, Hiller K, Franz G. Immunomodulatory and antitumoral effects of triterpenoid saponins. *Pharmazie.* 1997 Dec;52(12):953-7.

Poblocka-Olech L, Krauze-Baranowska M. SPE-HPTLC of procyanidins from the barks of different species and clones of Salix. *J Pharm Biomed Anal.* 2008 Nov 4;48(3):965-8.

Pohjavuori E, Viljanen M, Korpela R, Kuitunen M, Tiittanen M, Vaarala O, Savilahti E. Lactobacillus GG effect in increasing IFN-gamma production in infants with cow's milk allergy. *J Allergy Clin Immunol.* 2004 Jul;114(1):131-6.

Polito A, Aboab J, Annane D. The hypothalamic pituitary adrenal axis in sepsis. *Novartis Found Symp.* 2007;280:182-203.

Polk S, Sunyer J, Muñoz-Ortiz L, Barnes M, Torrent M, Figueroa C, Harris J, Vall O, Antó JM, Cullinan P. A prospective study of Fel d1 and Der p1 exposure in infancy and childhood wheezing. *Am J Respir Crit Care Med.* 2004 Aug 1;170(3):273-8.

Pollini F, Capristo C, Boner AL. Upper respiratory tract infections and atopy. *Int J Immunopathol Pharmacol.* 2010 Jan-Mar;23(1 Suppl):32-7.

Ponce J, Mearin F, Ponce M, Balboa A, Zapardiel J. Symptom profile in gastroesophageal reflux disease in untreated patients and those with persistent symptoms despite treatment. *Gastroenterol Hepatol.* 2010 Apr;33(4):271-9.

Ponsonby AL, McMichael A, van der Mei I. Ultraviolet radiation and autoimmune disease: insights from epidemiological research. *Toxicology.* 2002 Dec 27;181-182:71-8.

Postlethwait EM. Scavenger receptors clear the air. *J Clin Invest.* 2007 Mar;117(3):601-4.

Postma DS. Gender Differences in Asthma Development and Progression. *Gender Medicine.* 2007;4:S133-146.

Potterton D. (Ed.) *Culpeper's Color Herbal.* New York: Sterling, 1983.

Poulos LM, Waters AM, Correll PK, Loblay RH, Marks GB. Trends in hospitalizations for anaphylaxis, angioedema, and urticaria in Australia, 1993-1994 to 2004-2005. *J Allergy Clin Immunol.* 2007 Oct;120(4):878-84.

Pounder RE, Fraser AG. Gastric acid secretion and intragastric acidity: measurement in health and disease. *Baillieres Clin Gastroenterol.* 1993 Mar;7(1):55-80.

Prabha P, Karpagam T, Varalakshmi B, Packiavathy AS. Indigenous anti-ulcer activity of Musa sapientum on peptic ulcer. *Pharmacognosy Res.* 2011 Oct;3(4):232-8.

Pregun I, Herszényi L, Bakucz T, Banai J, Molnár L, Altorjay I, Orosz P, Csernay L, Tulassay Z. Novel aspects in the pathogenesis of gastroesophageal reflux disease. *Orv Hetil.* 2009 Oct 11;150(41):1883-7.

Prescott SL, Wickens K, Westcott L, Jung W, Currie H, Black PN, Stanley TV, Mitchell EA, Fitzharris P, Siebers R, Wu L, Crane J; Probiotic Study Group. Supplementation with Lactobacillus rhamnosus or Bifidobacterium lactis probiotics in pregnancy increases cord blood interferon-gamma and breast milk transforming growth factor-beta and immunoglobin A detection. *Clin Exp Allergy.* 2008 Oct;38(10):1606-14.

Priftis KN, Panagiotakos DB, Anthracopoulos MB, Papadimitriou A, Nicolaidou P. Aims, methods and preliminary findings of the Physical Activity, Nutrition and Allergies in Children Examined in Athens (PANACEA) epidemiological study. *BMC Public Health.* 2007 Jul 4;7:140.

Prioult G, Fliss I, Pecquet S. Effect of probiotic bacteria on induction and maintenance of oral tolerance to beta-lactoglobulin in gnotobiotic mice. *Clin Diagn Lab Immunol.* 2003 Sep;10(5):787-92.

Prucksunand C, Indrasukhsri B, Leethochawalit M, Hungspreugs K. Phase II clinical trial on effect of the long turmeric (Curcuma longa Linn) on healing of peptic ulcer. *Southeast Asian J Trop Med Public Health.* 2001 Mar;32(1):208-15.

REFERENCES

Pruthi S, Thapa MM. Infectious and inflammatory disorders. *Magn Reson Imaging Clin N Am.* 2009 Aug;17(3):423-38, v.

Qin HL, Zheng JJ, Tong DN, Chen WX, Fan XB, Hang XM, Jiang YQ. Effect of Lactobacillus plantarum enteral feeding on the gut permeability and septic complications in the patients with acute pancreatitis. *Eur J Clin Nutr.* 2008 Jul;62(7):923-30.

Qu C, Srivastava K, Ko J, Zhang TF, Sampson HA, Li XM. Induction of tolerance after establishment of peanut allergy by the food allergy herbal formula 2 is associated with up-regulation of interferon-gamma. *Clin Exp Allergy.* 2007 Jun;37(6):846-55.

Queiroz DM, Guerra JB, Rocha GA, Rocha AM, Santos A, De Oliveira AG, Cabral MM, Nogueira AM, De Oliveira CA. IL1B and IL1RN polymorphic genes and Helicobacter pylori cagA strains decrease the risk of reflux esophagitis. *Gastroenterology.* 2004 Jul;127(1):73-9.

Radon K, Danuser B, Iversen M, Jörres R, Monso E, Opravil U, Weber C, Donham KJ, Nowak D. Respiratory symptoms in European animal farmers. *Eur Respir J.* 2001 Apr;17(4):747-54.

Raherison C, Pénard-Morand C, Moreau D, Caillaud D, Charpin D, Kopferschmitt C, Lavaud F, Taytard A, Maesano IA. Smoking exposure and allergic sensitization in children according to maternal allergies. *Ann Allergy Asthma Immunol.* 2008 Apr;100(4):351-7.

Rahman MM, Bhattacharya A, Fernandes G. Docosahexaenoic acid is more potent inhibitor of osteoclast differentiation in RAW 264.7 cells than eicosapentaenoic acid. *J Cell Physiol.* 2008 Jan;214(1):201-9.

Raines D, Chester M, Diebold AE, Mamikunian P, Anthony CT, Mamikunian G, Woltering EA. A Prospective Evaluation of the Effect of Chronic Proton Pump Inhibitor Use on Plasma Biomarker Levels in Humans. *Pancreas.* 2012 Mar 28.

Raithel M, Weidenhiller M, Abel R, Baenkler HW, Hahn EG. Colorectal mucosal histamine release by mucosa oxygenation in comparison with other established clinical tests in patients with gastrointestinally mediated allergy. *World J Gastroenterol.* 2006 Aug 7;12(29):4699-705.

Rajendra S. Barrett's oesophagus in Asians—are ethnic differences due to genes or the environment? *J Intern Med.* 2011 Nov;270(5):421-7.

Raloff J. Ill Winds. *Science News.* 2001;160(14):218.

Ramieri V, Tarani L, Costantino F, Basile E, Liberati N, Rinna C, Cascone P, Colloridi F. Microdeletion 3q syndrome. *J Craniofac Surg.* 2011 Nov;22(6):2124-8.

Rampton DS, Murdoch RD, Sladen GE. Rectal mucosal histamine release in ulcerative colitis. *Clin Sci (Lond).* 1980 Nov;59(5):389-91.

Rancé F, Kanny G, Dutau G, Moneret-Vautrin DA. Food allergens in children. *Arch Pediatr.* 1999;6(Suppl 1):61S-66S.

Randal Bollinger R, Barbas AS, Bush EL, Lin SS, Parker W. Biofilms in the large bowel suggest an apparent function of the human vermiform appendix. *J Theor Biol.* 2007 Dec 21;249(4):826-31.

Ranjbaran Z, Keefer L, Stepanski E, Farhadi A, Keshavarzian A. The relevance of sleep abnormalities to chronic inflammatory conditions. *Inflamm Res.* 2007 Feb;56(2):51-7.

Rao NM. Protease inhibitors from ripened and unripened bananas. Biochem Int. 1991 May;24(1):13-22.

Rao SK, Rao PS, Rao BN. Preliminary investigation of the radiosensitizing activity of guduchi (Tinospora cordifolia) in tumor-bearing mice. *Phytother Res.* 2008 Nov;22(11):1482-9.

Rapin JR, Wiernsperger N. Possible links between intestinal permeablity and food processing: A potential therapeutic niche for glutamine. *Clinics (Sao Paulo).* 2010 Jun;65(6):635-43.

Rappoport J. Both sides of the pharmaceutical death coin. *Townsend Letter for Doctors and Patients.* 2006 Oct.

Rauha JP, Remes S, Heinonen M, Hopia A, Kähkönen M, Kujala T, Pihlaja K, Vuorela H, Vuorela P. Antimicrobial effects of Finnish plant extracts containing flavonoids and other phenolic compounds. *Int J Food Microbiol.* 2000 May 25;56(1):3-12.

Rauma A. Antioxidant status in vegetarians versus omnivores. *Nutrition.* 2003;16(2): 111-119.

Rautava S, Isolauri E. Cow's milk allergy in infants with atopic eczema is associated with aberrant production of interleukin-4 during oral cow's milk challenge. *J Pediatr Gastroenterol Nutr.* 2004 Nov;39(5):529-35.

Reavis KM. Management of the obese patient with gastroesophageal reflux disease. *Thorac Surg Clin.* 2011 Nov;21(4):489-98.

Recasens MA, Puig C, Ortiz-Santamaria V. Nutrition in systemic sclerosis.. *Reumatol Clin.* 2011 Dec 23.

Reger D, Goode S, Mercer E. *Chemistry: Principles & Practice.* Fort Worth, TX: Harcourt Brace, 1993.

Reha CM, Ebru A. Specific immunotherapy is effective in the prevention of new sensitivities. *Allergol Immunopathol (Madr).* 2007 Mar-Apr;35(2):44-51.

Remes-Troche JM, Ramírez-Cervantes KL, Vela ME. If no-acid, no-heartburn? New physiopathological mechanisms of the gastroesophageal reflux disease. *Rev Gastroenterol Mex.* 2011 Jul-Sep;76(3):237-46.

Reuter A, Lidholm J, Andersson K, Ostling J, Lundberg M, Scheurer S, Enrique E, Cistero-Bahima A, San Miguel-Moncin M, Ballmer-Weber BK, Vieths S. A critical assessment of allergen component-based in vitro diagnosis in cherry allergy across Europe. *Clin Exp Allergy.* 2006 Jun;36(6):815-23.

Reznik M, Sharif I, Ozuah PO. Rubbing ointments and asthma morbidity in adolescents. *J Altern Complement Med.* 2004 Dec;10(6):1097-9. Uu

Riccia DN, Bizzini F, Perilli MG, Polimeni A, Trinchieri V, Amicosante G, Cifone MG. Anti-inflammatory effects of Lactobacillus brevis (CD2) on periodontal disease. *Oral Dis.* 2007 Jul;13(4):376-85.

Riccioni G, Barbara M, Bucciarelli T, di Ilio C, D'Orazio N. Antioxidant vitamin supplementation in asthma. *Ann Clin Lab Sci.* 2007 Winter;37(1):96-101.

301

Riccioni G, Bucciarelli T, Mancini B, Di Ilio C, Della Vecchia R, D'Orazio N. Plasma lycopene and antioxidant vitamins in asthma: the PLAVA study. *J Asthma*. 2007 Jul-Aug;44(6):429-32.

Riccioni G, D'Orazio N. The role of selenium, zinc and antioxidant vitamin supplementation in the treatment of bronchial asthma: adjuvant therapy or not? *Expert Opin Investig Drugs*. 2005 Sep;14(9):1145-55.

Riccioni G, Di Stefano F, De Benedictis M, Verna N, Cavallucci E, Paolini F, Di Sciascio MB, Della Vecchia R, Schiavone C, Boscolo P, Conti P, Di Gioacchino M. Seasonal variability of non-specific bronchial responsiveness in asthmatic patients with allergy to house dust mites. *Allergy Asthma Proc*. 2001 Jan-Feb;22(1):5-9.

Rimkiene S, Ragazinskiene O, Savickiene N. The cumulation of Wild pansy (Viola tricolor L.) accessions: the possibility of species preservation and usage in medicine. *Medicina (Kaunas)*. 2003;39(4):411-6.

Rinne M, Kalliomaki M, Arvilommi H, Salminen S, Isolauri E. Effect of probiotics and breastfeeding on the bifidobacterium and lactobacillus/enterococcus microbiota and humoral immune responses. *J Pediatr*. 2005 Aug;147(2):186-91.

Río ME, Zago Beatriz L, Garcia H, Winter L. The nutritional status change the effectiveness of a dietary supplement of lactic bacteria on the emerging of respiratory tract diseases in children. *Arch Latinoam Nutr*. 2002 Mar;52(1):29-34.

Robert AM, Groult N, Six C, Robert L. The effect of procyanidolic oligomers on mesenchymal cells in culture II—Attachment of elastic fibers to the cells. *Pathol Biol*. 1990 Jun;38(6):601-7.

Roberts G, Lack G. Diagnosing peanut allergy with skin prick and specific IgE testing. *J Allergy Clin Immunol*. 2005 Jun;115(6):1291-6.

Robinson L, Cherewatenko VS, Reeves S. *Epicor: The Key to a Balanced Immune System*. Sherman Oaks, CA: Health Point, 2009.

Rodriguez J, Crespo JF, Burks W, Rivas-Plata C, Fernandez-Anaya S, Vives R, Daroca P. Randomized, double-blind, crossover challenge study in 53 subjects reporting adverse reactions to melon (Cucumis melo). *J Allergy Clin Immunol*. 2000 Nov;106(5):968-72.

Rodriguez-Fragoso L, Reyes-Esparza J, Burchiel SW, Herrera-Ruiz D, Torres E. Risks and benefits of commonly used herbal medicines in Mexico. *Toxicol Appl Pharmacol*. 2008 Feb 15;227(1):125-35.

Rodríguez-Ortiz PG, Muñoz-Mendoza D, Arias-Cruz A, González-Díaz SN, Herrera-Castro D, Vidaurri-Ojeda AC. Epidemiological characteristics of patients with food allergy assisted at Regional Center of Allergies and Clinical Immunology of Monterrey. *Rev Alerg Mex*. 2009 Nov-Dec;56(6):185-91.

Roduit C, Scholtens S, de Jongste JC, Wijga AH, Gerritsen J, Postma DS, Brunekreef B, Hoekstra MO, Aalberse R, Smit HA. Asthma at 8 years of age in children born by caesarean section. *Thorax*. 2009 Feb;64(2):107-13.

Roessler A, Friedrich U, Vogelsang H, Bauer A, Katz M, Hipler UC, Schmidt I, Jahreis G. The immune system in healthy adults and patients with atopic dermatitis seems to be affected differently by a probiotic intervention. *Clin Exp Allergy*. 2008 Jan;38(1):93-102.

Roger A, Justicia JL, Navarro LÁ, Eseverri JL, Ferrés J, Malet A, Alvà V. Observational study of the safety of an ultrarush sublingual immunotherapy regimen to treat rhinitis due to house dust mites. *Int Arch Allergy Immunol*. 2011;154(1):69-75. 2010 Jul 27.

Rohdewald P, Beil W. In vitro inhibition of Helicobacter pylori growth and adherence to gastric mucosal cells by Pycnogenol. *Phytother Res*. 2008 May;22(5):685-8.

Romeo J, Wärnberg J, Nova E, Díaz LE, González-Gross M, Marcos A. Changes in the immune system after moderate beer consumption. *Ann Nutr Metab*. 2007;51(4):359-66.

Romieu I, Barraza-Villarreal A, Escamilla-Núñez C, Texcalac-Sangrador JL, Hernandez-Cadena L, Díaz-Sánchez D, De Batlle J, Del Rio-Navarro BE. Dietary intake, lung function and airway inflammation in Mexico City school children exposed to air pollutants. *Respir Res*. 2009 Dec 10;10:122.

Ronteltap A, van Schaik J, Wensing M, Rynja FJ, Knulst AC, de Vries JH. Sensory testing of recipes masking peanut or hazelnut for double-blind placebo-controlled food challenges. *Allergy*. 2004 Apr;59(4):457-60. Clark S, Bock SA, Gaeta TJ, Brenner BE, Cydulka RK, Camargo CA; Multicenter Airway Research Collaboration-8 Investigators. Multicenter study of emergency department visits for food allergies. *J Allergy Clin Immunol*. 2004 Feb;113(2):347-52.

Rook GA, Hernandez-Pando R. Pathogenetic role, in human and murine tuberculosis, of changes in the peripheral metabolism of glucocorticoids and antiglucocorticoids. *Psychoneuroendocrinology*. 1997;22 Suppl 1:S109-13.

Ros E, Mataix J. Fatty acid composition of nuts—implications for cardiovascular health. *Br J Nutr*. 2006 Nov;96 Suppl 2:S29-35.

Rosenfeldt V, Benfeldt E, Valerius NH, Paerregaard A, Michaelsen KF. Effect of probiotics on gastrointestinal symptoms and small intestinal permeability in children with atopic dermatitis. *J Pediatr*. 2004 Nov;145(5):612-6.

Rosenkranz SK, Swain KE, Rosenkranz RR, Beckman B, Harms CA. Modifiable lifestyle factors impact airway health in non-asthmatic prepubescent boys but not girls. *Pediatr Pulmonol*. 2010 Dec 30.

Rozycki VR, Baigorria CM, Freyre MR, Bernard CM, Zannier MS, Charpentier M. Nutrient content in vegetable species from the Argentine Chaco. *Arch Latinoam Nutr*. 1997 Sep;47(3):265-70.

Rubin E., Farber JL. *Pathology*. 3rd Ed. Philadelphia: Lippincott-Raven, 1999.

Rudders SA, Espinola JA, Camargo CA Jr. North-south differences in US emergency department visits for acute allergic reactions. *Ann Allergy Asthma Immunol*. 2010 May;104(5):413-6.

Rynard PB, Palij B, Galloway CA, Roughley FR. Resperin inhalation treatment for chronic respiratory diseases. *Can Fam Physician*. 1968 Oct;14(10):70-1.

Saarinen KM, Juntunen-Backman K, Järvenpää AL, Klemetti P, Kuitunen P, Lope L, Renlund M, Siivola M, Vaarala O, Savilahti E. Breast-feeding and the development of cows' milk protein allergy. *Adv Exp Med Biol*. 2000;478:121-30.

REFERENCES

Sahagún-Flores JE, López-Peña LS, de la Cruz-Ramírez Jaimes J, García-Bravo MS, Peregrina-Gómez R, de Alba-García JE. Eradication of Helicobacter pylori: triple treatment scheme plus Lactobacillus vs. triple treatment alone. *Cir Cir.* 2007 Sep-Oct;75(5):333-6.

Sahakian NM, White SK, Park JH, Cox-Ganser JM, Kreiss K. Identification of mold and dampness-associated respiratory morbidity in 2 schools: comparison of questionnaire survey responses to national data. *J Sch Health.* 2008 Jan;78(1):32-7.

Sahin-Yilmaz A, Nocon CC, Corey JP. Immunoglobulin E-mediated food allergies among adults with allergic rhinitis. *Otolaryngol Head Neck Surg.* 2010 Sep;143(3):379-85.

Salem N, Wegher B, Mena P, Uauy R. Arachidonic and docosahexaenoic acids are biosynthesized from their 18-carbon precursors in human infants. *Proc Natl Acad Sci.* 1996;93:49-54.

Salim AS. Sulfhydryl-containing agents in the treatment of gastric bleeding induced by nonsteroidal anti-inflammatory drugs. *Can J Surg.* 1993 Feb;36(1):53-8.

Salmi H, Kuitunen M, Viljanen M, Lapatto R. Cow's milk allergy is associated with changes in urinary organic acid concentrations. *Pediatr Allergy Immunol.* 2010 Mar;21(2 Pt 2):e401-6.

Salminen S, Isolauri E, Salminen E. Clinical uses of probiotics for stabilizing the gut mucosal barrier: successful strains and future challenges. *Antonie Van Leeuwenhoek.* 1996 Oct;70(2-4):347-58.

Salom IL, Silvis SE, Doscherholmen A. Effect of cimetidine on the absorption of vitamin B12. *Scand J Gastroenterol.* 1982;17:129-31.

Salome CM, Marks GB. Sex, asthma and obesity: an intimate relationship? *Clin Exp Allergy.* 2011 Jan;41(1):6-8.

Salpietro CD, Gangemi S, Briuglia S, Meo A, Merlino MV, Muscolino G, Bisignano G, Trombetta D, Saija A. The almond milk: a new approach to the management of cow-milk allergy/intolerance in infants. *Minerva Pediatr.* 2005 Aug;57(4):173-80.

Salvi SS, Barnes PJ. Chronic obstructive pulmonary disease in non-smokers. *Lancet.* 2009 Aug 29;374(9691):733-43.

Sancho AI, Hoffmann-Sommergruber K, Alessandri S, Conti A, Giuffrida MG, Shewry P, Jensen BM, Skov P, Vieths S. Authentication of food allergen quality by physicochemical and immunological methods. *Clin Exp Allergy.* 2010 Jul;40(7):973-86.

Santos A, Dias A, Pinheiro JA. Predictive factors for the persistence of cow's milk allergy. *Pediatr Allergy Immunol.* 2010 Apr 27.

Sanz Ortega J, Martorell Aragonés A, Michavila Gómez A, Nieto García A; Grupo de Trabajo para el Estudio de la Alergia Alimentaria. Incidence of IgE-mediated allergy to cow's milk proteins in the first year of life. *An Esp Pediatr.* 2001 Jun;54(6):536-9.

Sato Y, Akiyama H, Matsuoka H, Sakata K, Nakamura R, Ishikawa S, Inakuma T, Totsuka M, Sugita-Konishi Y, Ebisawa M, Teshima R. Dietary carotenoids inhibit oral sensitization and the development of food allergy. *J Agric Food Chem.* 2010 Jun 23;58(12):7180-6.

Satyanarayana S, Sushruta K, Sarma GS, Srinivas N, Subba Raju GV. Antioxidant activity of the aqueous extracts of spicy food additives—evaluation and comparison with ascorbic acid in in-vitro systems. *J Herb Pharmacother.* 2004;4(2):1-10.

Savage JH, Kaeding AJ, Matsui EC, Wood RA. The natural history of soy allergy. *J Allergy Clin Immunol.* 2010 Mar;125(3):683-6.

Savilahti EM, Karinen S, Salo HM, Klemetti P, Saarinen KM, Klemola T, Kuitunen M, Hautaniemi S, Savilahti E, Vaarala O. Combined T regulatory cell and Th2 expression profile identifies children with cow's milk allergy. *Clin Immunol.* 2010 Jul;136(1):16-20.

Savilahti EM, Rantanen V, Lin JS, Karinen S, Saarinen KM, Goldis M, Mäkelä MJ, Hautaniemi S, Savilahti E, Sampson HA. Early recovery from cow's milk allergy is associated with decreasing IgE and increasing IgG4 binding to cow's milk epitopes. *J Allergy Clin Immunol.* 2010 Jun;125(6):1315-1321.e9.

Sazanova NE, Varnacheva LN, Novikova AV, Pletneva NB. Immunological aspects of food intolerance in children during first years of life. *Pediatriia.* 1992;(3):14-8.

Scadding G, Bjarnason I, Brostoff J, Levi AJ, Peters TJ. Intestinal permeability to 51Cr-labelled ethylenediaminetetraacetate in food-intolerant subjects. *Digestion.* 1989;42(2):104-9.

Scalabrin DM, Johnston WH, Hoffman DR, P'Pool VL, Harris CL, Mitmesser SH. Growth and tolerance of healthy term infants receiving hydrolyzed infant formulas supplemented with Lactobacillus rhamnosus GG: randomized, double-blind, controlled trial. *Clin Pediatr (Phila).* 2009 Sep;48(7):734-44.

Schauenberg P, Paris F. *Guide to Medicinal Plants.* New Canaan, CT: Keats Publ, 1977.

Schauss AG, Wu X, Prior RL, Ou B, Huang D, Owens J, Agarwal A, Jensen GS, Hart AN, Shanbrom E. Antioxidant capacity and other bioactivities of the freeze-dried Amazonian palm berry, Euterpe oleraceae mart. (acai). *J Agric Food Chem.* 2006 Nov 1;54(22):8604-10.

Schempp H, Weiser D, Elstner EF. Biochemical model reactions indicative of inflammatory processes. Activities of extracts from Fraxinus excelsior and Populus tremula. *Arzneimittelforschung.* 2000 Apr;50(4):362-72.

Schentag JJ, Goss TF. Pharmacokinetics and pharmacodynamics of acid-suppressive agents in patients with gastroesophageal reflux disease. *Am J Hosp Pharm.* 1993 Apr;50(4 Suppl 1):S7-10.

Schillaci D, Arizza V, Dayton T, Camarda L, Di Stefano V. In vitro anti-biofilm activity of Boswellia spp. oleogum resin essential oils. *Lett Appl Microbiol.* 2008 Nov;47(5):433-8.

Schmid B, Kötter I, Heide L. Pharmacokinetics of salicin after oral administration of a standardised willow bark extract. *Eur J Clin Pharmacol.* 2001 Aug;57(5):387-91.

Schmitt DA, Maleki SJ (2004) Comparing the effects of boiling, frying and roasting on the allergenicity of peanuts. *J Allergy Clin Immunol.* 113: S155.

Schmitz G, Ecker J. The opposing effects of n-3 and n-6 fatty acids. *Prog Lipid Res.* 2008 Mar;47(2):147-55.

Schnappinger M, Sausenthaler S, Linseisen J, Hauner H, Heinrich J. Fish consumption, allergic sensitisation and allergic diseases in adults. *Ann Nutr Metab.* 2009;54(1):67-74.

Schönfeld P. Phytanic Acid toxicity: implications for the permeability of the inner mitochondrial membrane to ions. *Toxicol Mech Methods.* 2004;14(1-2):47-52.

Schottner M, Gansser D, Spiteller G. Lignans from the roots of Urtica dioica and their metabolites bind to human sex hormone binding globulin (SHBG). *Planta Med.* 1997;65:529-532.

Schouten B, van Esch BC, Hofman GA, Boon L, Knippels LM, Willemsen LE, Garssen J. Oligosaccharide-induced whey-specific CD25(+) regulatory T-cells are involved in the suppression of cow milk allergy in mice. *J Nutr.* 2010 Apr;140(4):835-41.

Schroecksnadel S, Jenny M, Fuchs D. Sensitivity to sulphite additives. *Clin Exp Allergy.* 2010 Apr;40(4):688-9.

Schubert ML. Gastric secretion. *Curr Opin Gastroenterol.* 2003 Nov;19(6):519-25.

Schulick P. *Ginger: Common Spice & Wonder Drug.* Brattleboro, VT: Herbal Free Perss, 1996.

Schulz V, Hansel R, Tyler VE. *Rational Phytotherapy.* Berlin: Springer-Verlag; 1998.

Schumacher P. *Biophysical Therapy Of Allergies.* Stuttgart: Thieme, 2005.

Schütz K, Carle R, Schieber A. Taraxacum—a review on its phytochemical and pharmacological profile. *J Ethnopharmacol.* 2006 Oct 11;107(3):313-23.

Schwab D, Hahn EG, Raithel M. Enhanced histamine metabolism: a comparative analysis of collagenous colitis and food allergy with respect to the role of diet and NSAID use. *Inflamm Res.* 2003 Apr;52(4):142-7.

Schwab D, Müller S, Aigner T, Neureiter D, Kirchner T, Hahn EG, Raithel M. Functional and morphologic characterization of eosinophils in the lower intestinal mucosa of patients with food allergy. *Am J Gastroenterol.* 2003 Jul;98(7):1525-34.

Schwelberger HG. Histamine intolerance: a metabolic disease? *Inflamm Res.* 2010 Mar;59 Suppl 2:S219-21.

Scott-Taylor TH, O'B Hourihane J, Strobel S. Correlation of allergen-specific IgG subclass antibodies and T lymphocyte cytokine responses in children with multiple food allergies. *Pediatr Allergy Immunol.* 2010 Sep;21(6):935-44.

Scurlock AM, Jones SM. An update on immunotherapy for food allergy. *Curr Opin Allergy Clin Immunol.* 2010 Dec;10(6):587-93.

Sealey-Voyksner JA, Khosla C, Voyksner RD, Jorgenson JW. Novel aspects of quantitation of immunogenic wheat gluten peptides by liquid chromatography-mass spectrometry. *J Chromatogr A.* 2010 Jun 18;1217(25):4167-83.

Senapeschi Garita F, Pellicano R, Fagoonee S, Strona S, Cukier C, Magnoni CD. Obesity and gastro-esophageal reflux disease: a 2009 update. *Minerva Med.* 2009 Jun;100(3):213-9.

Senior F. Fallout. *New York Magazine.* Fall: 2003.

Senna G, Gani F, Leo G, Schiappoli M. Alternative tests in the diagnosis of food allergies. *Recenti Prog Med.* 2002 May;93(5):327-34.

Seo K, Jung S, Park M, Song Y, Choung S. Effects of leucocyanidines on activities of metabolizing enzymes and antioxidant enzymes. *Biol Pharm Bull.* 2001 May;24(5):592-3.

Seo SW, Koo HN, An HJ, Kwon KB, Lim BC, Seo EA, Ryu DG, Moon G, Kim HY, Kim HM, Hong SH. Taraxacum officinale protects against cholecystokinin-induced acute pancreatitis in rats. *World J Gastroenterol.* 2005 Jan 28;11(4):597-9.

Seppo L, Korpela R, Lönnerdal B, Metsäniitty L, Juntunen-Backman K, Klemola T, Paganus A, Vanto T. A follow-up study of nutrient intake, nutritional status, and growth in infants with cow milk allergy fed either a soy formula or an extensively hydrolyzed whey formula. *Am J Clin Nutr.* 2005 Jul;82(1):140-5.

Serra A, Cocuzza S, Poli G, La Mantia I, Messina A, Pavone P. Otologic findings in children with gastroesophageal reflux. *Int J Pediatr Otorhinolaryngol.* 2007 Nov;71(11):1693-7. 2007 Aug 22.

Sevar R. Audit of outcome in 455 consecutive patients treated with homeopathic medicines. *Homeopathy.* 2005 Oct;94(4):215-21.

Shahani KM, Meshbesher BF, Mangalampalli V. *Cultivate Health From Within.* Danbury, CT: Vital Health Publ, 2005.

Shaheen N, Provenzale D. The epidemiology of gastroesophageal reflux disease. *Am J Med Sci.* 2003 Nov;326(5):264-73.

Shaheen N, Ransohoff DF. Gastroesophageal reflux, barrett esophagus, and esophageal cancer: scientific. *JAMA.* 2002 Apr 17;287(15):1972-81.

Shaheen S, Potts J, Gnatiuc L, Makowska J, Kowalski ML, Joos G, van Zele T, van Durme Y, De Rudder I, Wöhrl S, Godnic-Cvar J, Skadhauge L, Thomsen G, Zuberbier T, Bergmann KC, Heinzerling L, Gjomarkaj M, Bruno A, Pace E, Bonini S, Fokkens W, Weersink EJ, Loureiro C, Todo-Bom A, Villanueva CM, Sanjuas C, Zock JP, Janson C, Burney P; Selenium and Asthma Research Integration project; GA2LEN. The relation between paracetamol use and asthma: a GA2LEN European case-control study. *Eur Respir J.* 2008 Nov;32(5):1231-6.

Shaheen SO, Newson RB, Rayman MP, Wong AP, Tumilty MK, Phillips JM, Potts JF, Kelly FJ, White PT, Burney PG. Randomised, double blind, placebo-controlled trial of selenium supplementation in adult asthma. *Thorax.* 2007 Jun;62(6):483-90.

Shakib F, Brown HM, Phelps A, Redhead R. Study of IgG sub-class antibodies in patients with milk intolerance. *Clin Allergy.* 1986 Sep;16(5):451-8.

Sharma P, Sharma BC, Puri V, Sarin SK. An open-label randomized controlled trial of lactulose and probiotics in the treatment of minimal hepatic encephalopathy. *Eur J Gastroent Hepatol.* 2008 Jun;20(6):506-11.

REFERENCES

Sharma SC, Sharma S, Gulati OP. Pycnogenol inhibits the release of histamine from mast cells. *Phytother Res.* 2003 Jan;17(1):66-9.

Sharnan J, Kumar I., Singh S. Comparison of results of skin prick tests, enzyme-linked immunosorbent assays and food challenges in children with respiratory allergy. *J Trop Pediatr.* 2001 Dec;47(6):367-8.

Shawcross DL, Wright G, Olde Damink SW, Jalan R. Role of ammonia and inflammation in minimal hepatic encephalopathy. *Metab Brain Dis.* 2007 Mar;22(1):125-38.

Shea KM, Trucker RT, Weber RW, Peden DB. Climate change and allergic disease. *Clin Rev Allergy Immunol.* 2008;6:443-453.

Shea-Donohue T, Stiltz J, Zhao A, Notari L. Mast Cells. *Curr Gastroenterol Rep.* 2010 Aug 14.

Shen FY, Lee MS, Jung SK. Effectiveness of pharmacopuncture for asthma: a systematic review and meta-analysis. *Evid Based Complement Alternat Med.* 2011;2011. pii: 678176.

Sheth SS, Waserman S, Kagan R, Alizadehfar R, Primeau MN, Elliot S, St Pierre Y, Wickett R, Joseph L, Harada L, Dufresne C, Allen M, Allen M, Godefroy SB, Clarke AE. Role of food labels in accidental exposures in food-allergic individuals in Canada. *Ann Allergy Asthma Immunol.* 2010 Jan;104(1):60-5.

Shi S, Zhao Y, Zhou H, Zhang Y, Jiang X, Huang K. Identification of antioxidants from Taraxacum mongolicum by high-performance liquid chromatography-diode array detection-radical-scavenging detection-electrospray ionization mass spectrometry and nuclear magnetic resonance experiments. *J Chromatogr A.* 2008 Oct 31;1209(1-2):145-52

Shi S, Zhou H, Zhang Y, Huang K, Liu S. Chemical constituents from Neo-Taraxacum siphonathum. *Zhongguo Zhong Yao Za Zhi.* 2009 Apr;34(8):1002-4.

Shi SY, Zhou CX, Xu Y, Tao QF, Bai H, Lu FS, Lin WY, Chen HY, Zheng W, Wang LW, Wu YH, Zeng S, Huang KX, Zhao Y, Li XK, Qu J. Studies on chemical constituents from herbs of Taraxacum mongolicum. *Zhongguo Zhong Yao Za Zhi.* 2008 May;33(10):1147-57.

Shibata H, Nabe T, Yamamura H, Kohno S. l-Ephedrine is a major constituent of Mao-Bushi-Saishin-To, one of the formulas of Chinese medicine, which shows immediate inhibition after oral administration of passive cutaneous anaphylaxis in rats. *Inflamm Res.* 2000 Aug;49(8):398-403.

Shichinohe K, Shimizu M, Kurokawa K. Effect of M-711 on experimental asthma in rats. *J Vet Med Sci.* 1996 Jan;58(1):55-9.

Shimauchi H, Mayanagi G, Nakaya S, Minamibuchi M, Ito Y, Yamaki K, Hirata H. Improvement of periodontal condition by probiotics with Lactobacillus salivarius WB21: a randomized, double-blind, placebo-controlled study. *J Clin Periodontol.* 2008 Oct;35(10):897-905.

Shimoi T, Ushiyama H, Kan K, Saito K, Kamata K, Hirokado M. Survey of glycoalkaloids content in the various potatoes. *Shokuhin Eiseigaku Zasshi.* 2007 Jun;48(3):77-82.

Shimoyama Y, Kusano M, Kawamura O, Zai H, Kuribayashi S, Higuchi T, Nagoshi A, Maeda M, Mori M. High-viscosity liquid meal accelerates gastric emptying. *Neurogastroenterol Motil.* 2007 Nov;19(11):879-86.

Shishehbor F, Behroo L, Ghafouriyan Broujerdnia M, Namjoyan F, Latifi SM. Quercetin effectively quells peanut-induced anaphylactic reactions in the peanut sensitized rats. *Iran J Allergy Asthma Immunol.* 2010 Mar;9(1):27-34.

Shishodia S, Harikumar KB, Dass S, Ramawat KG, Aggarwal BB. The guggul for chronic diseases: ancient medicine, modern targets. *Anticancer Res.* 2008 Nov-Dec;28(6A):3647-64.

Shivpuri DN, Menon MP, Parkash D. Preliminary studies in Tylophora indica in the treatment of asthma and allergic rhinitis. *J Assoc Physicians India.* 1968 Jan;16(1):9-15.

Shivpuri DN, Menon MP, Prakash D. A crossover double-blind study on Tylophora indica in the treatment of asthma and allergic rhinitis. *J Allergy.* 1969 Mar;43(3):145-50.

Shivpuri DN, Singhal SC, Parkash D. Treatment of asthma with an alcoholic extract of Tylophora indica: a cross-over, double-blind study. *Ann Allergy.* 1972; 30:407-12.

Shoaf, K., Muvey, G.L., Armstrong, G.D., Hutkins, R.W. (2006) Prebiotic galactooligosaccharides reduce adherence of enteropathogenic Escherichia coli to tissue culture cells. *Infect Immun.* Dec;74(12):6920-8.

Sicherer SH, Muñoz-Furlong A, Godbold JH, Sampson HA. US prevalence of self-reported peanut, tree nut, and sesame allergy: 11-year follow-up. *J Allergy Clin Immunol.* 2010 Jun;125(6):1322-6.

Sicherer SH, Noone SA, Koerner CB, Christie L, Burks AW, Sampson HA. Hypoallergenicity and efficacy of an amino acid-based formula in children with cow's milk and multiple food hypersensitivities. *J Pediatr.* 2001 May;138(5):688-93.

Sicherer SH, Sampson HA. Food allergy. *J Allergy Clin Immunol.* 2010 Feb;125(2 Suppl 2):S116-25.

Sidoroff V, Hyvärinen M, Piippo-Savolainen E, Korppi M. Lung function and overweight in school aged children after early childhood wheezing. *Pediatr Pulmonol.* 2010 Dec 30.

Sigstedt SC, Hooten CJ, Callewaert MC, Jenkins AR, Romero AE, Pullin MJ, Kornienko A, Lowrey TK, Slambrouck SV, Steelant WF. Evaluation of aqueous extracts of Taraxacum officinale on growth and invasion of breast and prostate cancer cells. *Int J Oncol.* 2008 May;32(5):1085-90.

Silman AJ, MacGregor AJ, Thomson W, Holligan S, Carthy D, Farhan A, Ollier WE. Twin concordance rates for rheumatoid arthritis: results from a nationwide study. *Br J Rheumatol.* 1993 Oct;32(10):903-7.

Silva MF, Kamphorst AO, Hayashi EA, Bellio M, Carvalho CR, Faria AM, Sabino KC, Coelho MG, Nobrega A, Tavares D, Silva AC. Innate profiles of cytokines implicated on oral tolerance correlate with low- or high-suppression of humoral response. *Immunology.* 2010 Jul;130(3):447-57.

Simeone D, Miele E, Boccia G, Marino A, Troncone R, Staiano A. Prevalence of atopy in children with chronic constipation. *Arch Dis Child.* 2008 Dec;93(12):1044-7.

Simões EA, Carbonell-Estrany X, Rieger CH, Mitchell I, Fredrick L, Groothuis JR; Palivizumab Long-Term Respiratory Outcomes Study Group. The effect of respiratory syncytial virus on subsequent recurrent wheezing in atopic and nonatopic children. *J Allergy Clin Immunol.* 2010 Aug;126(2):256-62. 2010 Jul 10.

Simons FER. What's in a name? The allergic rhinitis-asthma connection. *Clin Exp All Rev.* 2003;3:9-17.

Simonte SJ, Ma S, Mofidi S, Sicherer SH. Relevance of casual contact with peanut butter in children with peanut allergy. *J Allergy Clin Immunol.* 2003 Jul;112(1):180-2.

Simopoulos AP. Essential fatty acids in health and chronic disease. *Am J Clin Nutr.* 1999 Sep;70(3 Suppl):560S-569S.

Simpson A, Tan VY, Winn J, Svensén M, Bishop CM, Heckerman DE, Buchan I, Custovic A. Beyond atopy: multiple patterns of sensitization in relation to asthma in a birth cohort study. *Am J Respir Crit Care Med.* 2010 Jun 1;181(11):1200-6.

Simpson AB, Yousef E, Hossain J. Association between peanut allergy and asthma morbidity. *J Pediatr.* 2010 May;156(5):777-81.

Singer P, Shapiro H, Theilla M, Anbar R, Singer J, Cohen J. Anti-inflammatory properties of omega-3 fatty acids in critical illness: novel mechanisms and an integrative perspective. *Intensive Care Med.* 2008 Sep;34(9):1580-92.

Singh BB, Khorsan R, Vinjamury SP, Der-Martirosian C, Kizhakkeveettil A, Anderson TM. Herbal treatments of asthma: a systematic review. *J Asthma.* 2007 Nov;44(9):685-98.

Singh G, Triadafilopoulos G. Epidemiology of NSAID induced gastrointestinal complications. *J Rheumatol.* 1999;26 Suppl 56 :18-24.

Department of Medicine, Division of Immunology, Stanford University School of Medicine, Palo Alto, California 94304, USA.

Singh S, Khajuria A, Taneja SC, Johri RK, Singh J, Qazi GN. Boswellic acids: A leukotriene inhibitor also effective through topical application in inflammatory disorders. *Phytomedicine.* 2008 Jun;15(6-7):400-7.

Singh S, Khajuria A, Taneja SC, Khajuria RK, Singh J, Johri RK, Qazi GN. The gastric ulcer protective effect of boswellic acids, a leukotriene inhibitor from Boswellia serrata, in rats. *Phytomedicine.* 2008 Jun;15(6-7):408-15.

Singh V, Jain NK. Asthma as a cause for, rather than a result of, gastroesophageal reflux. *J Asthma.* 1983;20(4):241-3. 3.

Sirvent S, Palomares O, Vereda A, Villalba M, Cuesta-Herranz J, Rodríguez R. nsLTP and profilin are allergens in mustard seeds: cloning, sequencing and recombinant production of Sin a 3 and Sin a 4. *Clin Exp Allergy.* 2009 Dec;39(12):1929-36.

Skamstrup Hansen K, Vieths S, Vestergaard H, Skov PS, Bindslev-Jensen C, Poulsen LK. Seasonal variation in food allergy to apple. *J Chromatogr B Biomed Sci Appl.* 2001 May 25;756(1-2):19-32.

Skripak JM, Nash SD, Rowley H, Brereton NH, Oh S, Hamilton RG, Matsui EC, Burks AW, Wood RA. A randomized, double-blind, placebo-controlled study of milk oral immunotherapy for cow's milk allergy. *J Allergy Clin Immunol.* 2008 Dec;122(6):1154-60.

Sletten GB, Halvorsen R, Egaas E, Halstensen TS. Changes in humoral responses to beta-lactoglobulin in tolerant patients suggest a particular role for IgG4 in delayed, non-IgE-mediated cow's milk allergy. *Pediatr Allergy Immunol.* 2006 Sep;17(6):435-43.

Smith J. *Genetic Roulette: The Documented Health Risks of Genetically Engineered Foods.* White River Jct, Vermont: Chelsea Green, 2007.

Smith K, Warholak T, Armstrong E, Leib M, Rehfeld R, Malone D. Evaluation of risk factors and health outcomes among persons with asthma. *J Asthma.* 2009 Apr;46(3):234-7.

Smith LJ, Holbrook JT, Wise R, Blumenthal M, Dozor AJ, Mastronarde J, Williams L; American Lung Association Asthma Clinical Research Centers. Dietary intake of soy genistein is associated with lung function in patients with asthma. *J Asthma.* 2004;41(8):833-43.

Smith S, Sullivan K. Examining the influence of biological and psychological factors on cognitive performance in chronic fatigue syndrome: a randomized, double-blind, placebo-controlled, crossover study. *Int J Behav Med.* 2003;10(2):162-73.

Snow JM, Severson PA. Complications of adjustable gastric banding. *Surg Clin North Am.* 2011 Dec;91(6):1249-64, ix.

Sofic E, Denisova N, Youdim K, Vatrenjak-Velagic V, De Filippo C, Mehmedagic A, Causevic A, Cao G, Joseph JA, Prior RL. Antioxidant and pro-oxidant capacity of catecholamines and related compounds. Effects of hydrogen peroxide on glutathione and sphingomyelinase activity in pheochromocytoma PC12 cells: potential relevance to age-related diseases. *J Neural Transm.* 2001;108(5):541-57.

Soleo L, Colosio C, Alinovi R, Guarneri D, Russo A, Lovreglio P, Vimercati L, Birindelli S, Cortesi I, Flore C, Carta P, Colombi A, Parrinello G, Ambrosi L. Immunologic effects of exposure to low levels of inorganic mercury. *Med Lav.* 2002 May-Jun;93(3):225-32.

Sompamit K, Kukongviriyapan U, Nakmareong S, Pannangpetch P, Kukongviriyapan V. Curcumin improves vascular function and alleviates oxidative stress in non-lethal lipopolysaccharide-induced endotoxaemia in mice. *Eur J Pharmacol.* 2009 Aug 15;616(1-3):192-9.

Sonibare MA, Gbile ZO. Ethnobotanical survey of anti-asthmatic plants in South Western Nigeria. *Afr J Tradit Complement Altern Med.* 2008 Jun 18;5(4):340-5.

Sontag SJ, O'Connell S, Khandelwal S, Greenlee H, Schnell T, Nemchausky B, Chejfec G, Miller T, Seidel J, Sonnenberg A. Asthmatics with gastroesophageal reflux: long term results of a randomized trial of medical and surgical antireflux therapies. *Am J Gastroenterol.* 2003 May;98(5):987-99.

Sood MR, Rudolph CD. Gastroesophageal reflux in adolescents. *Adolesc Med Clin.* 2004 Feb;15(1):17-36, vii-viii.

Sosa M, Saavedra P, Valero C, Guañabens N, Nogués X, del Pino-Montes J, Mosquera J, Alegre J, Gómez-Alonso C, Muñoz-Torres M, Quesada M, Pérez-Cano R, Jódar E, Torrijos A, Lozano-Tonkin C, Díaz-Curiel M; GIUMO

REFERENCES

Study Group. Inhaled steroids do not decrease bone mineral density but increase risk of fractures: data from the GIUMO Study Group. J Clin Densitom. 2006 Apr-Jun;9(2):154-8.

Soyka F, Edmonds A. *The Ion Effect: How Air Electricity Rules your Life and Health*. Bantam, New York: Bantam, 1978.

Spence A. *Basic Human Anatomy*. Menlo Park, CA: Benjamin/Commings, 1986.

Spergel JM, Andrews T, Brown-Whitehorn TF, Beausoleil JL, Liacouras CA. Treatment of eosinophilic esophagitis with specific food elimination diet directed by a combination of skin prick and patch tests. *Ann Allergy Asthma Immunol*. 2005 Oct;95(4):336-43.

Spiller G. *The Super Pyramid*. New York: HRS Press, 1993.

Sporik R, Squillace SP, Ingram JM, Rakes G, Honsinger RW, Platts-Mills TA. Mite, cat, and cockroach exposure, allergen sensitisation, and asthma in children: a case-control study of three schools. *Thorax*. 1999 Aug;54(8):675-80.

Srivastava K, Zou ZM, Sampson HA, Dansky H, Li XM. Direct Modulation of Airway Reactivity by the Chinese Anti-Asthma Herbal Formula ASHMI. *J Allergy Clin Immunol*. 2005;115:S7.

Srivastava KD, Qu C, Zhang T, Goldfarb J, Sampson HA, Li XM. Food Allergy Herbal Formula-2 silences peanut-induced anaphylaxis for a prolonged posttreatment period via IFN-gamma-producing CD8+ T cells. *J Allergy Clin Immunol*. 2009 Feb;123(2):443-51.

Srivastava KD, Zhang TF, Qu C, Sampson HA, Li XM. Silencing Peanut Allergy: A Chinese Herbal Formula, FAHF-2, Completely Blocks Peanut-induced Anaphylaxis for up to 6 Months Following Therapy in a Murine Model Of Peanut Allergy. *J Allergy Clin Immunol*. 2006;117:S328.

Staden U, Rolinck-Werninghaus C, Brewe F, Wahn U, Niggemann B, Beyer K. Specific oral tolerance induction in food allergy in children: efficacy and clinical patterns of reaction. *Allergy*. 2007 Nov;62(11):1261-9.

Stahl SM. Selective histamine H1 antagonism: novel hypnotic and pharmacologic actions challenge classical notions of antihistamines. CNS Spectr. 2008 Dec;13(12):1027-38.

State Pharmacopoeia Commission of The People's Republic of China. *Pharmacopoeia of the People's Republic of China*. Beijing: Chemical Industry Press; 2005.

Steinman HA, Le Roux M, Potter PC. Sulphur dioxide sensitivity in South African asthmatic children. *S Afr Med J*. 1993 Jun;83(6):387-90.

Stenberg JA, Hambäck PA, Ericson L. Herbivore-induced "rent rise" in the host plant may drive a diet breadth enlargement in the tenant. *Ecology*. 2008 Jan;89(1):126-33.

Stengler M. *The Natural Physician's Healing Therapies*. Stamford, CT: Bottom Line Books, 2008.

Stensrud T, Carlsen KH. Can one single test protocol for provoking exercise-induced bronchoconstriction also be used for assessing aerobic capacity? *Clin Respir J*. 2008 Jan;2(1):47-53.

Steurer-Stey C, Russi EW, Steurer J: Complementary and alternative medicine in asthma: do they work? *Swiss Med Wkly*. 2002, 132:338-344.

Stillerman A, Nachtsheim C, Li W, Albrecht M, Waldman J. Efficacy of a novel air filtration pillow for avoidance of perennial allergens in symptomatic adults. *Ann Allergy Asthma Immunol*. 2010 May;104(5):440-9.

Stirapongsasuti P, Tanglertsampan C, Aunhachoke K, Sangasapaviliya A. Anaphylactic reaction to phuk-waan-ban in a patient with latex allergy. *J Med Assoc Thai*. 2010 May;93(5):616-9.

Stordal K, Johannesdottir GB, Bentsen BS, Knudsen PK, Carlsen KC, Closs O, Handeland M, Holm HK, Sandvik L. Acid suppression does not change respiratory symptoms in children with asthma and gastro-oesophageal reflux disease. *Arch Dis Child*. 2005 Sep;90(9):956-60.

Stratiki Z, Costalos C, Sevastiadou S, Kastanidou O, Skouroliakou M, Giakoumatou A, Petrohilou V. The effect of a bifidobacter supplemented bovine milk on intestinal permeability of preterm infants. *Early Hum Dev*. 2007 Sep;83(9):575-9.

Strinnholm A, Brulin C, Lindh V. Experiences of double-blind, placebo-controlled food challenges (DBPCFC): a qualitative analysis of mothers' experiences. *J Child Health Care*. 2010 Jun;14(2):179-88.

Stutius LM, Sheehan WJ, Rangsithienchai P, Bharmanee A, Scott JE, Young MC, Dioun AF, Schneider LC, Phipatanakul W. Characterizing the relationship between sesame, coconut, and nut allergy in children. *Pediatr Allergy Immunol*. 2010 Dec;21(8):1114-8.

Sugawara G, Nagino M, Nishio H, Ebata T, Takagi K, Asahara T, Nomoto K, Nimura Y. Perioperative synbiotic treatment to prevent postoperative infectious complications in biliary cancer surgery: a randomized controlled trial. *Ann Surg*. 2006 Nov;244(5):706-14.

Sulman FG, Levy D, Lunkan L, Pfeifer Y, Tal E. New methods in the treatment of weather sensitivity. *Fortschr Med*. 1977 Mar 17;95(11):746-52.

Sulman FG. Migraine and headache due to weather and allied causes and its specific treatment. *Ups J Med Sci Suppl*. 1980;31:41-4.

Sumantran VN, Kulkarni AA, Harsulkar A, Wele A, Koppikar SJ, Chandwaskar R, Gaire V, Dalvi M, Wagh UV. Hyaluronidase and collagenase inhibitory activities of the herbal formulation Triphala guggulu. *J Biosci*. 2007 Jun;32(4):755-61.

Sumiyoshi M, Sakanaka M, Kimura Y. Effects of Red Ginseng extract on allergic reactions to food in Balb/c mice. *J Ethnopharmacol*. 2010 Aug 14.

Sumona AA, Hossain MA, Musa AK, Shamsuzzaman AK, Mahmud MC, Khan MS, Ahmed S, Begum Z, Zahan NA, Ahmed MU, Debnath CR, Anne RA. Anti H.pylori IgM in symptomatic and asymptomatic population. *Mymensingh Med J*. 2009 Jan;18(1):18-20.

Sung JH, Lee JO, Son JK, Park NS, Kim MR, Kim JG, Moon DC. Cytotoxic constituents from Solidago virga-aurea var. gigantea MIQ. *Arch Pharm Res*. 1999 Dec;22(6):633-7.

Suomalainen H, Isolauri E. New concepts of allergy to cow's milk. *Ann Med.* 1994 Aug;26(4):289-96.

Sur S, Camara M, Buchmeier A, Morgan S, Nelson HS. Double-blind trial of pyridoxine (vitamin B6) in the treatment of steroid-dependent asthma. Ann Allergy. 1993 Feb;70(2):147-52.

Sütas Y, Kekki OM, Isolauri E. Late onset reactions to oral food challenge are linked to low serum interleukin-10 concentrations in patients with atopic dermatitis and food allergy. *Clin Exp Allergy.* 2000 Aug;30(8):1121-8.

Svanes C, Heinrich J, Jarvis D, Chinn S, Omenaas E, Gulsvik A, Künzli N, Burney P. Pet-keeping in childhood and adult asthma and hay fever: European community respiratory health survey. *J Allergy Clin Immunol.* 2003 Aug;112(2):289-300.

Svendsen AJ, Holm NV, Kyvik K, *et al.* Relative importance of genetic effects in rheumatoid arthritis: historical cohort study of Danish nationwide twin population. *BMJ* 2002;324(7332): 264-266.

Sweeney B, Vora M, Ulbricht C, Basch E. Evidence-based systematic review of dandelion (Taraxacum officinale) by natural standard research collaboration. *J Herb Pharmacother.* 2005;5(1):79-93.

Swiderska-Kielbik S, Krakowiak A, Wiszniewska M, Dudek W, Walusiak-Skorupa J, Krawczyk-Szulc P, Michowicz A, Palczyński C. Health hazards associated with occupational exposure to birds. *Med Pr.* 2010;61(2):213-22.

Szyf M, McGowan P, Meaney MJ. The social environment and the epigenome. *Environ Mol Mutagen.* 2008 Jan;49(1):46-60.

Tack J, Bisschops R, Koek G, Sifrim D, Lerut T, Janssens J. Dietary restrictions during ambulatory monitoring of duodenogastroesophageal reflux. *Dig Dis Sci.* 2003 Jul;48(7):1213-20.

Takada Y, Ichikawa H, Badmaev V, Aggarwal BB. Acetyl-11-keto-beta-boswellic acid potentiates apoptosis, inhibits invasion, and abolishes osteoclastogenesis by suppressing NF-kappa B and NF-kappa B-regulated gene expression. *J Immunol.* 2006 Mar 1;176(5):3127-40.

Takahashi N, Eisenhuth G, Lee I, Schachtele C, Laible N, Binion S. Nonspecific antibacterial factors in milk from cows immunized with human oral bacterial pathogens. *J Dairy Sci.* 1992 Jul;75(7):1810-20.

Takasaki M, Konoshima T, Tokuda H, Masuda K, Arai Y, Shiojima K, Ageta H. Anti-carcinogenic activity of Taraxacum plant. I. *Biol Pharm Bull.* 1999 Jun;22(6):602-5.

Takeda K, Suzuki T, Shimada SI, Shida K, Nanno M, Okumura K. Interleukin-12 is involved in the en-hancement of human natural killer cell activity by Lactobacillus casei Shirota. *Clin Exp Immunol.* 2006 Oct;146(1):109-15.

Tamaoki J, Chiyotani A, Sakai A, Takemura H, Konno K. Effect of menthol vapour on airway hyperresponsiveness in patients with mild asthma. *Respir Med.* 1995 Aug;89(7):503-4.

Tamura M, Shikina T, Morihana T, Hayama M, Kajimoto O, Sakamoto A, Kajimoto Y, Watanabe O, Nonaka C, Shida K, Nanno M. Effects of probiotics on allergic rhinitis induced by Japanese cedar pol-len: randomized double-blind, placebo-controlled clinical trial. *Int Arch Allergy Imml.* 2007;143(1):75-82.

Tan DX, Manchester LC, Reiter RJ, Qi WB, Karbownik M, Calvo JR. Significance of melatonin in antioxidative defense system: reactions and products. *Biol Signals Recept.* 2000 May-Aug;9(3-4):137-59.

Taniguchi C, Homma M, Takano O, Hirano T, Oka K, Aoyagi Y, Niitsuma T, Hayashi T. Pharmacological effects of urinary products obtained after treatment with saiboku-to, a herbal medicine for bronchial asthma, on type IV allergic reaction. *Planta Med.* 2000 Oct;66(7):607-11.

Tapiero H, Ba GN, Couvreur P, Tew KD. Polyunsaturated fatty acids (PUFA) and eicosanoids in human health and pathologies. *Biomed Pharmacother.* 2002 Jul;56(5):215-22.

Tapsell LC, Hemphill I, Cobiac L, Patch CS, Sullivan DR, Fenech M, Roodenrys S, Keogh JB, Clifton PM, Williams PG, Fazio VA, Inge KE. Health benefits of herbs and spices: the past, the present, the future. *Med J Aust.* 2006 Aug 21;185(4 Suppl):S4-24.

Tasli L, Mat C, De Simone C, Yazici H. Lactobacilli lozenges in the management of oral ulcers of Behçet's syndrome. *Clin Exp Rheumatol.* 2006 Sep-Oct;24(5 Suppl 42):S83-6.

Taussig SJ, Batkin S. Bromelain, the enzyme complex of pineapple (Ananas comosus) and its clinical application. An update. *J Ethnopharmacol.* 1988 Feb-Mar;22(2):191-203.

Taylor AL, Dunstan JA, Prescott SL. Probiotic supplementation for the first 6 months of life fails to reduce the risk of atopic dermatitis and increases the risk of allergen sensitization in high-risk children: a randomized controlled trial. *J Allergy Clin Immunol.* 2007 Jan;119(1):184-91.

Taylor AL, Hale J, Wiltschut J, Lehmann H, Dunstan JA, Prescott SL. Effects of probiotic supplementation for the first 6 months of life on allergen- and vaccine-specific immune responses. *Clin Exp Allergy.* 2006 Oct;36(10):1227-35.

Taylor RB, Lindquist N, Kubanek J, Hay ME. Intraspecific variation in palatability and defensive chemistry of brown seaweeds: effects on herbivore fitness. *Oecologia.* 2003 Aug;136(3):412-23.

Teitelbaum J. *From Fatigue to Fantastic.* New York: Avery, 2001.

Terheggen-Lagro SW, Khouw IM, Schaafsma A, Wauters EA. Safety of a new extensively hydrolysed formula in children with cow's milk protein allergy: a double blind crossover study. *BMC Pediatr.* 2002 Oct 14;2:10.

Terracciano L, Bouygue GR, Sarratud T, Veglia F, Martelli A, Fiocchi A. Impact of dietary regimen on the duration of cow's milk allergy: a random allocation study. *Clin Exp Allergy.* 2010 Apr;40(4):637-42.

Tesse R, Schieck M, Kabesch M. Asthma and endocrine disorders: Shared mechanisms and genetic pleiotropy. *Mol Cell Endocrinol.* 2010 Dec 4. [ahead of print] .

Thakkar K, Boatright RO, Gilger MA, El-Serag HB. Gastroesophageal reflux and asthma in children: a systematic. *Pediatrics.* 2010 Apr;125(4):e925-30.

Thakkar K, Boatright RO, Gilger MA, El-Serag HB. Gastroesophageal reflux and asthma in children: a systematic review. *Pediatrics.* 2010 Apr;125(4):e925-30. 2010 Mar 29.

Tham KW, Zuraimi MS, Koh D, Chew FT, Ooi PL. Associations between home dampness and presence of molds with asthma and allergic symptoms among young children in the tropics. *Pediatr Allergy Immunol.* 2007 Aug;18(5):418-24.

REFERENCES

Thampithak A, Jaisin Y, Meesarapee B, Chongthammakun S, Piyachaturawat P, Govitrapong P, Supavilai P, Sanvarinda Y. Transcriptional regulation of iNOS and COX-2 by a novel compound from Curcuma comosa in lipopolysaccharide-induced microglial activation. *Neurosci Lett.* 2009 Sep 22;462(2):171-5.

Theler B, Brockow K, Ballmer-Weber BK. Clinical presentation and diagnosis of meat allergy in Switzerland and Southern Germany. *Swiss Med Wkly.* 2009 May 2;139(17-18):264-70.

Theofilopoulos AN, Kono DH. The genes of systemic autoimmunity. *Proc Assoc Am Physicians.* 1999;111(3): 228-240.

Thiruvengadam KV, Haranath K, Sudarsan S, Sekar TS, Rajagopal KR, Zacharian MG, Devarajan TV. Tylophora indica in bronchial asthma (a controlled comparison with a standard anti-asthmatic drug). *J Indian Med Assoc.* 1978 Oct 1;71(7):172-6.

Thomas M. Are breathing exercises an effective strategy for people with asthma? *Nurs Times.* 2009 Mar 17-23;105(10):22-7.

Thomas, R.G., Gebhardt, S.E. 2008. Nutritive value of pomegranate fruit and juice. *Maryland Dietetic Association Annual Meeting, USDA-ARS.* 2008 April 11.

Thompson T, Lee AR, Grace T. Gluten contamination of grains, seeds, and flours in the United States: a pilot study. *J Am Diet Assoc.* 2010 Jun;110(6):937-40.

Tierra L. *The Herbs of Life.* Freedom, CA: Crossing Press, 1992.

Tierra M. *The Way of Herbs.* New York: Pocket Books, 1990.

Tisserand R. *The Art of Aromatherapy.* New York: Inner Traditions, 1979.

Tiwari M. *Ayurveda: A Life of Balance.* Rochester, VT: Healing Arts, 1995.

Tlaskalová-Hogenová H, Stepánková R, Hudcovic T, Tucková L, Cukrowska B, Lodinová-Zádníková R, Kozáková H, Rossmann P, Bártová J, Sokol D, Funda DP, Borovská D, Reháková Z, Sinkora J, Hofman J, Drastich P, Kokesová A. Commensal bacteria (normal microflora), mucosal immunity and chronic inflammatory and autoimmune diseases. *Immunol Lett.* 2004 May 15;93(2-3):97-108.

Todd GR, Acerini CL, Ross-Russell R, Zahra S, Warner JT, McCance D. Survey of adrenal crisis associated with inhaled corticosteroids in the United Kingdom. *Arch Dis Child.* 2002 Dec;87(6):457-61.

Tolia V, Lin CH, Kuhns LR. Gastric emptying using three different formulas in infants with gastroesophageal reflux. *J Pediatr Gastroenterol Nutr.* 1992 Oct;15(3):297-301.

Tolín Hernani M, Crespo Medina M, Luengo Herrero V, Martínez López C, Salcedo Posadas A, Alvarez Calatayud G, Morales Pérez JL, Sánchez Sánchez C. Comparison between conventional ph measurement and multichannel intraluminal esophageal impedance in children with respiratory disorders.. *An Pediatr (Barc).* 2011 Nov 25.

Tominaga K, Iwakiri R, Fujimoto K, Fujiwara Y, Tanaka M, Shimoyama Y, Umegaki E, Higuchi K, Kusano M, Arakawa T; and the GERD 4 Study Group. Rikkunshito improves symptoms in PPI-refractory GERD patients: a prospective, randomized, multicenter trial in Japan. *J Gastroenterol.* 2011 Nov 15.

Tonkal AM, Morsy TA. An update review on Commiphora molmol and related species. *J Egypt Soc Parasitol.* 2008 Dec;38(3):763-96.

Topçu G, Erenler R, Cakmak O, Johansson CB, Celik C, Chai HB, Pezzuto JM. Diterpenes from the berries of Juniperus excelsa. *Phytochemistry.* 1999 Apr;50(7):1195-9.

Tordesillas L, Pacios LF, Palacín A, Cuesta-Herranz J, Madero M, Díaz-Perales A. Characterization of IgE epitopes of Cuc m 2, the major melon allergen, and their role in cross-reactivity with pollen profilins. *Clin Exp Allergy.* 2010 Jan;40(1):174-81.

Torrent M, Sunyer J, Muñoz L, Cullinan P, Iturriaga MV, Figueroa C, Vall O, Taylor AN, Anto JM. Early-life domestic aeroallergen exposure and IgE sensitization at age 4 years. *J Allergy Clin Immunol.* 2006 Sep;118(3):742-8.

Towers GH. FAHF-1 purporting to block peanut-induced anaphylaxis. *J Allergy Clin Immunol.* 2003 May;111(5):1140; author reply 1140-1.

Towle A. *Modern Biology.* Austin: Harcourt Brace, 1993.

Trojanová I, Rada V, Kokoska L, Vlková E. The bifidogenic effect of Taraxacum officinale root. *Fitoterapia.* 2004 Dec;75(7-8):760-3.

Troncone R, Caputo N, Florio G, Finelli E. Increased intestinal sugar permeability after challenge in children with cow's milk allergy or intolerance. *Allergy.* 1994 Mar;49(3):142-6.

Trout L, King M, Feng W, Inglis SK, Ballard ST. Inhibition of airway liquid secretion and its effect on the physical properties of airway mucus. *Am J Physiol.* 1998 Feb;274(2 Pt 1):L258-63.

Tsai JC, Tsai S, Chang WC. Comparison of two Chinese medical herbs, Huangbai and Qianniuzi, on influence of short circuit current across the rat intestinal epithelia. *J Ethnopharmacol.* 2004 Jul;93(1):21-5.

Tsong T. Deciphering the language of cells. *Trends in Biochem Sci.* 1989;14:89-92.

Tsou VM, Bishop PR. Gastroesophageal reflux in children. *Otolaryngol Clin North Am.* 1998 Jun;31(3):419-34.

Tucker KL, Olson B, Bakun P, Dallal GE, Selhub J, Rosenberg IH. Breakfast cereal fortified with folic acid, vitamin B-6, and vitamin B-12 increases vitamin concentrations and reduces homocysteine concentrations: a randomized trial. *Am J Clin Nutr.* 2004 May;79(5):805-11.

Tulk HM, Robinson LE. Modifying the n-6/n-3 polyunsaturated fatty acid ratio of a high-saturated fat challenge does not acutely attenuate postprandial changes in inflammatory markers in men with meta-bolic syndrome. *Metabolism.* 2009 Jul 20.

Tunnicliffe WS, Burge PS, Ayres JG. Effect of domestic concentrations of nitrogen dioxide on airway responses to inhaled allergen in asthmatic patients. *Lancet.* 1994 Dec 24-31;344(8939-8940):1733-6.

Tunnicliffe WS, Fletcher TJ, Hammond K, Roberts K, Custovic A, Simpson A, Woodcock A, Ayres JG. Sensitivity and exposure to indoor allergens in adults with differing asthma severity. *Eur Respir J.* 1999 Mar;13(3):654-9.

309

Tursi A, Brandimarte G, Giorgetti GM, Elisei W. Mesalazine and/or Lactobacillus casei in maintaining long-term remission of symptomatic uncomplicated diverticular disease of the colon. *Hepatogastroenterology.* 2008 May-Jun;55(84):916-20.

U.S. Food and Drug Administration *Guidance for Industry Botanical Drug Products.* CfDEaR. 2000

Uddenfeldt M, Janson C, Lampa E, Leander M, Norbäck D, Larsson L, Rask-Andersen A. High BMI is related to higher incidence of asthma, while a fish and fruit diet is related to a lower- Results from a long-term follow-up study of three age groups in Sweden. *Respir Med.* 2010 Jul;104(7):972-80.

Udupa AL, Udupa SL, Guruswamy MN. The possible site of anti-asthmatic action of Tylophora asthmatica on pituitary-adrenal axis in albino rats. *Planta Med.* 1991 Oct;57(5):409-13.

Ueno H, Yoshioka K, Matsumoto T. Usefulness of the skin index in predicting the outcome of oral challenges in children. *J Investig Allergol Clin Immunol.* 2007;17(4):207-10.

Ueno M, Adachi A, Fukumoto T, Nishitani N, Fujiwara N, Matsuo H, Kohno K, Morita E. Analysis of causative allergen of the patient with baker's asthma and wheat-dependent exercise-induced anaphylaxis (WDEIA). *Arerugi.* 2010 May;59(5):552-7.

Ukabam SO, Mann RJ, Cooper BT. Small intestinal permeability to sugars in patients with atopic eczema. *Br J Dermatol.* 1984 Jun;110(6):649-52.

Ulrich RS, Simons RF, Losito BD, Fiorito E, Miles MA, Zelson M. Stress recovery during exposure to natural and urban environments. *J Envir Psychol.* 1991;11:201-30.

Ulualp SO, Toohill RJ, Hoffmann R, Shaker R. Possible relationship of gastroesophagopharyngeal acid reflux with pathogenesis of chronic sinusitis. *Am J Rhinol.* 1999 May-Jun;13(3):197-202.

Uno K, Iijima K, Hatta W, Koike T, Abe Y, Asano N, Kusaka G, Shimosegawa T. Direct measurement of gastroesophageal reflux episodes in patients with squamous cell carcinoma by 24-h pH-impedance monitoring. *Am J Gastroenterol.* 2011 Nov;106(11):1923-9.

Unsel M, Sin AZ, Ardeniz O, Erdem N, Ersoy R, Gulbahar O, Mete N, Kokuludağ A. New onset egg allergy in an adult. *J Investig Allergol Clin Immunol.* 2007;17(1):55-8.

Upadhyay AK, Kumar K, Kumar A, Mishra HS. Tinospora cordifolia (Willd.) Hook. f. and Thoms. (Guduchi) - validation of the Ayurvedic pharmacology through experimental and clinical studies. *Int J Ayurveda Res.* 2010 Apr;1(2):112-21.

Urata Y, Yoshida S, Irie Y, Tanigawa T, Amayasu H, Nakabayashi M, Akahori K. Treatment of asthma patients with herbal medicine TJ-96: a randomized controlled trial. *Respir Med.* 2002 Jun;96(6):469-74.

Usai P, Manca R, Cuomo R, Lai MA, Russo L, Boi MF. Effect of gluten-free diet on preventing recurrence of gastroesophageal reflux disease-related symptoms in adult celiac patients with nonerosive reflux disease. *J Gastroenterol Hepatol.* 2008 Sep;23(9):1368-72.

Vally H, Thompson PJ, Misso NL. Changes in bronchial hyperresponsiveness following high- and low-sulphite wine challenges in wine-sensitive asthmatic patients. *Clin Exp Allergy.* 2007 Jul;37(7):1062-6.

van Beelen VA, Roeleveld J, Mooibroek H, Sijtsma L, Bino RJ, Bosch D, Rietjens IM, Alink GM. A comparative study on the effect of algal and fish oil on viability and cell proliferation in Caco-2 cells. *Food Chem Toxicol.* 2007 May;45(5):716-24.

Van den Bulck J, Eggermont S. Media use as a reason for meal skipping and fast eating in secondary school children. *J Hum Nutr Diet.* 2006 Apr;19(2):91-100.

van Elburg RM, Uil JJ, de Monchy JG, Heymans HS. Intestinal permeability in pediatric gastroenterology. *Scand J Gastroenterol Suppl.* 1992;194:19-24.

van Huisstede A, Braunstahl GJ. Obesity and asthma: co-morbidity or causal relationship? *Monaldi Arch Chest Dis.* 2010 Sep;73(3):116-23.

van Kampen V, Merget R, Rabstein S, Sander I, Bruening T, Broding HC, Keller C, Muesken H, Overlack A, Schultze-Werninghaus G, Walusiak J, Raulf-Heimsoth M. Comparison of wheat and rye flour solutions for skin prick testing: a multi-centre study (Stad 1). *Clin Exp Allergy.* 2009 Dec;39(12):1896-902.

van Odijk J, Peterson CG, Ahlstedt S, Bengtsson U, Borres MP, Hulthén L, Magnusson J, Hansson T. Measurements of eosinophil activation before and after food challenges in adults with food hypersensitivity. *Int Arch Allergy Immunol.* 2006;140(4):334-41.

van Zwol A, Moll HA, Fetter WP, van Elburg RM. Glutamine-enriched enteral nutrition in very low birthweight infants and allergic and infectious diseases at 6 years of age. *Paediatr Perinat Epidemiol.* 2011 Jan;25(1):60-6.

Vanderhoof JA, Moran JR, Harris CL, Merkel KL, Orenstein SR. Efficacy of a pre-thickened infant formula: a multicenter, double-blind, randomized, placebo-controlled parallel group trial in 104 infants with symptomatic gastroesophageal reflux. *Clin Pediatr (Phila).* 2003 Jul-Aug;42(6):483-95.

Vanderhoof JA. Probiotics in allergy management. *J Pediatr Gastroenterol Nutr.* 2008 Nov;47 Suppl 2:S38-40.

VanHaitsma TA, Mickleborough T, Stager JM, Koceja DM, Lindley MR, Chapman R. Comparative effects of caffeine and albuterol on the bronchoconstrictor response to exercise in asthmatic athletes. *Int J Sports Med.* 2010 Apr;31(4):231-6.

Vanto T, Helppilä S, Juntunen-Backman K, Kalimo K, Klemola T, Korpela R, Koskinen P. Prediction of the development of tolerance to milk in children with cow's milk hypersensitivity. *J Pediatr.* 2004 Feb;144(2):218-22.

Vargas C, Bustos P, Diaz PV, Amigo H, Rona RJ. Childhood environment and atopic conditions, with emphasis on asthma in a Chilean agricultural area. *J Asthma.* 2008 Jan-Feb;45(1):73-8.

Varonier HS, de Haller J, Schopfer C. Prevalence of allergies in children and adolescents. *Helv Paediatr Acta.* 1984;39:129-136.

REFERENCES

Varraso R, Fung TT, Barr RG, Hu FB, Willett W, Camargo CA Jr. Prospective study of dietary patterns and chronic obstructive pulmonary disease among US women. *Am J Clin Nutr.* 2007 Aug;86(2):488-95.

Varraso R, Fung TT, Hu FB, Willett W, Camargo CA. Prospective study of dietary patterns and chronic obstructive pulmonary disease among US men. *Thorax.* 2007 Sep;62(9):786-91. 2007 May 15.

Varraso R, Jiang R, Barr RG, Willett WC, Camargo CA Jr. Prospective study of cured meats consumption and risk of chronic obstructive pulmonary disease in men. *Am J Epidemiol.* 2007 Dec 15;166(12):1438-45. 2007 Sep 4. 17785711; .

Vassallo MF, Banerji A, Rudders SA, Clark S, Mullins RJ, Camargo CA Jr. Season of birth and food allergy in children. *Ann Allergy Asthma Immunol.* 2010 Apr;104(4):307-13.

Vempati R, Bijlani RL, Deepak KK. The efficacy of a comprehensive lifestyle modification programme based on yoga in the management of bronchial asthma: a randomized controlled trial. *BMC Pulm Med.* 2009 Jul 30;9:37.

Vendt N, Grünberg H, Tuure T, Malminiemi O, Wuolijoki E, Tillmann V, Sepp E, Korpela R. Growth during the first 6 months of life in infants using formula enriched with Lactobacillus rhamnosus GG: double-blind, randomized trial. *J Hum Nutr Diet.* 2006 Feb;19(1):51-8.

Venkatachalam KV. Human 3'-phosphoadenosine 5'-phosphosulfate (PAPS) synthase: biochemistry, molecular biology and genetic deficiency. *IUBMB Life.* 2003 Jan;55(1):1-11.

Venkatesan N, Punithavathi D, Babu M. Protection from acute and chronic lung diseases by curcumin. *Adv Exp Med Biol.* 2007;595:379-405.

Venter C, Hasan Arshad S, Grundy J, Pereira B, Bernie Clayton C, Voigt K, Higgins B, Dean T. Time trends in the prevalence of peanut allergy: three cohorts of children from the same geographical location in the UK. *Allergy.* 2010 Jan;65(1):103-8.

Venter C, Meyer R. Session 1: Allergic disease: The challenges of managing food hypersensitivity. *Proc Nutr Soc.* 2010 Feb;69(1):11-24.

Venter C, Pereira B, Grundy J, Clayton CB, Arshad SH, Dean T. Prevalence of sensitization reported and objectively assessed food hypersensitivity amongst six-year-old children: A population-based study. *Pediatr Allergy Immunol.* 2006;17: 356-363.

Venter C, Pereira B, Grundy J, Clayton CB, Roberts G, Higgins B, Dean T. Incidence of parentally reported and clinically diagnosed food hypersensitivity in the first year of life. *J Allergy Clin Immunol.* 2006;117: 1118-1124.

Ventura MT, Polimeno L, Amoruso AC, Gatti F, Annoscia E, Marinaro M, Di Leo E, Matino MG, Buquicchio R, Bonini S, Tursi A, Francavilla A. Intestinal permeability in patients with adverse reactions to food. *Dig Liver Dis.* 2006 Oct;38(10):732-6.

Venturi A, Gionchetti P, Rizzello F, Johansson R, Zucconi E, Brigidi P, Matteuzzi D, Campieri M. Impact on the composition of the faecal flora by a new probiotic preparation: preliminary data on maintenance treatment of patients with ulcerative colitis. *Aliment Pharmacol Ther.* 1999 Aug;13(8):1103-8.

Vera FM, Manzaneque JM, Maldonado EF, Carranque GA, Rodriguez FM, Blanca MJ, Morell M. Subjective Sleep Quality and hormonal modulation in long-term yoga practitioners. *Biol Psychol.* 2009 Jul;81(3):164-8.

Verhasselt V. Oral tolerance in neonates: from basics to potential prevention of allergic disease. *Mucosal Immunol.* 2010 Jul;3(4):326-33.

Verstege A, Mehl A, Rolinck-Werninghaus C, Staden U, Nocon M, Beyer K, Niggemann B. The predictive value of the skin prick test weal size for the outcome of oral food challenges. Clin Exp Allergy. 2005 Sep;35(9):1220-6. Rolinck-Werninghaus C, Staden U, Mehl A, Hamelmann E, Beyer K, Niggemann B. Specific oral tolerance induction with food in children: transient or persistent effect on food allergy? *Allergy.* 2005 Oct;60(10):1320-2.

Vidgren HM, Agren JJ, Schwab U, Rissanen T, Hanninen O, Uusitupa MI. Incorporation of n-3 fatty acids into plasma lipid fractions, and erythrocyte membranes and platelets during dietary supplementation with fish, fish oil, and docosahexaenoic acid-rich oil among healthy young men. *Lipids.* 1997 Jul;32(7):697-705.

Viinanen A, Munhbayarlah S, Zevgee T, Narantsetseg L, Naidansuren Ts, Koskenvuo M, Helenius H, Terho EO. Prevalence of asthma, allergic rhinoconjuctivitis and allergic sensitization in Mongolia. *Allergy.* 2005;60:1370-1377.

Vila R, Mundina M, Tomi F, Furlán R, Zacchino S, Casanova J, Cañigueral S. Composition and antifungal activity of the essential oil of Solidago chilensis. *Planta Med.* 2002 Feb;68(2):164-7.

Viljanen M, Kuitunen M, Haahtela T, Juntunen-Backman K, Korpela R, Savilahti E. Probiotic effects on faecal inflammatory markers and on faecal IgA in food allergic atopic eczema/dermatitis syndrome infants. *Pediatr Allergy Immunol.* 2005 Feb;16(1):65-71.

Viljanen M, Savilahti E, Haahtela T, Juntunen-Backman K, Korpela R, Poussa T, Tuure T, Kuitunen M. Probiotics in the treatment of atopic eczema/dermatitis syndrome in infants: a double-blind placebo-controlled trial. *Allergy.* 2005 Apr;60(4):494-500.

Vinson JA, Proch J, Bose P. MegaNatural((R)) Gold Grapeseed Extract: In Vitro Antioxidant and In Vivo Human Supplementation Studies. *J Med Food.* 2001 Spring;4(1):17-26.

Visitsunthorn N, Pacharn P, Jirapongsananuruk O, Weeravejsukit S, Sripramong C, Sookrung N, Bunnag C. Comparison between Siriraj mite allergen vaccine and standardized commercial mite vaccine by skin prick testing in normal Thai adults. *Asian Pac J Allergy Immunol.* 2010 Mar;28(1):41-5.

Visness CM, London SJ, Daniels JL, Kaufman JS, Yeatts KB, Siega-Riz AM, Liu AH, Calatroni A, Zeldin DC. Association of obesity with IgE levels and allergy symptoms in children and adolescents: results from the National Health and Nutrition Examination Survey 2005-2006. *J Allergy Clin Immunol.* 2009 May;123(5):1163-9, 1169.e1-4.

Visness CM, London SJ, Daniels JL, Kaufman JS, Yeatts KB, Siega-Riz AM, Calatroni A, Zeldin DC. Association of childhood obesity with atopic and nonatopic asthma: results from the National Health and Nutrition Examination Survey 1999-2006. *J Asthma.* 2010 Sep;47(7):822-9.

Vlieg-Boerstra BJ, Dubois AE, van der Heide S, Bijleveld CM, Wolt-Plompen SA, Oude Elberink JN, Kukler J, Jansen DF, Venter C, Duiverman EJ. Ready-to-use introduction schedules for first exposure to allergenic foods in children at home. *Allergy.* 2008 Jul;63(7):903-9.

Vlieg-Boerstra BJ, van der Heide S, Bijleveld CM, Kukler J, Duiverman EJ, Wolt-Plompen SA, Dubois AE. Dietary assessment in children adhering to a food allergen avoidance diet for allergy prevention. *Eur J Clin Nutr.* 2006 Dec;60(12):1384-90.

Voicekovska JG, Orlikov GA, Karpov IuG, Teibe U, Ivanov AD, Baidekalne I, Voicehovskis NV, Maulins E. External respiration function and quality of life in patients with bronchial asthma in correction of selenium deficiency. *Ter Arkh.* 2007;79(8):38-41.

Voïtsekhovskaia IuG, Skesters A, Orlikov GA, Silova AA, Rusakova NE, Larmane LT, Karpov IuG, Ivanov AD, Maulins E. Assessment of some oxidative stress parameters in bronchial asthma patients beyond add-on selenium supplementation. *Biomed Khim.* 2007 Sep-Oct;53(5):577-84.

Vojdani A. Antibodies as predictors of complex autoimmune diseases. *Int J Immunopathol Pharmacol.* 2008 Apr-Jun;21(2):267-78.

von Berg A, Filipiak-Pittroff B, Krämer U, Link E, Bollrath C, Brockow I, Koletzko S, Grübl A, Heinrich J, Wichmann HE, Bauer CP, Reinhardt D, Berdel D; GINIplus study group. Preventive effect of hydrolyzed infant formulas persists until age 6 years: long-term results from the German Infant Nutritional Intervention Study (GINI). *J Allergy Clin Immunol.* 2008 Jun;121(6):1442-7.

von Berg A, Koletzko S, Grübl A, Filipiak-Pittroff B, Wichmann HE, Bauer CP, Reinhardt D, Berdel D; German Infant Nutritional Intervention Study Group. The effect of hydrolyzed cow's milk formula for allergy prevention in the first year of life: the German Infant Nutritional Intervention Study, a randomized double-blind trial. *J Allergy Clin Immunol.* 2003 Mar;111(3):533-40.

von Kruedener S, Schneider W, Elstner EF. A combination of Populus tremula, Solidago virgaurea and Fraxinus excelsior as an anti-inflammatory and antirheumatic drug. A short review. *Arzneimittelforschung.* 1995 Feb;45(2):169-71.

von Mutius E, Vercelli D. Farm living: effects on childhood asthma and allergy. *Nat Rev Immunol.* 2010 Dec;10(12):861-8. 2010 Nov 9.

Vulevic J, Drakoularakou A, Yaqoob P, Tzortzis G and Gibson GR; Modulation of the fecal microflora profile and immune function by a novel trans-galactooligosaccharide mixture (B-GOS) in healthy elderly volunteers. *Am J Clin Nutr.* 1988 88;1438-1446.

Waddell L. Food allergies in children: the difference between cow's milk protein allergy and food intolerance. *J Fam Health Care.* 2010;20(3):104.

Wagner JS, DiBonaventura MD, Balu S, Buchner D. The burden of diurnal and nocturnal gastroesophageal reflux disease symptoms. *Expert Rev Pharmacoecon Outcomes Res.* 2011 Dec;11(6):739-49.

Wahler D, Gronover CS, Richter C, Foucu F, Twyman RM, Moerschbacher BM, Fischer R, Muth J, Prufer D. Polyphenoloxidase silencing affects latex coagulation in Taraxacum spp. *Plant Physiol.* 2009 Jul 15.

Waite DA, Eyles EF, Tonkin SL, O'Donnell TV. Asthma prevalence in Tokelauan children in two environments. *Clin Allergy.* 1980;10:71-75.

Walker S, Wing A. Allergies in children. *J Fam Health Care.* 2010;20(1):24-6.

Walker WA. Antigen absorption from the small intestine and gastrointestinal disease. *Pediatr Clin North Am.* 1975 Nov;22(4):731-46.

Walker WA. Antigen handling by the small intestine. *Clin Gastroenterol.* 1986 Jan;15(1):1-20.

Walle UK, Walle T. Transport of the cooked-food mutagen 2-amino-1-methyl-6-phenylimidazo- 4,5-b pyridine (PhIP) across the human intestinal Caco-2 cell monolayer: role of efflux pumps. *Carcinogenesis.* 1999 Nov;20(11):2153-7.

Walsh MG. Toxocara infection and diminished lung function in a nationally representative sample from the United States population. *Int J Parasitol.* 2010 Nov 8.

Walsh SJ, Rau LM: Autoimmune diseases: a leading cause of death among young and middle-aged women in the United States. *Am J Public Health* 2000, 90(9): 1463-1466.

Wang G, Liu CT, Wang ZL, Yan CL, Luo FM, Wang L, Li TQ. Effects of Astragalus membranaceus in promoting T-helper cell type 1 polarization and interferon-gamma production by up-regulating T-bet expression in patients with asthma. *Chin J Integr Med.* 2006 Dec;12(4):262-7.

Wang H, Chang B, Wang B. The effect of herbal medicine including astragalus membranaceus (fisch) bge, codonpsis pilosula and glycyrrhiza uralensis fisch on airway responsiveness. *Zhonghua Jie He He Hu Xi Za Zhi.* 1998 May;21(5):287-8.

Wang H, Liu B, Jiang JL. Clinical features of gastroesophageal reflux disease in geriatric patients. *Zhongguo Yi Xue Ke Xue Yuan Xue Bao.* 2002 Apr;24(2):178-80.

Wang J, Lin J, Bardina L, Goldis M, Nowak-Wegrzyn A, Shreffler WG, Sampson HA. Correlation of IgE/IgG4 milk epitopes and affinity of milk-specific IgE antibodies with different phenotypes of clinical milk allergy. *J Allergy Clin Immunol.* 2010 Mar;125(3):695-702, 702.e1-702.e6.

Wang J, Patil SP, Yang N, Ko J, Lee J, Noone S, Sampson HA, Li XM. Safety, tolerability, and immunologic effects of a food allergy herbal formula in food allergic individuals: a randomized, double-blinded, placebo-controlled, dose escalation, phase 1 study. *Ann Allergy Asthma Immunol.* 2010 Jul;105(1):75-84.

Wang J. Management of the patient with multiple food allergies. *Curr Allergy Asthma Rep.* 2010 Jul;10(4):271-7.

REFERENCES

Wang JL, Shaw NS, Kao MD. Magnesium deficiency and its lack of association with asthma in Taiwanese elementary school children. *Asia Pac J Clin Nutr.* 2007;16 Suppl 2:579-84.

Wang JS, Hung WP. The effects of a swimming intervention for children with asthma. *Respirology.* 2009 Aug;14(6):838-42.

Wang KY, Li SN, Liu CS, Perng DS, Su YC, Wu DC, Jan CM, Lai CH, Wang TN, Wang WM. Effects of ingesting Lacto-bacillus- and Bifidobacterium-containing yogurt in subjects with colonized Helicobacter pylori. *Am J Clin Nutr.* 2004 Sep;80(3):737-41.

Wang X, Kang GH, Campan M, Weisenberger DJ, Long TI, Cozen W, Bernstein L, Wu AH, Siegmund KD, Shibata D, Laird PW. Epigenetic subgroups of esophageal and gastric adenocarcinoma with differential GATA5 DNA methylation associated with clinical and lifestyle factors. *PLoS One.* 2011;6(10):e25985.

Wang YH, Yang CP, Ku MS, Sun HL, Lue KH. Efficacy of nasal irrigation in the treatment of acute sinusitis in children. *Int J Pediatr Otorhinolaryngol.* 2009 Dec;73(12):1696-701. 2009 Sep 27.

Wang YM, Huan GX. *Utilization of Classical Formulas.* Beijing, China: Chinese Medicine and Pharmacology Publishing Co, 1998.

Waring G, Levy D. Challenging adverse reactions in children with food allergies. *Paediatr Nurs.* 2010 Jul;22(6):16-22.

Waser M, Michels KB, Bieli C, Flöistrup H, Pershagen G, von Mutius E, Ege M, Riedler J, Schram-Bijkerk D, Brunekreef B, van Hage M, Lauener R, Braun-Fahrländer C; PARSIFAL Study team. Inverse association of farm milk consumption with asthma and allergy in rural and suburban populations across Europe. *Clin Exp Allergy.* 2007 May;37(5):661-70.

Watkins BA, Hannon K, Ferruzzi M, Li Y. Dietary PUFA and flavonoids as deterrents for environmental pollutants. *J Nutr Biochem.* 2007 Mar;18(3):196-205.

Watson R. Preedy VR. Botanical Medicine in Clinical Practice. Oxfordshire: CABI, 2008.

Watzl B, Bub A, Blockhaus M, Herbert BM, Lührmann PM, Neuhäuser-Berthold M, Rechkemmer G. Prolonged tomato juice consumption has no effect on cell-mediated immunity of well-nourished elderly men and women. *J Nutr.* 2000 Jul;130(7):1719-23.

Webber CM, England RW. Oral allergy syndrome: a clinical, diagnostic, and therapeutic challenge. *Ann Allergy Asthma Immunol.* 2010 Feb;104(2):101-8; quiz 109-10, 117.

Webster D, Taschereau P, Belland RJ, Sand C, Rennie RP. Antifungal activity of medicinal plant extracts; preliminary screening studies. *J Ethnopharmacol.* 2008 Jan 4;115(1):140-6.

Wei A, Shibamoto T. Antioxidant activities and volatile constituents of various essential oils. *J Agric Food Chem.* 2007 Mar 7;55(5):1737-42.

Wei WI, Lam KH, Choi S, Wong J. Late problems after pharyngolaryngoesophagectomy and pharyngogastric anastomosis for cancer of the larynx and hypopharynx. Am J Surg. 1984 Oct;148(4):509-13.

Weiler JM, Layton T, Hunt M. Asthma in United States Olympic athletes who participated in the 1996 Summer Games. J Allergy Clin Immunol. 1998 Nov;102(5):722-6. 7.

Weiner MA. *Secrets of Fijian Medicine.* Berkeley, CA: Univ. of Calif., 1969.

Weisgerber M, Webber K, Meurer J, Danduran M, Berger S, Flores G. Moderate and vigorous exercise programs in children with asthma: safety, parental satisfaction, and asthma outcomes. Pediatr Pulmonol. 2008 Dec;43(12):1175-82.

Weiss RF. *Herbal Medicine.* Gothenburg, Sweden: Beaconsfield, 1988.

Wen MC, Huang CK, Srivastava KD, Zhang TF, Schofield B, Sampson HA, Li XM. Ku-Shen (Sophora flavescens Ait), a single Chinese herb, abrogates airway hyperreactivity in a murine model of asthma. *J Allergy Clin Immunol.* 2004;113:218.

Wen MC, Taper A, Srivastava KD, Huang CK, Schofield B, Li XM. Immunology of T cells by the Chinese Herbal Medicine Ling Zhi (Ganoderma lucidum) *J Allergy Clin Immunol.* 2003;111:S320.

Wen MC, Wei CH, Hu ZQ, Srivastava K, Ko J, Xi ST, Mu DZ, Du JB, Li GH, Wallenstein S, Sampson H, Kattan M, Li XM. Efficacy and tolerability of anti-asthma herbal medicine intervention in adult patients with moderate-severe allergic asthma. *J Allergy Clin Immunol.* 2005;116:517-24.

Werbach M. *Nutritional Influences on Illness.* Tarzana, CA: Third Line Press, 1996.

Werbach MR. Melatonin for the treatment of gastroesophageal reflux disease. *Altern Ther Health Med.* 2008 Jul-Aug;14(4):54-8.

West CE, Hammarström ML, Hernell O. Probiotics during weaning reduce the incidence of eczema. *Pediatr Allergy Immunol.* 2009 Aug;20(5):430-7.

West R. Risk of death in meat and non-meat eaters. *BMJ.* 1994 Oct 8;309(6959):955.

Westerholm-Ormio M, Vaarala O, Tiittanen M, Savilahti E. Infiltration of Foxp3- and Toll-like receptor-4-positive cells in the intestines of children with food allergy. *J Pediatr Gastroenterol Nutr.* 2010 Apr;50(4):367-76.

Wheeler JG, Shema SJ, Bogle ML, Shirrell MA, Burks AW, Pittler A, Helm RM. Immune and clinical impact of *Lactobacillus acidophilus* on asthma. *Ann Allergy Asthma Immunol.* 1997 Sep;79(3):229-33.

White LB, Foster S. The Herbal Drugstore. Emmaus, PA: Rodale, 2000.

Whitfield KE, Wiggins SA, Belue R, Brandon DT. Genetic and environmental influences on forced expiratory volume in African Americans: the Carolina African-American Twin Study of Aging. *Ethn Dis.* 2004 Spring;14(2):206-11.

WHO. *Guidelines for Drinking-water Quality.* 2nd ed, vol. 2. Geneva: World Health Organization, 1996.

WHO. Health effects of the removal of substances occurring naturally in drinking water, with special reference to demineralized and desalinated water. Report on a working group (Brussels, 20-23 March 1978). *EURO Reports and Studies.* 1979;16.

WHO. How trace elements in water contribute to health. *WHO Chronicle.* 1978;32:382-385.

WHO. *INFOSAN Food Allergies. Information Note No. 3.* Geneva, Switzerland: World Health Organization, 2006.

Wickbom G, Bushkin FL, Woodward ER. Alkaline reflux esophagitis. *Surg Gynecol Obstet.* 1974 Aug;139(2):267-71.

Widdicombe JG, Ernst E. Clinical cough V: complementary and alternative medicine: therapy of cough. *Handb Exp Pharmacol.* 2009;(187):321-42.

Wilkens H, Wilkens JH, Uffmann J, Bövers J, Fröhlich JC, Fabel H. Effect of the platelet-activating factor antagonist BN 52063 on exertional asthma. *Pneumologie.* 1990 Feb;44 Suppl 1:347-8.

Willard T, Jones K. *Reishi Mushroom: Herb of Spiritual Potency and Medical Wonder.* Issaquah, Washington: Sylvan Press, 1990.

Willard T. *Edible and Medicinal Plants of the Rocky Mountains and Neighbouring Territories.* Calgary: 1992.

Willemsen LE, Koetsier MA, Balvers M, Beermann C, Stahl B, van Tol EA. Polyunsaturated fatty acids support epithelial barrier integrity and reduce IL-4 mediated permeability in vitro. *Eur J Nutr.* 2008 Jun;47(4):183-91.

Williams DM. Considerations in the long-term management of asthma in ambulatory patients. *AM J Health Sits Pham.* 2006;63:S14-21.

Wilson D, Evans M, Guthrie N, Sharma P, Baisley J, Schonlau F, Burki C. A randomized, double-blind, placebo-controlled exploratory study to evaluate the potential of pycnogenol for improving allergic rhinitis symptoms. *Phytother Res.* 2010 Aug;24(8):1115-9.

Wilson K, McDowall L, Hodge D, Chetcuti P, Cartledge P. Cow's milk protein allergy. *Community Pract.* 2010 May;83(5):40-1.

Wilson L. *Nutritional Balancing and Hair Mineral Analysis.* Prescott, AZ: LD Wilson, 1998.

Wilson NM, Charette L, Thomson AH, Silverman M. Gastro-oesophageal reflux and childhood asthma: the acid test. *Thorax.* 1985 Aug;40(8):592-7.

Winchester AM. *Biology and its Relation to Mankind.* New York: Van Nostrand Reinhold, 1969.

Wittenberg JS. *The Rebellious Body.* New York: Insight, 1996.

Woessner KM, Simon RA, Stevenson DD. Monosodium glutamate sensitivity in asthma. *J Allergy Clin Immunol.* 1999 Aug;104(2 Pt 1):305-10.

Wöhrl S, Hemmer W, Focke M, Rappersberger K, Jarisch R. Histamine intolerance-like symptoms in healthy volunteers after oral provocation with liquid histamine. *Allergy Asthma Proc.* 2004 Sep-Oct;25(5):305-11.

Wolvers DA, van Herpen-Broekmans WM, Logman MH, van der Wielen RP, Albers R. Effect of a mixture of micronutrients, but not of bovine colostrum concentrate, on immune function parameters in healthy volunteers: a randomized placebo-controlled study. *Nutr J.* 2006 Nov 21;5:28.

Wolverton BC. *How to grow fresh air: 50 houseplants that purify your home or office.* New York: Penguin, 1997.

Wong GWK, Hui DSC, Chan HH, Fox TF, Leung R, Zhong NS, Chen YZ, Lai CKW. Prevalence of respiratory and atopic disorders in Chinese schoolchildren. *Clinical and Experimental Allergy.* 2001;31:1125-1231.

Wong WM, Lai KC, Lam KF, Hui WM, Hu WH, Lam CL, Xia HH, Huang JQ, Chan CK, Lam SK, Wong BC. Prevalence, clinical spectrum and health care utilization of gastro-oesophageal reflux disease in a Chinese population: a population-based study. *Aliment Pharmacol Ther.* 2003 Sep 15;18(6):595-604.

Wood M. *The Book of Herbal Wisdom.* Berkeley, CA: North Atlantic, 1997.

Wood RA, Kraynak J. *Food Allergies for Dummies.* Hoboken, NJ: Wiley Publ, 2007.

Woods RK, Abramson M, Bailey M, Walters EH. International prevalences of reported food allergies and intolerances. Comparisons arising from the European Community Respiratory Health Survey (ECRHS) 1991-1994. *Eur J Clin Nutr* 2001;55:298-304.

Woods RK, Abramson M, Bailey M, Walters EH. International prevalences of reported food allergies and intolerances. Comparisons arising from the European Community Respiratory Health Survey (ECRHS) 1991-1994. *Eur J Clin Nutr.* 2001 Apr;55(4):298-304.

Woods RK, Abramson M, Raven JM, Bailey M, Weiner JM, Walters EH. Reported food intolerance and respiratory symptoms in young adults. *Eur Respir J.* 1998;11: 151-155.

Wouters EF, Reynaert NL, Dentener MA, Vernooy JH. Systemic and local inflammation in asthma and chronic obstructive pulmonary disease: is there a connection? *Proc Am Thorac Soc.* 2009 Dec;6(8):638-47.

Wright A, Lavoie KL, Jacob A, Rizk A, Bacon SL. Effect of body mass index on self-reported exercise-triggered asthma. *Phys Sportsmed.* 2010 Dec;38(4):61-6.

Wright GR, Howieson S, McSharry C, McMahon AD, Chaudhuri R, Thompson J, Donnelly I, Brooks RG, Lawson A, Jolly L, McAlpine L, King EM, Chapman MD, Wood S, Thomson NC. Effect of improved home ventilation on asthma control and house dust mite allergen levels. *Allergy.* 2009 Nov;64(11):1671-80.

Wright RA, Goldsmith LJ, Ameen V, D'Angelo A, Kirby SL, Prakash S. Transdermal nicotine patches do not cause clinically significant gastroesophageal reflux or esophageal motor disorders. *Nicotine Tob Res.* 1999 Dec;1(4):371-4.

Wright RJ. Epidemiology of stress and asthma: from constricting communities and fragile families to epigenetics. *Immunol Allergy Clin North Am.* 2011 Feb;31(1):19-39.

Wu B, Yu J, Wang Y. Effect of Chinese herbs for tonifying Shen on balance of Th1 /Th2 in children with asthma in remission stage. *Zhongguo Zhong Xi Yi Jie He Za Zhi.* 2007 Feb;27(2):120-2.

Xenos ES. The role of esophageal motility and hiatal hernia in esophageal exposure to acid. *Surg Endosc.* 2002 Jun;16(6):914-20.

Xia HH, Talley NJ. Helicobacter pylori infection, reflux esophagitis, and atrophic gastritis: an unexplored triangle. *Am J Gastroenterol.* 1998 Mar;93(3):394-400.

Xiao P, Kubo H, Ohsawa M, Higashiyama K, Nagase H, Yan YN, Li JS, Kamei J, Ohmiya S. kappa-Opioid receptor-mediated antinociceptive effects of stereoisomers and derivatives of (+)-matrine in mice. *Planta Med.* 1999 Apr;65(3):230-3.

REFERENCES

Xie JY, Dong JC, Gong ZH. Effects on herba epimedii and radix Astragali on tumor necrosis factor-alpha and nuclear factor-kappa B in asthmatic rats. *Zhongguo Zhong Xi Yi Jie He Za Zhi.* 2006 Aug;26(8):723-7.

Xu X, Zhang D, Zhang H, Wolters PJ, Killeen NP, Sullivan BM, Locksley RM, Lowell CA, Caughey GH. Neutrophil histamine contributes to inflammation in mycoplasma pneumonia. *J Exp Med.* 2006 Dec 25;203(13):2907-17.

Yadav RK, Ray RB, Vempati R, Bijlani RL. Effect of a comprehensive yoga-based lifestyle modification program on lipid peroxidation. *Indian J Physiol Pharmacol.* 2005 Jul-Sep;49(3):358-62.

Yadav VS, Mishra KP, Singh DP, Mehrotra S, Singh VK. Immunomodulatory effects of curcumin. *Immunopharmacol Immunotoxicol.* 2005;27(3):485-97.

Yadzir ZH, Misnan R, Abdullah N, Bakhtiar F, Arip M, Murad S. Identification of Ige-binding proteins of raw and cooked extracts of Loligo edulis (white squid). *Southeast Asian J Trop Med Public Health.* 2010 May;41(3):653-9.

Yang YX, Lewis JD, Epstein S, Metz DC. Long-term proton pump inhibitor therapy and risk of hip fracture. *JAMA.* 2006 Dec 27;296(24):2947-53.

Yang Z. Are peanut allergies a concern for using peanut-based formulated foods in developing countries? *Food Nutr Bull.* 2010 Jun;31(2 Suppl):S147-53.

Yeager S. *The Doctor's Book of Food Remedies.* Emmaus, PA: Rodale Press, 1998.

Yeh CC, Lin CC, Wang SD, Chen YS, Su BH, Kao ST. Protective and anti-inflammatory effect of a traditional Chinese medicine, Xia-Bai-San, by modulating lung local cytokine in a murine model of acute lung injury. *Int Immunopharmacol.* 2006 Sep;6(9):1506-14.

Yu L, Zhang Y, Chen C, Cui HF, Yan XK. Meta-analysis on randomized controlled clinical trials of acupuncture for asthma. *Zhongguo Zhen Jiu.* 2010 Sep;30(9):787-92.

Yu LC. The epithelial gatekeeper against food allergy. *Pediatr Neonatol.* 2009 Dec;50(6):247-54.

Yuan Y, Chen LQ. Does fundoplication really reduce deoxyribonucleic acid methylation of Barrett esophagus? *Ann Surg.* 2011 Dec;254(6):1077; author reply 1077-8.

Yusoff NA, Hampton SM, Dickerson JW, Morgan JB. The effects of exclusion of dietary egg and milk in the management of asthmatic children: a pilot study. *J R Soc Promot Health.* 2004 Mar;124(2):74-80.

Zanjanian MH. The intestine in allergic diseases. *Ann Allergy.* 1976 Sep;37(3):208-18.

Zarkadas M, Scott FW, Salminen J, Ham Pong A. Common Allergenic Foods and Their Labelling in Canada. *Can J Allergy Clin Immun.* 1999; 4:118-141.

Zeiger RS, Heller S. The development and prediction of atopy in high-risk children: follow-up at age seven years in a prospective randomized study of combined maternal and infant food allergen avoidance. *J Allergy Clin Immunol.* 1995 Jun;95(6):1179-90.

Zerbib F, Bruley Des Varannes S, Scarpignato C, Leray V, D'Amato M, Rozé C, Galmiche JP. Endogenous cholecystokinin in postprandial lower esophageal sphincter function and fundic tone in humans. *Am J Physiol.* 1998 Dec;275(6 Pt 1):G1266-73.

Zerbib F. Gastroesophageal reflux in the adult: what are the results of medical treatments? (II). *Gastroenterol Clin Biol.* 1999 Jan;23(1 Pt 2):S255-73.

Zhang J, Lam SP, Li SX, Li AM, Wing YK. The longitudinal course and impact of non-restorative sleep: A five-year community-based follow-up study. *Sleep Med.* 2012 Mar 23.

Zhang T, Srivastava K, Wen MC, Yang N, Cao J, Busse P, Birmingham N, Goldfarb J, Li XM. Pharmacology and immunological actions of a herbal medicine ASHMI on allergic asthma. *Phytother Res.* 2010 Jul;24(7):1047-55.

Zhang Z, Lai HJ, Roberg KA, Gangnon RE, Evans MD, Anderson EL, Pappas TE, Dasilva DF, Tisler CJ, Salazar LP, Gern JE, Lemanske RF Jr. Early childhood weight status in relation to asthma development in high-risk children. *J Allergy Clin Immunol.* 2010 Dec;126(6):1157-62. 2010 Nov 4.

Zhao FD, Dong JC, Xie JY. Effects of Chinese herbs for replenishing shen and strengthening qi on some indexes of neuro-endocrino-immune network in asthmatic rats. *Zhongguo Zhong Xi Yi Jie He Za Zhi.* 2007 Aug;27(8):715-9.

Zhao J, Bai J, Shen K, Xiang L, Huang S, Chen A, Huang Y, Wang J, Ye R. Self-reported prevalence of childhood allergic diseases in three cities of China: a multicenter study. *BMC Public Health.* 2010 Sep 13;10:551.

Zheng M. Experimental study of 472 herbs with antiviral action against the herpes simplex virus. *Zhong Xi Yi Jie He Za Zhi.* 1990 Jan;10(1):39-41, 6.

Zhou Q, Zhang B, Verne GN. Intestinal membrane permeability and hypersensitivity in the irritable bowel syndrome. *Pain.* 2009 Nov;146(1-2):41-6.

Zhu HH, Chen YP, Yu JE, Wu M, Li Z. Therapeutic effect of Xincang Decoction on chronic airway inflammation in children with bronchial asthma in remission stage. *Zhong Xi Yi Jie He Xue Bao.* 2005 Jan;3(1):23-7.

Ziaei Kajbaf T, Asar S, Alipoor MR. Relationship between obesity and asthma symptoms among children in Ahvaz, Iran:A cross sectional study. *Ital J Pediatr.* 2011 Jan 6;37(1):1.

Zielen S, Kardos P, Madonini E. Steroid-sparing effects with allergen-specific immunotherapy in children with asthma: a randomized controlled trial. *J Allergy Clin Immunol.* 2010 Nov;126(5):942-9. 2010 Jul 10.

Ziment I, Tashkin DP. Alternative medicine for allergy and asthma. *J Allergy Clin Immunol.* 2000 Oct;106(4):603-14.

Ziment I. Alternative therapies for asthma. *Curr Opin Pulm Med.* 1997 Jan;3(1):61-71.

Zizza, C. The nutrient content of the Italian food supply 1961-1992. *Euro J Clin Nutr.* 1997;51: 259-265.

Zoccatelli G, Pokoj S, Foetisch K, Bartra J, Valero A, Del Mar San Miguel-Moncin M, Vieths S, Scheurer S. Identification and characterization of the major allergen of green bean (Phaseolus vulgaris) as a non-specific lipid transfer protein (Pha v 3). *Mol Immunol.* 2010 Apr;47(7-8):1561-8.

315

Index

(too many remedies to list all)

cytokines, 104, 126, 161, 211, 251, 270, 290
dandelion, 219, 220
dehydration, 223
delta brainwaves, 345
dental erosion, 22
depression, 291, 342
dermatitis, 105
detergents, 165
detoxification, 202, 204, 213
diabetes, 225, 238
diaphragm, 158
diarrhea, 5, 14, 31, 32, 34, 36, 105, 125, 126, 176, 178, 179, 230
diphtheria, 119
dust mites, 185
dysphagia, 24
ear infection, 130
eczema, 104, 130, 176
eicosapentaenoic acid (EPA), 76, 78
emphysema, 187
endocrine, 202
endothelium-derived relaxing factor (EDRF), 82
endotoxins, 182, 192, 320
Enterococcus faecalis, 119
eosinophilia, 135
eosinophilic esophagitis, 21
epinephrine, 212
Escherichia coli, 113, 126, 127, 128, 166, 167, 320
esophageal adenocarcinoma, 14, 22, 25
esophageal carcinoma, 24
esophageal pH, 9, 14, 15, 21, 150, 153, 240, 260

esophageal sphincters, 15, 43, 107, 147, 148, 151, 239, 279, 285, 324, 331
essential fatty acids, 76, 308
fever, 167, 176, 202
fibrin, 231
flatulence, 126
flavonoids, 319
folic acid, 308
food allergies, 27
forced expiratory volume (FEV), 185, 233, 251, 252
forests, 164
formaldehyde, 140, 189, 190, 191, 192
fragrances, 187, 188
free radicals, 205, 231
fructooligosachharides, 318
galactooligosaccharide, 318
galactooligosaccharides (GOS), 313
gallbladder, 225, 238
gamma-linolenic acid, 76
garlic, 319
gas, 14, 44, 184, 185, 187, 189, 190, 209, 217, 221
gastric acid, 37, 48
gastrin, 60, 117, 172
gastritis, 174, 205, 230
German Commission E, 230
ginger, 200, 221, 222, 223, 237, 238
gingivitis, 126, 168
glutathione, 205, 219
glycerophosphatidylcholines, 79
goblet cells, 59, 60, 93, 108
green, 344

niacin, 308
nitric oxide (NO), 82, 233
nitrogen, 63, 185, 187, 191
NSAIDs, 171, 172, 177, 179,
 197, 226, 231
nutrition, 319, 320
obesity, 5, 23, 149, 150
oil, 164
oligosaccharides, 318
oral plaque, 122, 126
organic foods, 294, 313
overdose, 196
oxidation, 77
oxygen, 125, 127, 164
ozone, 191
palmitic acid, 218
pantothenic acid, 308
papain, 323
paracrine, 76, 77
paracrines, 76, 77
parietal cells, 16, 30, 48, 53,
 60, 67, 117, 278, 288, 289
pathobiotic, 309
pectin, 218
peptidase, 322
periodontal disease, 122, 126,
 132
pharmaceuticals, 127, 163
phenol, 203
photosensitivity, 177
phytanic acid, 192
phytonutrients, 320
pink, 345
pneumonia, 129, 131, 134,
 167
pollen, 192, 235, 300
polyphenols, 308, 319
polysaccharide, 305

Porphyromonas gingivalis,
 168
potassium, 204, 218, 219
prebiotics, 318, 319
preservatives, 182
propellants, 188
prostaglandins, 75, 77, 78, 79,
 80, 81, 171, 173, 175, 203,
 204, 220, 269
proteinuria, 305
Proteus sp., 119
Pseudomonas aeruginosa,
 120, 130, 134
purple, 345
pyloric sphincter valve, 49
pyridoxine, 308
quercetin, 213
reactive oxygen species, 252,
 256
refined sugars, 145, 281, 282,
 313
regurgitation, 12, 13, 14, 37,
 83, 112, 143, 157, 336
relaxation, 341, 342, 346
reservatrol, 319
Rett syndrome, 22
Reye's syndrome, 174
rhinosinusitis, 22
riboflavin, 308
rivers, 164
root canals, 168
rotavirus, 125, 128, 129
Saccharomyces boulardii, 116
salicin, 172, 202, 204, 230
salivaricin, 123
salmonella, 318
Salmonella sp., 126, 127
sauerkraut, 130, 310

(NOTES)

(NOTES)